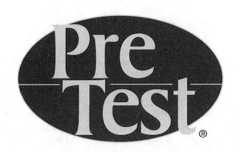

Family Medicine

PreTest® Self-Assessment and Review

Notice

Medicine is an ever-changing science. As new research and clinical experience broaden our knowledge, changes in treatment and drug therapy are required. The authors and the publisher of this work have checked with sources believed to be reliable in their efforts to provide information that is complete and generally in accord with the standards accepted at the time of publication. However, in view of the possibility of human error or changes in medical sciences, neither the authors nor the publisher nor any other party who has been involved in the preparation or publication of this work warrants that the information contained herein is in every respect accurate or complete, and they disclaim all responsibility for any errors or omissions or for the results obtained from use of the information contained in this work. Readers are encouraged to confirm the information contained herein with other sources. For example, and in particular, readers are advised to check the product information sheet included in the package of each drug they plan to administer to be certain that the information contained in this work is accurate and that changes have not been made in the recommended dose or in the contraindications for administration. This recommendation is of particular importance in connection with new or infrequently used drugs.

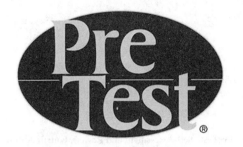

Family Medicine

PreTest® Self-Assessment and Review

Fourth Edition

Doug Knutson, MD
Vice President, Academic Affairs
Chief Academic Officer
OhioHealth
Columbus, Ohio

Robin Devine, DO
Assistant Program Director, Family Medicine Residency
Grant Medical Center
Medical Director, Academic Research
OhioHealth Research and Innovation Institute
Columbus, Ohio

New York   Chicago   San Francisco   Athens   London   Madrid   Mexico City
Milan   New Delhi   Singapore   Sydney   Toronto

Family Medicine: PreTest® Self-Assessment and Review, Fourth Edition

Copyright © 2019 by McGraw-Hill Education. All rights reserved. Printed in the United States of America. Except as permitted under the United States Copyright Act of 1976, no part of this publication may be reproduced or distributed in any form or by any means, or stored in a data base or retrieval system, without the prior written permission of the publisher.

Previous editions copyright © 2012, 2009, 2008 by The McGraw-Hill Companies, Inc.

PreTest® is a registered trademark of McGraw-Hill Education Global Holdings, LLC. All rights reserved.

2 3 4 5 6 7 8 9   LCR   23 22 21 20

ISBN 978-1-260-14358-4
MHID 1-260-14358-9

This book was set in Minion pro by Cenveo® Publisher Services.
The editors were Bob Boehringer and Rhiannon Wong.
The production supervisor was Richard Ruzycka.
Project management was provided by Ishan Chaudhary, Cenveo Publisher Services.

Library of Congress Cataloging-in-Publication Data

Names: Knutson, Doug, editor.
Title: Family medicine preTest self-assessment and review / editor, Doug
    Knutson, MD, Vice President, Academic Affairs, Chief Academic Officer,
    OhioHealth, Columbus, Ohio, Robin Devine, DO, Assistant Program Director,
    Family Medicine Residency, Grant Medical Center, Medical Director,
    Academic Research, OhioHealth Research and Innovation Institute, Columbus, Ohio.
Description: Fourth edition. | New York : McGraw-Hill Education, [2019]
    Identifiers: LCCN 2018046746 | ISBN 9781260143584 (paperback)
Subjects: LCSH: Family medicine—Examinations, questions, etc. |
    Medicine—Examinations, questions, etc. | BISAC: MEDICAL / Clinical Medicine.
Classification: LCC RC58 .F34 2019 | DDC 610.76—dc23 LC record available

McGraw-Hill Education books are available at special quantity discounts to use as premiums and sales promotions, or for use in corporate training programs. To contact a representative, please visit the Contact Us pages at www.mhprofessional.com.

Student Reviewers

Asad S. Akhter, MD
Resident Physician
Department of Neurosurgery, PGY-1
The Ohio State University

Blake Arthurs
Fourth Year Medical Student
Wayne State School of Medicine
Class of 2019

Contents

Acknowledgments

Special thanks to all clinicians who take time from their busy practices and devote themselves to teaching the next generation of physicians. And, thanks to our families for allowing us the time and space to complete this edition.

Introduction

Family Medicine: PreTest® Self-Assessment and Review, Fourth Edition, is intended to provide medical students, as well as house officers and physicians, with a convenient tool for assessing and improving their knowledge of family medicine. The 500 questions in this book are similar in format and complexity to those included in Step 2 of the United States Medical Licensing Examination (USMLE). They may also be a useful study tool for Step 3.

For multiple-choice questions, the *one best* response to each question should be selected. For matching sets, a group of questions will be preceded by a list of lettered options. For each question in the matching set, select *one* lettered option that is *most* closely associated with the question. Each question in this book has a corresponding answer and a short discussion of various issues raised by the question and its answer. Recommended reading and references follow each section within the chapter, or each chapter.

To simulate the time constraints imposed by the qualifying examinations for which this book is intended as a practice guide, the student or physician should allot about 1 minute for each question. After answering all questions in a chapter, as much time as necessary should be spent in reviewing the explanations for each question at the end of the chapter. Attention should be given to all explanations, even if the examinee answered the question correctly. Those seeking more information on a subject should refer to the reference materials listed or to other standard texts in medicine.

Preventive Medicine

Questions

Immunizations

1. You are examining a normal-term newborn whose mother is hepatitis B virus (HBV) surface antigen positive. Which of the following protocols is recommended for the child?

a. Hepatitis B vaccination at 0 to 2 months, a second dose at 1 to 4 months, and a third dose at 6 to 18 months of age.

b. Hepatitis B vaccination within 12 hours of birth, with the timing of the second and third doses based on the mother's hepatitis B viral load at the time of delivery.

c. Hepatitis B vaccination and hepatitis B immune globulin within 12 hours of birth, a second dose of hepatitis B vaccine at 1 to 2 months, and a third dose of vaccine at 6 months.

d. Hepatitis B vaccination and hepatitis B immune globulin within 12 hours of birth, a second dose of the vaccine and immune globulin at 1 to 2 months, and a third dose of the vaccine and immune globulin at 6 months.

e. Hepatitis B vaccination at birth, with serologic testing of the baby before additional vaccinations are given.

2. You are counseling a mother about her child's immunization schedule. She asks specifically if her child would benefit from the *Haemophilus influenzae* type b (Hib) vaccine. Which of the following statements is true about this vaccine?

a. Unvaccinated infants who develop invasive Hib disease before the age of two should receive the vaccine.

b. The vaccine will help to prevent otitis media caused by *H influenzae*.

c. Adverse reactions to the vaccine include an unusual high-pitched cry, high fevers, and seizures.

d. The first vaccine should be administered at birth.

e. The vaccine cannot be given concurrently with other vaccines.

3. You are discussing varicella-zoster vaccination with a 24-year-old US-born male health care worker who does not ever remember having chicken pox. He does not have any contraindications to vaccine administration. Which of the following statements is true?

a. Based on his age, he is considered immune.
b. Based on his age, only one dose of vaccine is required.
c. Serologic testing for varicella antibodies is necessary before vaccination.
d. If his wife is pregnant, vaccination should be avoided until after she delivers.
e. After vaccination, he may develop a varicella infection, but when it occurs, it does not appear to be contagious.

4. You are caring for a 23-year-old pregnant patient (G0P0) with an active substance use disorder. She has actively injected heroin during this pregnancy and presents for her first prenatal visit at 18 weeks' gestation. Initial physical examination is normal, the baby has normal fetal heart tones and activity, and mom is well-appearing but has mild symptoms of withdrawal. She was last seen 13 months ago in your clinic and received her first dose of hepatitis B vaccine. Regarding hepatitis B testing and vaccination, what would be the most appropriate action?

a. Readminister the first dose of hepatitis B vaccine now without serologic testing since the schedule has been interrupted.
b. Administer the second dose of hepatitis B vaccine now prior to serologic testing.
c. Counsel the patient regarding the need to complete this series and recommend she receive it after she delivers.
d. Order serologic testing for hepatitis and administer the vaccine only if her HBsAg is negative.
e. Administer the second dose of hepatitis vaccine immediately after obtaining serologic testing for hepatitis.

5. You are caring for a 27-year-old healthy gay man who works as an accountant and lives alone. He had the "typical childhood vaccinations" and provides documentation of his immunization record. He is up-to-date on tetanus, and was primarily immunized against diphtheria, pertussis, polio, hepatitis B, measles, mumps, rubella, and *H influenzae* type b. Which of the following vaccinations is indicated for this patient?

a. Human papillomavirus (HPV)
b. Meningococcus
c. Hepatitis A
d. Pneumococcus
e. A booster of the measles-mumps-rubella (MMR) vaccine

6. In the prenatal workup for a 24-year-old patient, you discover she is not immune to rubella. When is the best time to vaccinate her against rubella?

a. Immediately
b. In the second trimester of pregnancy
c. In the third trimester of pregnancy
d. In the early postpartum period
e. At least 4 weeks postpartum

7. A 32-year-old woman comes to your office for a complete physical examination. When discussing her vaccinations, you discover that she received her primary tetanus series as a child, and her last tetanus booster was 11 years ago. Which of the following is true?

a. No vaccination is required.
b. The patient should receive a tetanus-diphtheria (Td) booster.
c. The patient should receive tetanus immune globulin.
d. The patient should receive a diphtheria-tetanus-pertussis (DTaP) immunization.
e. The patient should receive tetanus, diphtheria, and acellular pertussis (Tdap) immunization.

8. You are caring for a family and find that the mother would like her children to be vaccinated against influenza. Her children are aged 4 months, 24 months, and 5 years. Which of the following represents current immunization recommendations for influenza?

a. None of her children should be vaccinated.
b. The 4-month-old and the 24-month-old should be vaccinated.
c. The 24-month-old and the 5-year-old should be vaccinated.
d. Only the 24-month-old should be vaccinated.
e. All the children should be vaccinated.

9. You care for a child whose mother wants him immunized against influenza. He is currently 18 months old and has never had the influenza vaccine in the past. Which of the following is correct regarding this situation?

a. He should not be immunized against influenza.
b. He should receive one dose of the live, attenuated influenza vaccine (LAIV).
c. He should receive two doses of LAIV.
d. He should receive one dose of the trivalent inactivated influenza vaccine (TIV).
e. He should receive two doses of TIV.

10. You are caring for a 2 1/2-year-old boy who is coming to your office for the first time. Reviewing his immunization record, you find that he has never received vaccination for invasive pneumococcal disease using the 13-valent pneumococcal conjugate vaccine. Which of the following is true regarding recommendations in his case?

a. He is no longer at risk for invasive pneumococcal disease and does not need to be vaccinated.
b. He should only be vaccinated if he has an immunocompromising condition.
c. He should only be vaccinated if he has a congenital or genetic pulmonary condition.
d. He should be vaccinated and should start the usual series for primary vaccination.
e. He should be vaccinated, but with a modified schedule for immunization.

11. You are caring for a 30-year-old woman who asks you about the HPV vaccination. She is recently divorced and not in a monogamous relationship. She has a history of genital warts, and had an abnormal Papanicolaou (Pap) test 2 years ago, for which she underwent colposcopy, biopsy, and cryotherapy. Subsequent Pap tests have been normal. Which of the following is true?

a. She is unable to be vaccinated because she has a history of genital warts.
b. She is unable to be vaccinated because she has a history of an abnormal Pap test.
c. She is unable to be vaccinated because she is not in a monogamous relationship.
d. Vaccination is not recommended for 30-year-old women.
e. She should be vaccinated.

12. You are determining which of the patients in your practice should receive the quadrivalent HPV vaccination. This vaccine is inappropriate for which of the following patients?

a. An 18-year-old woman with an abnormal Pap test that has yet to be followed up appropriately
b. A 16-year-old girl who recently delivered her first child and is currently breast-feeding
c. A pregnant 14-year-old
d. A 12-year-old boy with asthma currently taking steroids for an exacerbation
e. An 11-year-old victim of sexual abuse

13. A recently retired 67-year-old woman presents to you to establish care. She was a smoker for a long time but quit 5 years ago. She is generally healthy, but her prior physician told her that she has "emphysema". She was prescribed an "inhaler" to use as needed and only uses it rarely. She asks about necessary immunizations. Her social history indicates that she lives with her daughter and often cares for her infant granddaughter. Her chart indicates that she had a pneumococcal polysaccharide vaccine at age 63 and a Td shot at age 63. Which of the following vaccines should she receive?

a. Pneumococcal conjugate vaccine followed by pneumococcal polysaccharide vaccine 8 weeks later
b. Pneumococcal polysaccharide vaccine followed by pneumococcal conjugate vaccine 8 weeks later
c. Pneumococcal conjugate vaccine followed by pneumococcal polysaccharide vaccine at least 5 years after the previous dose
d. Pneumococcal conjugate vaccine followed by pneumococcal polysaccharide vaccine in 5 years
e. Intranasal influenza

14. Based on the Advisory Committee on Immunization Practices (ACIP), which patient would be considered the most appropriate candidate for vaccination against herpes zoster?

a. A 53-year-old man with a history of chicken pox as a child and a personal history of diabetes mellitus
b. A 48-year-old woman who recently underwent successful surgery for colon cancer
c. A 33-year-old man who was recently diagnosed with human immunodeficiency virus (HIV)
d. A 22-year-old with a personal history of sickle-cell disease
e. A 66-year-old man with a personal history of shingles at age 56

15. You are seeing adolescent siblings in the office for their well-child examinations. A 16-year-old boy and a 14-year-old girl, both are healthy and without medical problems. Mom asks if they are due for their HPV vaccines. The 16-year-old began his series at the age of 11 and received his second dose 2 months later but has yet to receive his third dose. The 14-year-old received her first and only dose at age 12. Which of the following statements is true regarding the dose schedule for HPV vaccine?

a. The 14-year-old requires two more doses of HPV vaccine, one today and another at least 5 months later.
b. The 16-year-old does not require any further doses of HPV vaccine since he admits he is already sexually active.
c. Both siblings are adequately immunized since they both began the series prior to the age of 15 years of age.
d. The 14-year-old and the 16-year-old both require one dose of vaccine today to complete the series.
e. The 14-year-old girl should have a pregnancy test prior to administration of the vaccine.

16. You are seeing an 18-year-old male patient for his physical examination prior to starting college. He has a past medical history of allergic rhinitis and eczema that are both well controlled. He currently lives at home but will be living in a dormitory at the university. The forms he brought with him indicate that several immunizations are required prior to moving in, including proof of meningococcal vaccination. This patient received a dose of MPSV4 at the age of 16. What do you recommend for him today?

a. He should receive a second dose of MPSV4 today.
b. He does not need any further meningococcal vaccination because he is not at elevated risk for infection.
c. He does not need any further meningococcal vaccination because he was vaccinated at 16 years of age or older.
d. He should receive a single dose of MenACWY vaccine today and, unless he develops additional risk factors for infection, does not require any more doses.
e. He should have serologic titers drawn, and if they are positive, this will serve as proof of immunity.

Screening Tests

17. You are seeing a husband and wife for their routine physicals. They have received a flyer in the mail suggesting they have ultrasonography to screen for abdominal aortic aneurysm (AAA). According to the United States Preventive Services Task Force (USPSTF), which of the following individuals should receive this screening?

a. A 76-year-old man with hypertension and a 25-pack-year smoking history
b. A 65-year-old woman with a 30-pack-year smoking history
c. A 67-year-old man with a 10-pack-year smoking history
d. A 70-year-old man with hypertension who has never smoked
e. A 57-year-old woman with a 20-pack-year smoking history

18. You are seeing a patient with a smoking history for a routine health examination. Which of the following attributes would exclude this patient from the current USPSTF lung cancer screening recommendations with low-dose computed tomography (LDCT) of the chest?

a. A 79-year-old man who quit smoking 10 years ago
b. A 65-year-old woman who quit smoking 20 years ago
c. A 56-year-old man with a 30-pack-year smoking history
d. A 75-year-old woman who continues to smoke
e. A 71-year-old woman who has signed a Do Not Resuscitate (DNR) order

19. You are seeing a healthy 26-year-old woman for a routine health visit. She mentions that she and her husband are thinking about starting a family soon. She has never been pregnant before. Which of the following interventions, if done prior to pregnancy, has been shown to have a clear beneficial outcome for this woman and her potential child?

a. Blood typing and antibody testing
b. Screening for HIV
c. Screening for *Chlamydia*
d. Screening for asymptomatic bacteriuria
e. Prescribing 0.4 to 0.8 mg of folic acid daily

20. You are discussing options for colorectal cancer screening for a 51-year-old patient. Although several options exist, which of the following choices and screening intervals is most appropriate for asymptomatic individuals aged 50 to 75 at average risk?

a. Guaiac-based fecal occult blood test (gFOBT) every 2 years
b. Flexible sigmoidoscopy every 3 years
c. Fecal immunochemical tests (FIT) every year
d. Colonoscopy every 5 years
e. Computed tomography (CT) colonography every year

21. You are discussing cancer screening with a female patient. She has no family history of breast cancer, and routine risk analysis indicates that she is not at increased risk for the disease. According to the USPSTF, at what age should she start getting routine mammograms?

a. 30 years
b. 35 years
c. 40 years
d. 45 years
e. 50 years

22. In a routine examination, a 33-year-old woman asks you about breast self-examination (BSE) as a breast cancer screening method. Which of the following best represents the current American Academy of Family Physicians (AAFP) recommendations regarding BSE in average-risk females?

a. There is strong evidence that BSE is an appropriate screening modality.
b. There is limited evidence that BSE is an appropriate screening modality.
c. Available evidence shows that BSE reduces the need for additional testing or biopsy.
d. There is insufficient evidence to recommend for or against BSE.
e. Clinicians should not teach their female patients how to perform effective BSE.

23. During a routine appointment to discuss an upper respiratory infection, you find that your 17-year-old female patient has become sexually active for the first time. According to current guidelines, when should you begin cervical cancer screening on this patient?

a. At the current time.
b. At the age of 19.
c. At the age of 20.
d. At the age of 21.
e. Cervical cancer screening is not recommended.

24. You are seeing a 60-year-old patient for her annual physical examination. She has been married to her husband for 32 years and reports that both have been monogamous. Records indicate that she has had normal Pap smears every 1 to 2 years for the last 20 years, and has one abnormal pap with colposcopy indicating CIN I but regressed spontaneously without treatment 10 years prior. At what age is it appropriate to discontinue Pap screening on this patient?

a. 55 years
b. 60 years
c. 65 years
d. 70 years
e. Never discontinue screening

25. You are caring for a healthy woman whose cousin was just diagnosed with unilateral breast cancer at age 33. Your patient has no other relatives with known histories of breast or ovarian cancer. Which of the following is true regarding the current recommendations for genetic screening for breast cancer mutations?

a. The patient should not be offered genetic testing.
b. The patient should be tested only if she is of Ashkenazi Jewish descent.
c. The patient should be screened with a breastcancer–specific risk prediction tool to determine if she should be referred for genetic testing.
d. The patient should be tested if her cousin with breast cancer is male.
e. The patient should be offered testing regardless of her ethnicity.

The Well Child

26. You are seeing a 5-day-old female infant for a newborn well-child check. Mom reports the child is doing well. She is breast-feeding and the child is latching without difficulty and nursing for 10 to 15 minutes per side. Which of the following statements is true regarding breast-feeding and the newborn?

a. Breast-fed newborns should be given supplemental drops with Vitamin D and iron since these are not supplied in breast milk.
b. Breast-fed newborns should be given supplemental Vitamin D drops.
c. Breast-fed newborns should be screened for iron deficiency since iron is not supplied in breast milk.
d. It is best for parents to assign a schedule to feeding the newborn so that they can keep track of feedings.
e. Breast-fed infants should receive fluoride supplementation as soon as tooth eruption occurs.

27. You are seeing a 4-week-old male infant for a well-child checkup. Mom notes that the baby has been fussy for the last week, crying excessively, pulling up his legs, and passing flatus. Which of the following is true regarding infantile colic?

a. Symptoms are typically worse in the early morning hours.
b. Colic is more common in male versus female infants.
c. The incidence of colic peaks around 3 to 4 weeks of age.
d. Colic typically is present for several months and resolve around 6 to 7 months of age.
e. An organic cause is identified in about 15% of cases.

28. Developmental assessment is an important component of the well-child examination. Which of the following are considered developmental "red flags"?

a. An infant who does not turn toward sights or sounds by 2 months of age
b. A 6-month-old infant who does not respond to his/her own name
c. An infant who is unable to sit up unassisted by age 4 months of age
d. A 3-month-old infant who is not reaching for objects
e. A 3-month-old infant who has trouble maneuvering items to his/her mouth

29. A 7-day-old newborn male is at your office for a 1-week well-child examination. The child's mother is a 26-year-old G1P1 without any medical problems. Her pregnancy was uncomplicated, and the infant was born via vaginal delivery at 38 weeks and 6 days of gestation. He was circumcised prior to discharge from the hospital, and mom is breast-feeding. She states he is latching well and eating on demand, but she is concerned about the volume of milk she is producing. Which of the following is criteria for failure to thrive in an infant?

a. Weight below the 10th percentile for age
b. A weight loss of 6% from birth to the 1-week well-child visit
c. A weight loss that crosses a major percentile line on the appropriate growth chart
d. The infant's weight is less than 75% of the median weight for age
e. Failure to regain birth weight by one week of age

30. During a well-child examination for a 3-year-old male patient, you have difficulty palpating both testicles. Dad states that sometimes, the left one can be seen after a warm bath, but they have never felt or seen the right testicle. If left untreated, which of the following is a risk of cryptorchidism?

a. Hydrocele
b. Testicular cancer
c. Hypogonadism
d. Epididymitis
e. Small stature

31. The American Academy of Pediatrics recommends universal lead screening for all children at 12 and 24 months. However, if the child is at high risk, it should begin at 6 months. Which of the following patients should receive screening starting at 12 months instead of 6 months?

a. A child whose 5-year-old brother is being treated for high lead levels
b. A child that lives in a home built in 1976
c. A child whose father is a licensed plumber
d. A child who lives in a mid-century house that is being renovated
e. A child whose mother works as a nail technician

32. Your last patient of the day is a 15-year-old male child who needs his sports preparticipation physical completed so he can participate in football practice tomorrow. Past medical history includes allergic rhinitis and obesity. Upon review of his chart, you notice that he was seen a month ago by one of your partners and his blood pressure was elevated at the time. The physician recommended an increase in physical activity, healthy dietary changes, and a follow-up in 1 month. The boy states he signed up for football so he could be more active. Today, two blood pressure readings taken 15 minutes apart fall just below the 90th percentile category for his age and height. How would you categorize his blood pressure?

a. This is a normal blood pressure for his age and height.
b. This is prehypertension.
c. This is stage 1 hypertension.
d. This is stage 2 hypertension.
e. This is hypotension.

33. You have volunteered to perform preparticipation physical examinations at your local middle school and high school. Understanding that the goal of these screenings is to ensure safe participation in sports, you review the American Academy of Pediatrics guidelines for the preparticipation examination. Based on these guidelines, which of the following scenarios would disqualify a patient from sports participation?

a. A 16-year-old male weightlifter with epilepsy
b. A 13-year-old female runner with an eating disorder who has been receiving treatment and has a normal BMI
c. A 15-year-old male football player with a blood pressure in the 90th to 95th percentile range
d. A 13-year-old volleyball player who has a systolic murmur on examination that increases with Valsalva maneuver and decreases with squatting
e. A 17-year-old female soccer player with a wasp allergy

The Preoperative Evaluation

34. You are completing a preoperative evaluation on a 46-year-old woman who has recently been diagnosed with gallstones. She is generally healthy, and besides being obese has no chronic medical problems. Given her history, what is the potential surgical complication that would be most likely be lethal for her?

a. Infectious complications
b. Cardiac complications
c. Pulmonary complications
d. Thrombosis
e. Adverse reaction to anesthesia

35. You are doing a preoperative history and physical examination on a 58-year-old woman who will be undergoing a thyroidectomy later in the month. She is obese, sedentary with type 2 diabetes, and has hyperlipidemia. She reports that she is unable to walk two blocks without stopping to rest. She denies chest pain with activity. What type of cardiac evaluation should she have prior to undergoing her surgical procedure?

a. No cardiac evaluation is necessary.
b. She should have an electrocardiogram (ECG) prior to surgery, but if that is normal, she needs no other cardiac evaluation.
c. She should have a noninvasive stress test prior to surgery.
d. She should have a heart catheterization prior to surgery.
e. Surgery should be deferred, as her risk is too great.

36. You are doing a preoperative clearance for a 60-year-old man undergoing an elective knee replacement. He has diabetes, hyperlipidemia, and a history of a prior myocardial infarction (MI) 4 months ago. After his heart attack, he had triple-vessel bypass surgery. Since that time, he has done well and has been asymptomatic from a cardiac standpoint. Which of the following is true in this case?

a. Prior to surgery, no cardiac evaluation is necessary given his recent revascularization.
b. He should have an ECG prior to surgery. If that is normal, he needs no other cardiac evaluation.
c. He should have a stress test prior to surgery.
d. He should have a heart catheterization prior to surgery.
e. Surgery should be deferred.

37. A 59-year-old male patient is presenting for preoperative testing before undergoing a hernia repair. He has a history of coronary artery disease and hyperlipidemia, but no other significant medical history. He had a positive stress test 4 years ago that was followed by an angioplasty. He has been asymptomatic ever since. Which of the following is the best answer regarding the type of cardiac evaluation he should have prior to undergoing his procedure?

a. No cardiac evaluation is necessary.
b. He should have an echocardiogram prior to surgery.
c. He should have a stress test prior to surgery.
d. He should have a heart catheterization prior to surgery.
e. Surgery should be deferred.

38. You are completing a preoperative evaluation on a 66-year-old man who will be undergoing prostate surgery. He has hypertension but no other diagnosed medical problems. He has smoked half pack of cigarettes daily since he was 21 years old. He denies dyspnea or cough. Which of the following is true regarding his preoperative evaluation?

a. No pulmonary evaluation is necessary.
b. He should have a routine baseline chest x-ray prior to surgery.
c. He should have pulmonary function testing prior to surgery.
d. He should have a baseline pulse oximetry reading prior to surgery.
e. He should have arterial blood gasses done prior to surgery.

Travel Medicine

39. You are seeing a patient who is traveling to Japan for business and is concerned about the risk of blood clots during his travels. Which of the following has been shown to reduce the risk of deep vein thrombosis (DVT) in prolonged air travel?

a. Sitting in a window seat
b. Wearing compression hose during the flight
c. 81 mg aspirin 4 hours prior to the flight
d. 325 mg aspirin 4 hours prior to the flight
e. Low-molecular-weight heparin on the day of travel

40. You are performing a physical examination on a student traveling to Mexico with her college Spanish class. She is well and has no chronic conditions. She is concerned about traveler's diarrhea and asks about prevention strategies. Which of the following is consistent with the current guideline from the Centers for Disease Control and Prevention (CDC) for prevention of traveler's diarrhea?

a. The CDC does not recommend routine antibiotic prophylaxis for traveler's diarrhea.
b. The traveler should take trimethoprim-sulfamethoxazole.
c. The traveler should take ciprofloxacin.
d. The traveler should take rifaximin.
e. The traveler should take bismuth subsalicylate (BSS).

41. A 36-year-old male patient comes to see you for a travel medicine visit. He is traveling to South America for a 3-week leisure trip and notes that the countries he is visiting require the yellow fever vaccine. Which of the following is true regarding yellow fever vaccination?

a. It is a live, attenuated vaccine.
b. Is only recommended for individuals less than 60 years of age due to a high rate of adverse events.
c. Booster dosing is only needed for travelers to West Africa due to resistance.
d. Individuals with myasthenia gravis are at higher risk for complications of yellow fever and should receive booster dosing every 10 years if they continue to travel.
e. Vaccination must occur at an authorized site and be completed at least 28 days prior to travel to an endemic area.

42. A 28-year-old female patient is planning a trip to her hometown in Africa to visit her family. She will be gone for 4 weeks and will be staying with her family and friends in small villages. She is healthy with no past medical history and takes no medications. What do you tell her regarding Malaria chemoprophylaxis?

a. She would not benefit from chemoprophylaxis since she spent her childhood in the same country and is likely immune.

b. She is at lower risk for acquiring malaria because she is staying with friends and family.

c. Chemoprophylaxis does not confer additional benefit if she utilizes an aerosol repellent containing DEET (*N, N*-diethyl-*meta*-toluamide) in her hotel room.

d. If she is staying in an area more than 2500 m above sea level, she is at low risk for malaria because transmission does not occur at this elevation.

e. If she is traveling anywhere in a country that has malaria activity, she is at high risk for acquiring the disease and would benefit from chemoprophylaxis.

43. A 23-year-old female patient presents to your office prior to leaving on a trip to Peru. She is healthy and an avid exerciser but is concerned about the possibility of altitude sickness during her trip. She will be embarking on a 2-week-long hiking/backpacking trip when she arrives at the airport and will climb to an elevation of 2000 m above sea level before descending again. What advice do you give her?

a. Acetazolamide taken at the first signs of altitude sickness reduces the risk of altitude sickness.

b. She does not need to worry about altitude sickness, because she is flying to her destination.

c. She should plan to arrive a few days early to acclimatize to the environment before ascending.

d. She is unlikely to experience altitude sickness at altitudes less than 2400 m.

e. There is no effective therapy for altitude sickness except descending to a lower altitude.

Contraception

44. You are counseling a 28-year-old woman on contraceptive options during a well-woman examination. She is a G0P0 and is not sure she wants children. She has never been diagnosed with a sexually transmitted disease and has had two sexual partners in the last year and five sexual partners in her lifetime. Her menses are regular but heavy and crampy. She is interested in something to help with this as well as provide contraception. Which of the following is true regarding intrauterine devices (IUDs)?

a. This patient would not be a good candidate for an IUD because of her history of multiple sexual partners.
b. This patient would not be a good candidate for an IUD because of her nulliparity.
c. This patient would benefit from a copper IUD to help lighten her bleeding and cramping.
d. The rate of expulsion of IUDs is low, but her nulliparity increases this risk.
e. The levonorgestrel IUD is associated with a higher rate of pelvic inflammatory disease (PID) due to its effects on cervical mucous.

45. You are reevaluating a 32-year-old woman in your office. You started her on combination oral contraceptives (COCs) 3 months ago, and at each of three visits since then, her blood pressure has been elevated. Which of the following is the most appropriate next step?

a. Discontinue the oral contraceptive and recommend a barrier method
b. Change to a pill with a higher estrogen component
c. Change to a pill with a lower estrogen component
d. Change to a pill with a lower progestin component
e. Change to a progestin-only pill

46. You started a 20-year-old woman on COCs 2 months ago. She returns to your office asking to discontinue their use because of side effects. Statistically speaking, which side effect of COCs is most frequently cited as the reason for discontinuing their use?

a. Nausea
b. Breast tenderness
c. Fluid retention
d. Headache
e. Irregular bleeding

47. A 19-year-old woman has come to see you for contraception advice. She is in college and has recently become sexually active. She saw a physician and is currently taking COC pills, but has an erratic schedule and is having trouble remembering to take them. She is interested in learning about other options. Which of the following is true regarding the side effects of depot-medroxyprogesterone acetate (DMPA) injections?

a. Ninety percent of women will experience amenorrhea while using DMPA.
b. Women should not use DMPA for more than 3 years due to its effects on fertility.
c. The use of DMPA is associated with decreased bone mineral density.
d. DMPA is a weight-neutral option for contraception.
e. Women greater than 35 years of age who smoke should not use DMPA due to the increased risk of blood clots.

48. You are counseling a 23-year-old woman who is interested in starting COC pills. Which of the following is true regarding risks associated with COC use?

a. Users of COC pills have an increased risk of ovarian cancer.
b. Users of COC pills have an increased risk of endometrial cancer.
c. Users of COC pills have an increased risk of venous thromboembolism.
d. Users of COC pills have an increased risk of hemorrhagic stroke.
e. Users of COC pills have an increased risk of diabetes mellitus.

49. You are counseling a patient over the phone who has been taking oral contraceptives regularly for 2 years. Her husband surprised her with a weekend "get away" vacation, and she forgot to bring her pills. She therefore missed taking one active pill. She and her husband had intercourse during their trip and are not interested in being pregnant at this time. Which of the following is most correct?

a. She should ignore the one missed pill.
b. She should take two pills immediately.
c. She should take two pills immediately and use a backup method of contraception for 7 days.
d. She should use emergency contraception immediately and restart her pills on the following day.
e. She should use emergency contraception immediately and use a different form of birth control for the remainder of her cycle.

50. A 29-year-old obese woman with type 2 diabetes mellitus is asking you about progestin-only pills as a method of contraception. Which of the following is true?

a. Progestin-only pills are contraindicated in women with diabetes.
b. Progestin-only pills would increase her risk of thromboembolic events.
c. Progestin-only pills are only Food and Drug Administration (FDA) approved for nursing women.
d. Progestin-only pills increase her risk for ectopic pregnancy.
e. Progestin-only pills should be taken every day of the month, without a hormone-free period.

51. You are counseling a patient regarding contraception options. She is 36 years old, smokes one pack of cigarettes daily, weighs 215 pounds, and has no medical illnesses. She is sexually active but is not in a monogamous relationship. Which of the following is her best contraception option?

a. COC pills.
b. An intravaginal ring system delivering estrogen and progestin.
c. A transdermal contraceptive patch delivering estrogen and progestin.
d. An injectable form of long-acting progestin.
e. Condoms are her only option.

52. A 28-year-old monogamous married woman comes to you for emergency contraception. She and her husband typically use condoms to prevent pregnancy, but when they had sex approximately 36 hours ago, the condom broke. She does not want to start a family at this time. Which of the following statements is true regarding the use of emergency contraception pills (ECPs)?

a. She is too late to use ECPs in this case.
b. ECPs are 90% to 100% effective when used correctly.
c. There are no medical contraindications to the use of ECPs, other than allergy or hypersensitivity to the pill components.
d. ECPs disrupt the pregnancy, if given within days of implantation.
e. Clinicians should perform a pregnancy test before prescribing ECPs.

Genetics

53. Consider the following pedigree:

Pedigree 1

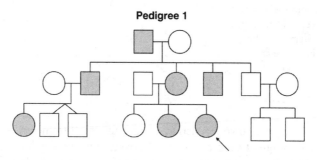

Assuming that the solid circles indicate that the persons are affected with the condition in question, which of the following is true regarding this condition?

a. It is autosomal dominant.
b. It is autosomal recessive.
c. It is X-linked recessive.
d. It is X-linked dominant.
e. It is unlikely to be a genetic disorder.

54. Consider the following pedigree:

Pedigree 2

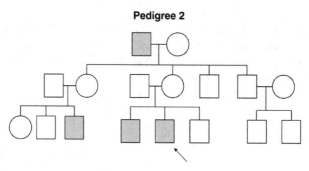

Assuming that the solid squares indicate that the persons are affected with the condition in question, which of the following is true regarding this condition?

a. It is autosomal dominant.
b. It is autosomal recessive.
c. It is X-linked recessive.
d. It is X-linked dominant.
e. It is unlikely to be a genetic disorder.

55. You are caring for a young family who just had a child with multiple malformations of unknown etiology. What type of testing would be best for identifying the diagnosis?

a. Chromosome/karyotype analysis
b. Direct DNA testing
c. Biochemical testing
d. Linkage analysis
e. Protein-specific testing

Biostatistics

56. You note that in your practice, a large number of women with a family history of breast cancer in a first-degree relative develop breast cancer themselves. You evaluate a number of charts and find that 5% of the women in your practice who have breast cancer have a family history, but only 2% of women without breast cancer have a family history. Given this information, what is the sensitivity of using family history as a predictor of breast cancer in your patient population?

a. 2%
b. 5%
c. 93%
d. 95%
e. 98%

57. You are reading a population study that reports 90% of people with lung cancer are smokers. Thirty percent of the people without lung cancer are also smokers. Given this information, what is the specificity using smoking as a predictor of lung cancer?

a. 10%
b. 30%
c. 40%
d. 70%
e. 90%

58. You are determining whether or not to use a rapid streptococcal antigen test to screen for streptococcal pharyngitis. The package insert cites a study with an N of 310 where they evaluated the screen compared to the gold standard throat culture. Among them, 210 patients had a positive throat culture and 100 had a negative throat culture. Of the 100 people who had a negative throat culture, the screen was negative in 98 of them. Of the 210 patients who had a positive throat culture, the screen was negative in 2 of them. Which of the following statements best describes this situation?

a. The sensitivity of the test is 2%.
b. The specificity of the test is 98%.
c. The test has a 2% false-negative rate.
d. The test has a 98% false-positive rate.
e. The test has a positive predictive value of 2%.

59. You are evaluating a clinical trial for an experimental lung cancer drug. You learn that 250 subjects received the experimental drug while 150 subjects received the control drug. At the end of the year-long trial, 50 patients in the intervention arm died and 50 patients in the control arm died. Which of the following is true about risk reduction?

a. The relative risk reduction (RRR) of the drug is 13%.
b. The RRR is 40%.
c. The absolute risk reduction (ARR) is 20%.
d. The ARR is 33%.
e. The ARR is 40%.

60. In a study evaluating a new heart failure drug, 100 patients participated in a 6-month clinical trial to evaluate its effect on mortality. Among them, 60 patients received the intervention drug and 40 patients received the control drug. At the end of the study, 8 patients in the control group had died and 6 patients in the intervention group had died. From this information, how many patients would you need to treat in order to save one life?

a. 6
b. 10
c. 14
d. 20
e. 25

61. You are reading a medical journal and come across an article about diabetes. The study followed 10,000 patients over 3 years. At the start of the study, 2000 people had diabetes. At the end of the study, 1000 additional people developed diabetes. What was the incidence of diabetes during the study?

a. 10%
b. 12.5%
c. 20%
d. 30%
e. 50%

62. You are reading a study that compares cholesterol levels in children whose fathers died from an MI with cholesterol levels in children whose fathers died from other causes. The p value obtained in the test was less than 0.001. What does this value indicate?

a. There was no difference in cholesterol levels between the two groups.
b. The difference in the cholesterol levels was less than 0.1%.
c. There is a less than 0.1% probability that the results obtained in this study were incorrect.
d. There is a less than 0.1% probability that the results obtained in this study occurred because of a sampling error.
e. If the null hypothesis is true, there is a less than 0.1% probability of obtaining a test statistic equal to or more extreme than the one obtained.

63. You are considering using a new influenza screening test. You find a study that evaluated 1000 patients with this new test. Of these 1000 patients, 400 had the disease. Three hundred of those had positive tests, and 100 of those had a negative test. Of the 600 who did not have the disease, 200 had positive tests and 400 had negative tests. What is the positive predictive value of this test?

a. 50%
b. 60%
c. 66%
d. 75%
e. 80%

64. You find that many of your patients who have gone to the emergency department with chest pain have a negative set of initial cardiac enzymes. Most of those with a negative set of initial enzymes did not have a heart attack. You decide to evaluate 100 of your patients who have gone to the emergency department with chest pain to find out if an initial set of negative enzymes by itself is a good predictor of those that are not having an MI. Of those 100 patients, 20 of them had acute MIs. Of those 20, 10 had a positive set of enzymes initially. Of the 80 who did not have an acute MI, none of them had a positive set of initial enzymes. Given this information, what is the negative predictive value of the initial set of cardiac enzymes in your patient population?

a. 20%
b. 22%
c. 50%
d. 89%
e. 100%

Preventive Medicine

Answers

Immunizations

1. The answer is c. Hepatitis B infects approximately 1.25 million people in the United States and more than 450 million people globally. It is transmitted more efficiently than hepatitis C or HIV, and the likelihood of transmission increases with the level of HBV DNA in the serum. In high-prevalence areas, hepatitis B is most often vertically transmitted, but because of screening and immunization practices, it's most often transmitted horizontally in the United States. Young age is a risk factor for the development of chronic hepatitis B, with more than 90% of children who contract the disease before 5 years of age developing chronic disease. Studies have shown that compared to no intervention, treating the infant of a hepatitis B-positive mother with hepatitis B immune globulin within 12 hours of birth, and vaccination, substantially reduces the transmission rate. Therefore, all mothers should be screened for hepatitis B surface antigen, and if positive, the babies should be treated as described in this question. If the hepatitis status of the mother is unknown, the child should get the vaccine, and the mother should be tested. If the mother is found to be positive, the baby should receive immune globulin within 7 days.

2. The answer is a. Prior to the introduction of an effective vaccine, 1 in 200 children developed invasive Haemophilus disease before age 5, often leading to meningitis, hearing loss, or intellectual disability. Vaccines against Hib have been 95% to 100% effective in preventing invasive Hib disease. Before the introduction of the Hib vaccine, infection with *H influenzae* led to 20,000 invasive cases per year and about 1000 deaths per year. The most common manifestations of invasive disease are meningitis, epiglottis, pneumonia, arthritis, and cellulitis. The vaccine does not reduce the rate of otitis media, as most cases are caused by nontypeable *H influenzae*. Invasive disease does not always result in adequate antibody production, and therefore, unvaccinated children under the age of 2 who develop invasive Hib should be vaccinated as soon as possible after convalescence. Adverse reactions to the vaccine are very rare. In fact, no serious reactions have been linked to the vaccine, and systemic reactions like fever and irritability are infrequent. The most common side effects are limited to mild fever, local redness, swelling, or warmth. The vaccine should not be administered before 6 weeks of age, as immune tolerance to the antigen may be induced. The vaccine may be given with other vaccines.

3. The answer is e. Varicella immunization is recommended for adults who have not had evidence of infection or immunization. US-born people born before 1980 are generally considered immune, with the exception of health care workers and pregnant women. Two doses of vaccine are required, 4 to 8 weeks apart, regardless of a person's age, unless they have evidence of receiving one vaccine dose in the past. While many people who do not remember having chicken pox have serologic evidence of immunity, testing is not necessary, as the vaccine is well-tolerated in those already immune. While nonimmune pregnant women should not receive the vaccine until after delivery, household contacts of immunocompetent pregnant women do not need to delay vaccination. Rarely, given that the vaccine is a live-attenuated virus, people receiving the vaccine may develop infection. This occurs in approximately 1% of people vaccinated. However, the case is mild and does not appear to be contagious. Individuals with malignancy, including blood or lymphatic, should not receive the varicella vaccination. Adults with HIV infection and a CD4 count more than or equal to 200 cells/μL may receive the vaccination.

4. The answer is e. The dosing schedule for HBV vaccination is 0, 1, and 6 months. When the second or third dose is delayed, there is no need to restart the series and the subsequent dose can be administered as long as there is an 8-week gap between the second and third dose of vaccine. The vaccine is not a live virus, so it can be administered to pregnant or lactating women. Routine prenatal care does not call for administration of hepatitis B vaccine, but women who are at high risk for hepatitis B should be vaccinated, including women who are being evaluated or treated for a sexually transmitted infection (STI), have recent or current injection-drug use, have had a hepatitis B virus surface antigen (HBsAg)-positive sexual partner, or have had more than one sexual partner in the past 6 months. It is recommended that administration of the HBV vaccine in any high-risk patient occur immediately after serologic testing is obtained and counseling is provided. Waiting for serology is not necessary as duplicate immunization is not associated with adverse events nor is the presence of past or current infection. However, some patients with risk factors for HBV are at risk for not following up and waiting may result in a failure of the patient to receive appropriate vaccination.

5. The answer is c. Hepatitis A vaccination is indicated for men who have sex with men or users of injection drugs. Occupational indications include persons working with hepatitis A virus (HAV)-infected primates or with HAV in a research laboratory setting. Medical indications include chronic liver disease and persons that receive clotting factor concentrates. The HPV vaccine is recommended for gay, bisexual, and other men who have sex with men through the age of 26. Meningitis vaccination is indicated for those with functional asplenia, travelers to endemic areas, or those within an area of identified outbreak. College students can be counseled about the vaccination, especially if they are living in a dormitory. Pneumococcal vaccination is only indicated for those with chronic diseases, functional asplenia, smokers, or residents of long-term care facilities. An MMR booster is not indicated.

6. The answer is d. Rubella is normally a mild self-limited illness, but infection during pregnancy can result in fetal death or congenital defects known as congenital rubella syndrome (CRS). CRS is devastating, and rubella immunity is important for women considering pregnancy. The risk of CRS is greatest during the first trimester, so ideally, nonimmunity to rubella should be identified as part of preconception counseling. If a woman is found to be rubella nonimmune, vaccination should not occur if she is pregnant or planning pregnancy in the next 4 weeks. Although the vaccine is contraindicated in pregnancy, inadvertent vaccination is not an indication for therapeutic abortion. If the patient is currently pregnant and nonimmune, she should be vaccinated as early in the postpartum period as possible.

7. The answer is e. Increasing reports of pertussis among US adults has stimulated vaccine development for adults. A tetanus-diphtheria 5-component acellular pertussis vaccine (Tdap) is available. Adults aged 19 to 64 should receive a single dose, regardless of the interval since the last tetanus or diphtheria-toxoid–containing vaccine. Subsequently, they should receive a booster with Td every 10 years. Adults with close contact to babies under 12 months should be encouraged to receive the vaccine due to the high mortality rates for infants who contract pertussis. Pregnant women should receive one dose of TdaP with each pregnancy, preferably during weeks 27 to 36. The DTaP formulation of pertussis vaccination is indicated only for children under 7 years of age. Td, with coverage only for tetanus and diphtheria, should be administered instead of TdaP when a child has had a moderately severe reaction to TdaP, including uncontrollable crying for more than 3 hours after TdaP vaccination, fever more than 102°F, or seizure within 72 hours of vaccination with TdaP.

8. The answer is c. Influenza is a highly contagious viral infection. Vaccination is between 30% and 90% effective in preventing influenza or complications from influenza. Influenza vaccination is recommended annually for children aged 6 months and older. The minimum age for vaccination with the TIV is 6 months. ACIP does not currently recommend the use of the live, attenuated influenza vaccination (LAIV) for children aged 2 to 17 due to a lack of effectiveness against certain subtypes of H1N1 influenza in this group. In this case, since the mother wishes all her children be vaccinated, only the 4-month-old should be excluded because of age.

9. The answer is e. The influenza vaccine is recommended for all persons aged 6 months and older. The minimum age for LAIV is 2 years, so that vaccine would be inappropriate for the child in this question. Also, ACIP does not currently recommend the use of the LAIV for children aged 2 to 17 due to a lack of effectiveness against certain subtypes of H1N1 influenza in this group. The minimum age for TIV is 6 months. It is recommended that practitioners administer two doses of vaccine (separated by at least 4 weeks) to children between the ages of 6 months and 8 years who are receiving the seasonal influenza vaccine for the first time, or who were vaccinated for the first time during the previous influenza season but received only one dose. Since this is the child's first vaccination, he should receive two doses.

10. The answer is e. The CDC's ACIP recommendation states that all healthy children aged 24 to 59 months who have not completed their primary immunization for pneumococcal disease be given one dose of PCV13. If the child had received less than three doses of the PCV13 during his/her primary immunization series, two doses should be given at least 8 weeks apart. The usual schedule for the series is one vaccination at 2, 4, 6, and 12 to 15 months.

11. The answer is d. The HPV vaccination is recommended for all adult women younger than 26 years of age who have not completed the vaccine series. History of genital warts or an abnormal Pap test are not, by themselves, evidence of prior infection with all HPV subtypes, and are not reasons to avoid vaccination. Persons who are sexually active but not in monogamous relationships are at risk for infection, and should therefore be immunized if they meet criteria.

12. The answer is c. The quadrivalent HPV vaccination has been shown to be highly immunogenic, safe, and well-tolerated in male and female individuals aged 9 to 26 in studies. To be most effective, the vaccine should be given before an adolescent becomes sexually active. It can be administered when a patient has an abnormal Pap test, genital warts, or when a woman is breast-feeding. It can also be given when a patient is immunocompromised because of a disease or medication. It is not recommended for use during pregnancy.

13. The answer is c. According to 2015 guidelines, adults 65 years or above should receive one dose of pneumococcal conjugate vaccine and one dose of pneumococcal polysaccharide vaccine. The pneumococcal conjugate vaccine should be given before the polysaccharide vaccine if they are both due at the same time. After giving the conjugate vaccine, the polysaccharide vaccine should be given at least a year later in immunocompetent individuals. In patients 65 years or older who also have immunocompromising conditions, the next dose of polysaccharide vaccine can be given 8 or more weeks later as long as it is 5 years from the previous dose of polysaccharide vaccine. If either vaccine is given earlier than recommended, however, it is not necessary to repeat the dose. Although she has a medical indication for the pneumococcal polysaccharide vaccine, she had her first shot before the age of 65. Therefore, she should receive the pneumococcal conjugate vaccine now and get a one-time revaccination of the polysaccharide vaccine 5 years after her initial vaccination. Intranasal influenza should only be used in healthy adults younger than the age of 50.

14. The answer is e. The herpes zoster vaccination is currently recommended by ACIP and the CDC for adults 60 years or older regardless of whether or not they report a prior episode of herpes zoster. The vaccination is FDA approved for persons younger than 60. ACIP continues to recommend the vaccination only for individuals 60 years of age or greater. Adults with malignant conditions and those with immunodeficiency (including HIV) or who are receiving immunosuppressive therapies should not receive the Zostavax vaccine but may receive the newly released recombinant zoster vaccine, Shingrix.

15. The answer is d. ACIP recommends the HPV vaccine for administration as a two-dose series to all adolescents at ages 11 or 12. When the vaccine first became available, it was given as a three-dose series at times 0, 1-2 months, and 6 months. Recently, ACIP and the FDA approved the use of a two-dose series for anyone who initiates vaccination before the age of 15. The dosing interval is 0, then 6-12 months with a minimum of 5 months in between dose 1 and 2. Therefore, the 14-year-old can complete her series today with the second dose since it has been more than 5 months since she received the first vaccine. The 16-year-old is not adequately immunized because, although he initiated the series before the age of 15, the interval between the first and second immunization was less than 5 months. Although it is recommended to immunize adolescents before the onset of sexual activity, it is not a contraindication to immunization.

16. The answer is d. Individuals at high risk of meningococcal disease are those with certain immunocompromising conditions (HIV) involving the terminal complement component, functional asplenia, individuals traveling to areas with endemic meningococcal disease, and those living in close quarters—including college students up to the age of 21. Two types of meningococcal vaccination are in use today, MPSV4 and MenACWY. MPSV4 is a polysaccharide vaccine that was approved in 1974. Due to poor sustained immune response, it is not the preferred form of vaccination today. The MenACWY vaccine is a conjugate vaccine that provides protection against the A, C, W, and Y serotypes and produces documented "serologic memory" but immunity does wane after 3 to 5 years. It is the preferred choice of vaccination. For adolescents, the current recommendation is to administer two doses of MenACWY at 11 or 12 years with a booster at age 16. Adolescents who receive their first dose of MenACWY at 16 do not need any additional vaccination unless they develop additional risk factors for disease. Booster is not recommended for college students over the age of 21. This patient has not received any MenACWY vaccine, and therefore, should receive a single dose today.

Screening Tests

17. The answer is c. Risk factors for AAA include male gender, age, hypertension, and tobacco use. The USPSTF recommends a one-time ultrasonography screening for males aged 65 to 75 years of age who have *ever* smoked. This current recommendation is not based on pack-year history. The USPSTF recommends against the universal screening of women who have never smoked and finds insufficient evidence to recommend screening in women aged 65 to 75 years who have ever smoked.

18. The answer is b. The USPSTF has concluded that screening for lung cancer with LDCT is of moderate net benefit in asymptomatic individuals at high risk for lung cancer. They recommend screening in individuals "aged 55 to 80 who have a more than or equal to 30-pack-year smoking history and currently smoke or have quit within the past 15 years." The task force recommends discontinuing screening once a patient has not smoked for 15 years, and recommend not screening if the patient has a condition resulting in a limited life-expectancy, or would not be able or willing to undergo curative lung surgery. This recommendation is somewhat controversial, due to the concerns for radiation exposure over the 25-year span based on a study that occurred over a 3-year period of time.

19. The answer is e. Of the interventions listed above, only prescribing folic acid has been shown to be beneficial *prior* to pregnancy. It will decrease the chance of neural tube defects in the baby. The other interventions should be done early in the pregnancy to ensure good pregnancy outcomes.

20. The answer is c. Both the AAFP and the USPSTF recommend screening for colorectal cancer in individuals of average risk between the ages of 50 and 75. The most useful screening for low risk individuals is usually colonoscopy every 10 years; however, this option may not be available for all patients. Decisions to screen between the ages of 76 and 85 years should be individualized and should consider benefits and risks in this population. Screening can be accomplished through indirect tests such as gFOBT, FIT, CT colonography, or with direct visualization tests such as flexible sigmoidoscopy. Optimal screening intervals based on surveillance models and life-years gained indicate the gFOBT and FIT should be performed yearly, while CT colonography and flexible sigmoidoscopy should be performed every 5 years. For a similar benefit, colonoscopy has a longer screening interval at once every 10 years. FIT and colonoscopy have similar efficacy on reduction of mortality, but colonoscopy is associated with greater risks. When polyps or colorectal cancer are diagnosed in a patient by one of these measures, surveillance is no longer considered screening and these intervals no longer apply.

21. The answer is e. Mammographic screening has been shown to decrease mortality from breast cancer. However, screening interval and recommendations have changed based on evidence review. As recently as 2009, the USPSTF developed evidence-based recommendations to help guide physicians and patients. Those guidelines include recommendations that decisions to conduct screening before the age of 50 should be individualized, and take into account patient's risks and preferences. There is a stronger recommendation that women between the age of 50 and 74 years should get screening mammograms every 2 years. Therefore, in this question, the correct answer is to begin routine screening at age 50.

22. The answer is e. The issues surrounding BSE remain controversial. While it is true that most breast cancers are found by women (not by mammography or by clinical breast examination), the AAFP and the USPSTF have reviewed the evidence and found that a significant number of additional imaging procedures and biopsies were performed for women performing BSE than control participants. The increased number of negative procedures and costs associated with this led the USPSTF and the AAFP to recommend *against* the performance of BSE for women at average risk for breast cancer. Prior to 2009, there was insufficient evidence to recommend for or against teaching or performing BSE.

23. The answer is d. There is a strong recommendation from AAFP for cervical cancer screening at least every 3 years for women between the ages of 21 and 65 who have a cervix. Initiation of screening has been postponed from earlier recommendations based on data showing spontaneous disease remission is common in younger patients with dysplasia. The USPSTF and AAFP currently recommend against screening for cervical cancer in women younger than 21 years of age.

24. The answer is c. Current guidelines indicate that screening for cervical cancer should be conducted with cytology (pap smear) every 3 years in women aged 21 to 65. In women aged 30 to 65 who wish to lengthen the interval, screening with cytology and HPV testing should occur every 5 years. Women should be informed, however, that screening with HPV testing may increase positive screens and subsequent interventions. Screening should end at age 65 in women with adequate screening, which is described by the American Cancer Society/American Society for Colposcopy and Cervical Pathology/American Society for Clinical Pathology (ACS/ASCCP/ASCP) guidelines as three consecutive negative cytology results or two consecutive negative HPV results within 10 years prior. In a women with a history of a high-grade lesion (CIN II or greater), whether they have had spontaneous regression or appropriate treatment, screening should continue for 20 years even if this means screening past the age of 65. For this question, the best answer is age 65.

25. The answer is c. The AAFP and the USPSTF recommend against routine referral for genetic counseling or routine genetic testing for breast cancer mutations when women do not meet specific high-risk criteria. For a woman with at least one family member with breast, ovarian, or other BRCA-related cancer, clinicians should use one of several breast cancer risk prediction screening tools to determine if the individual should have in-depth genetic testing. Family history characteristics associated with an increased likelihood of BRCA mutations include:

- Breast cancer diagnosis before age 50
- Bilateral breast cancer
- Both breast and ovarian cancer in the family
- Presence of male breast cancer
- Multiple cases of breast cancer
- One or more family members with two primary types of BRCA-related cancer
- Ashkenazi Jewish ethnicity

The Well Child

26. The answer is b. Well-child visits in the newborn period are critical to ensure the infant is receiving adequate nutrition and is demonstrating adequate growth. In the first 6 months, the infant should gain about 1oz/day. Infants should feed "on-demand," meaning whenever they exhibit signs of hunger or at least every 3 hours. Exclusive breast-feeding for the first 6 months of life is recommended for all infants. However, breast milk does not supply adequate amounts of vitamin D or iron. Vitamin D supplementation (400 U/day) is recommended for all breast-fed newborns. Iron supplementation is not recommended in full-term breast-fed infants until 4 months of age, when they are felt to deplete their iron stores. Infants who are formula fed receive enough vitamin D and iron in the formula and, therefore, do not require supplementation. Fluoride supplementation should begin at age 6 to 9 months in high-risk children, not with tooth eruption.

27. The answer is c. Infantile colic is a term used to describe infants who are excessively fussy despite a normal examination. Specifically, infants with 3 or more hours of crying or fussing at least 3 times a week for at least 3 weeks meet the criteria for colic. The exact etiology is unclear, but it occurs equally in male and female infants, peaks around 3 to 4 weeks of age, and is typically resolved by 3 to 4 months of age. Symptoms include fussiness with eating, pulling up of the legs, passing flatus, facial expressions of pain or discomfort, and difficulty falling or staying asleep. Symptoms are typically worse in the evening hours. An organic cause is only identified in less than 5% of cases.

28. The answer is a. History and physical examination during the well-child visit is important for early detection of many developmental disabilities. While every child develops on a unique timeline, normal timeframes have been developed as to when most children will achieve certain milestones. Failure to meet certain timelines are agreed to as "red flags." An infant that does not turn toward-sights and sounds by 2 months of age should be a red flag to a provider and necessitate further evaluation and/or referral for further evaluation. By 4 months of age, a child should watch or track things, smile and coo, and reach for items nearby. A 6-month-old child should be able to maneuver items into his/her mouth and roll over. A 9-month-old child should be able to transfer toys from hand to hand, sit without assistance, and recognize his/her own name.

29. The answer is d. Failure to thrive does not have a single, agreed upon definition. Several criteria are used and should be considered when a physician encounters a child with weight loss or failure to gain weight. A weight less than 3 to 5 percentile, weight that crosses two major percentiles downward, or less than 75% of the median weight for age are all accepted definitions. It is typical for infants to lose weight in the first week of life as feeding patterns and milk production are developing. However, a weight loss of more than 8% merits close follow-up visits. Most newborns regain their birthweight by the end of the second week of life.

30. The answer is b. Cryptorchidism, or failure of one or both testicles to descend into the scrotum, occurs in 2% to 5% of full-term infants and 30% of premature male infants. In many male infants, the missing testicle is caused by muscular contraction and can be palpated after a warm bath. In infants with a persistent absence of testicle(s), orchiopexy is recommended between 6 months and 1 year of age to avoid the increased risks of testicular neoplasms, infertility, testicular torsion, and inguinal hernia. Hydrocele, hypogonadism, epididymitis, and small stature are not associated with cryptorchidism.

31. The answer is e. Risk factors for childhood lead poisoning include significant exposure to lead in the environment. Lead paint was commonly used in homes prior to 1950 and homes built after 1978 are unlikely to contain lead. In older homes with lead paint, additional coats of paint effectively "seal" off the lead and reduce the risk of exposure. However, an older home that has chipping, peeling paint or is under renovation also raises the likelihood of lead poisoning. Small children who crawl on the floor, tend to put nonfood items in their mouth, and suck their thumbs are likely to have increased exposures to lead if it is in their home or environment. Having close contact with an adult with high lead exposure, such as someone in the plumbing, construction, or manufacturing industries, is a risk factor for high lead levels. Nail products are not sources of lead exposure. If one sibling has high lead levels, other siblings in the same home are at increased risk.

32. The answer is a. Hypertension in children is often overlooked. It is more often due to secondary causes than in adults and can lead to hypertension in adulthood. Normal pediatric blood pressure values in children increase with body size, age, and height. Abnormal blood pressure values are defined by the National High Blood Pressure Education Program (NHBPEP) and are based on tables produced by the National Institutes of Health. Normal blood pressure is defined as systolic or diastolic blood pressure that is less than 90th percentile based on age and height. Prehypertension is blood pressure in the 90th to less than 95th percentile (or $\geq$ 120/80 mm Hg). Stage 1 hypertension is blood pressure between the 95th to less than

99th percentile plus 5 mm Hg, and stage 2 hypertension is blood pressure more than 99th percentile plus 5 mm Hg.

33. The answer is d. The American Academy of Pediatrics provides guidelines on the preparticipation physical examination. This examination is intended to detect conditions which could cause injury or illness through sports participation. A systolic murmur that increases with Valsalva maneuver and decreases with squatting is concerning for left ventricular outflow obstruction or hypertrophic cardiomyopathy (HCOM). Individuals with this type of systolic murmur should not be cleared for athletics until they have a more thorough cardiovascular workup, including echocardiogram, and those with confirmed HCOM are disqualified from athletics. Having a chronic medical condition such as epilepsy or asthma does not necessarily disqualify a child from athletics if the condition is well controlled or the particular sport does not pose an additional risk to their condition. For example, it would be dangerous to allow a weightlifter with uncontrolled epilepsy to lift heavy weights, but if the condition is controlled the risks are acceptable. Similarly, a child with asthma or an eating disorder can compete if the condition is controlled. Exercise is helpful in the treatment of hypertension and should be encouraged unless it is severe.

The Preoperative Evaluation

34. The answer is b. The purpose of the preoperative evaluation is to identify and manage risk. The primary care physician is frequently asked to perform this evaluation on surgical patients. All surgeries involve some level of risk, and the evaluation allows the patient to balance the risks involved in surgery against the potential benefits, and allows the physician to minimize risks before, during, and after the procedure. Potential surgical complications involve infectious (wound infections, pneumonia, urinary tract infections, bacterial endocarditis, and sepsis), cardiac (MI, cardiac arrest, pulmonary edema, and complications of congestive heart failure [CHF]), pulmonary (pneumonia, atelectasis, bronchitis, respiratory failure, pulmonary embolus), thrombosis (peripheral venous thromboembolism, arterial thrombosis) adverse reactions to anesthesia, gastrointestinal (ulcer disease, ileus, hyperemesis), and psychologic (delirium, exacerbation of existing psychiatric disease) complications. Of the complications listed, cardiac events are the events that are most likely to be lethal.

Pulmonary complications are most likely to be seen in children and are common in obese patients, but are less likely to be lethal.

35. The answer is c. The American College of Cardiology and the American Heart Association have printed guidelines for preoperative cardiac evaluation. If a patient has no known heart disease, the evaluator should look at clinical predictors for heart disease. Major clinical predictors would require coronary artery evaluation prior to surgery, and include unstable coronary syndromes, decompensated CHF, significant arrhythmias, or severe valvular disease. Intermediate clinical predictors include mild angina, a prior MI, compensated CHF, diabetes, and renal insufficiency. Intermediate clinical predictors require the evaluator to look at the patient's functional capacity to determine level of preoperative cardiac testing. In a patient with poor functional capacity, noninvasive testing is recommended. In the question above, the patient has diabetes (an intermediate clinical predictor) and poor functional capacity. Therefore, stress testing is recommended.

36. The answer is e. Recent coronary revascularization is a risk for poor perioperative outcomes. People with clinically important coronary artery disease should defer noncardiac procedures until 6 months after revascularization, when possible. If surgery is necessary within 6 months after revascularization, repeated evaluation of the coronary arteries is necessary prior to surgery. In this case, because the surgery is elective, the patient should defer the surgery until 6 months has elapsed from the time of coronary revascularization. If the patient is asymptomatic at that time, the patient may be able to proceed to surgery without reassessment.

37. The answer is a. Asymptomatic patients who have had a normal stress test in the past 2 years, bypass surgery in the past 5 years, or angioplasty in the past 5 years are unlikely to have developed significant new disease. Current recommendations are that these people may proceed to surgery without further cardiac workup. However, some experts suggest screening ECG should be done in patients older than 65. Assessment of left ventricular function (such as an echocardiogram) is not recommended, as it will unlikely change the perioperative management of the patient.

38. The answer is a. Pulmonary complications from surgery are most common in surgeries that are anatomically close to the diaphragm.

Preexisting respiratory disease increases the change of bad outcomes, and smoking is a risk factor for pulmonary problems after surgery. Despite this, chest x-ray is not indicated as a routine baseline test for patients undergoing surgery. It may be indicated for the evaluation of physical examination abnormalities or reported symptoms of dyspnea or cough, but it is unhelpful in the absence of these symptoms. Pulmonary function testing is useful for demonstrating the status of asthma or chronic obstructive pulmonary disease (COPD) prior to surgery, but would not be an effective routine test in the absence of these diagnoses or symptoms leading one to suspect these diagnoses. Pulse oximetry or arterial blood gases are rarely useful in the preoperative patient without symptoms.

Travel Medicine

39. The answer is b. While rare, there is an increased risk for DVT and pulmonary emboli with prolonged air travel. Wearing compression hose, walking, or stretching have all demonstrated a benefit in the prevention of DVT. Aspirin has not been shown to reduce the risk of blood clots and low-molecular-weight heparin has not been adequately studied in this setting. Sitting in a window seat is unlikely to be beneficial as it would make walking and movement more difficult than other seating choices.

40. The answer is a. The CDC does not recommend antibiotic chemoprophylaxis for traveler's diarrhea because of the development of resistant organisms. Most times, the condition is self-limited. However, they do suggest that antibiotic prophylaxis can be considered in those who are immunocompromised or in those in which illness would be catastrophic for their travel. In this case, ciprofloxacin or rifaximin is recommended and effective in preventing traveler's diarrhea. BSS may also be used for the prevention of traveler's diarrhea. The CDC does recommend using common sense regarding food and water, eating nothing unless it is boiled, peeled, or cooked.

41. The answer is a. Yellow fever is a mosquito-borne illness endemic to parts of Sub-Saharan Africa and South America. While the disease is rarely acquired by travelers, the length of travel and the types of activities can affect an individual's risk. Countries can require proof of vaccination prior to entry. The vaccine can only be administered by authorized sites and the completion of a World Health Organization yellow card is required by many countries at least 10 days prior to entry. The vaccine is a live-attenuated formulation with uncommon side effects. However, the likelihood of serious adverse events increases with age, with those over 60 at higher risk of side effects. Administration of the vaccine should be based on consideration of the benefits versus risks; there is no age-related cutoff. Myasthenia gravis or diseases affecting the thymus increase the risk of side effects from the vaccine itself, not the disease. As of 2016, the vaccine is considered effective for life unless certain high-risk situations exist: long-term travel, travel to West Africa, and traveling to an area with a current yellow fever outbreak.

42. The answer is d. The decision of whether or not to use malaria chemoprophylaxis should be based on information provided by the CDC and their online malaria maps. Because activity within a country can vary significantly, information about where and how long an individual will travel is essential for estimating exposure risk. Transmission varies between urban/rural environments and resistance to various regimens does exist and should affect which agent is used. Chloroquine, doxycycline, atovaquone-proguanil (Malarone), and mefloquine (Larium) are commonly used regimens. Using DEET in her hotel room is effective at reducing transmission, but only lasts 6 to 8 hours and will not protect her when she ventures outside. Interestingly, there is no transmission of malaria in altitudes more than 2500 m. Malaria is the most common cause of fever in returning travelers to the United States and individuals returning to their malaria-endemic homeland are major sources for malaria in the United States, because these individuals often do not use chemoprophylaxis. Clinicians should not assume immunity to malaria just because a person has visited or lived in a malaria-affected region or country.

43. The answer is d. Altitude sickness is a preventable and possibly fatal illness. Rapid ascent to altitudes more than 2400 m are associated with the illness, which often presents with dyspnea, nausea, vomiting, headache, and altered mental status. Air travel allows travelers to arrive at high-altitude destinations suddenly, without time for acclimatization. Acetazolamide is an effective prevention therapy, but should be started 1 day prior to ascent and continued twice daily until the individual has been at their final altitude for 2 to 3 days. Ascent rates less than 300 m/day may also reduce the risk of the sickness. While the only definitive treatment for altitude sickness is descent, increasing hydration, rest, and limiting exertion can aid with the acclimatization process and reduce the possibility of altitude sickness.

This patient is only traveling to a final altitude of 2000 m and will have a week to slowly acclimatize, so she does not need to arrive early and she is unlikely to experience altitude sickness in these conditions.

Contraception

44. The answer is d. The IUD is the most common form of contraception in the world, but the rates of use in the United States are much lower. Before the development of modern-day IUDs, nulliparity, multiple sexual partners, and age less than 25 were considered contraindications. However, the newer IUDs may be used in these populations due to smaller size and improved design. The risk of PID is greatest in the first 20 days after insertion and then returns to baseline, indicating that the infection is likely due to the introduction of bacteria during insertion, not the IUD itself. The levonorgestrel IUD appears to lower the risk of PID by thickening the cervical mucous. However, women who have multiple sexual partners should be counseled to use condoms to protect against STDs. Expulsion occurs in 2% to 10% of women and this rate is increased in women of nulliparity and when the IUD is inserted during menses. Two main categories of IUD are available in the United States. The copper IUD is approved for 10 years of use; it may increase menstrual bleeding and cramping. The levonorgestrel IUD, depending on the brand, are approved for 3 to 5 years of use. The progesterone in the levonorgestrel IUD reduces menstrual blood flow and can be used to treat heavy menstrual bleeding.

45. The answer is a. In some patients, COCs cause a small increase in blood pressure. This risk increases with age. Both estrogen and progestin are known to cause blood pressure elevations, so changing formulations of COC or using progestin-only pills may not lead to problem resolution. Once COCs are discontinued, blood pressure usually returns to normal within 3 months.

46. The answer is e. Side effects of COCs include androgenic effects (hair growth, male pattern baldness, nausea) and estrogenic effects (nausea, breast tenderness, and fluid retention). Weight gain is thought to be a common side effect, but multiple studies have failed to show it to be a statistically significant side effect. The side effect most frequently cited as the reason for stopping the use of COCs is irregular bleeding. It is common in the first 3 months of use and generally diminishes over time.

47. The answer is c. DMPA is an injectable long-acting contraception given every 3 months by intramuscular injection. It eliminates the need for daily medication and can be self-administered in many women. DMPA inhibits ovulation and has a comparable failure rate to levonorgestrel implants, sterilization, and copper IUDs. The most common side effect of DMPA is menstrual changes, with around 75% of women experiencing amenorrhea by 1 year. Fertility can be delayed after cessation of DMPA, but there is no permanent effect. Most women successfully conceive within 10 months of the last injection. DMPA does cause a decrease in bone mass density (BMD) and for this reason, use beyond 2 years is no longer recommended. However, newer studies have shown reversal of the decrease in BMD after cessation of DMPA. Weight gain is a significant side effect of DMPA. However, it can be used safely in woman more than 35 years of age who smoke or are at increased risk of arterial or venous clots.

48. The answer is c. The use of COC pills is associated with a threefold risk of venous thromboembolism. COCs have a protective effect against ovarian cancer and endometrial cancer. The risk of hemorrhagic stroke is not increased by the use of COCs, and they have not been shown in studies to impact carbohydrate metabolism in a statistically significant way.

49. The answer is d. It is important to counsel patients appropriately if they miss an oral contraceptive pill. If an active pill is missed at any time, and no intercourse has occurred in the past 5 days, two pills should be taken immediately and a backup method should be used for 7 days. If intercourse occurred in the previous 5 days, emergency contraception should be used immediately and pills should be restarted the following day. A backup method should be used for 5 days. There is no need to change contraceptive method.

50. The answer is e. Progestin-only pills prevent conception through suppression of ovulation, thickening of cervical mucus, alteration of the endometrium, and inhibition of tubal transport. The effectiveness of this method is dependent on consistency of use. In fact, if a pill is taken even 3 hours late, an alternative form of contraception should be used for 48 hours. There is no hormone-free period with these pills, and they should be taken every day. The pills do not carry an increased risk for thromboembolism, and the World Health Organization has reported this form of contraception to be safe for women with a history of venous thrombosis, pulmonary embolism, diabetes, obesity, or hypertension. Nursing women can use this pill, but there is FDA approval for use in others as well.

In general, progestin-only pills protect against ectopic pregnancy by lowering the chance of conception. However, if progestin-only pill users get pregnant, the chance of ectopic pregnancy is 6% to 10% higher than the rate found in women not using contraception. Therefore, users should be aware of the symptoms for ectopic pregnancy.

51. The answer is d. Oral contraceptive pills containing estrogen and progestin components are contraindicated in smokers older than 35 years, because of an increased risk of thromboembolic events. An intravaginal ring or transdermal patch that releases estrogen and progestin is also contraindicated in smokers older than 35 years for the same reason. Additionally, pregnancy is more likely to occur in women who use the transdermal patch and weigh more than 189 pounds. Injectable progestin can be safely used in women more than 35 years of age who smoke or otherwise at risk for arterial or venous thromboembolism. An injectable long-acting progestin would therefore be the best choice in this woman.

52. The answer is c. Emergency contraception is appropriate when no contraception was used (including cases of sexual assault), or when there is contraceptive failure. They should be used less than 5 days after intercourse. ECPs involve limited hormonal exposure, and therefore have not been shown to increase the risk of venous thromboembolism, stroke, or MI. In fact, there are no medical contraindications to the use of ECPs. They do not disrupt an already implanted pregnancy and do not cause birth defects. Progestin ECPs prevent 85% of expected pregnancies when used correctly, and combined ECPs prevent 75% of expected pregnancies. They are not 100% effective in pregnancy prevention. There is no need to perform a pregnancy test when prescribing.

Genetics

53. The answer is a. The pedigree shown is for an autosomal dominant condition. As the pedigree shows, males and females in the family are equally affected, and parents are transmitting the gene to their offspring (vertical inheritance). If this were an autosomal recessive trait, horizontal inheritance would be more present, with multiple children being affected from unaffected parents. X-linked recessive traits affect more males than females, and X-linked dominant traits affect more females than males.

54. The answer is c. The pedigree shown is for an X-linked recessive condition. As the pedigree shows, the condition affects more males than females, and inheritance is through the maternal side of the family (diagonal inheritance). Female carriers have a 50% risk for each daughter to be a carrier and a 50% risk for each son to be affected. All daughters of an affected male are carriers, and none of his sons are affected. If this were an autosomal dominant condition, males and females would be equally affected, and parents would transmit the gene to their offspring. If this were an autosomal recessive trait, horizontal inheritance would be present, with multiple children being affected from unaffected parents. If it were X-linked dominant, more females would be affected than males.

55. The answer is a. Chromosome/karyotype analysis is a microscopic study of the chromosomes and is used to identify abnormalities in chromosome number, size, or structure. It is commonly ordered when patients are suspected of having a recognizable chromosomal syndrome (trisomy 21) and in newborns with multiple malformations of unknown etiology or with ambiguous genitalia. Direct DNA testing is indicated for patients affected or predisposed to a condition for which the gene change that causes the condition has been identified (cystic fibrosis). Biochemical tests identify or quantify metabolites or enzymes to measure activity, and are commonly used to diagnose and monitor disorders of metabolism. Linkage analyses identify genetic sequences that are physically in close proximity to a disease gene of interest.

Biostatistics

56. The answer is b. Sensitivity is thought of as the probability that a symptom is present given that the person has the disease. In the above example, the "symptom" in question is a family history (fmx) of breast cancer. Of women that have breast cancer, 5% have a family history; therefore, the sensitivity of using family history as a predictor of breast cancer is 5%.

	Disease Present	**Disease Absent**
Test Positive (fmx +)	A (5)	B
Test Negative (fmx-)	C (95)	D
Sensitivity = A/(A + C) × 100 = 5/(95 + 5) × 100 = 5%		

57. The answer is d. Specificity can be thought of as the probability that the symptom is *not* present given that a person does not have a disease. In the above example, the "symptom" is smoking. Of people who do not have lung cancer, 30% of them are smokers, indicating that 70% of them are not smokers. Of the people who do not have lung cancer, 70% of them do not smoke.

	Disease Present	Disease Absent
Test Positive (smoking)	A	B (30)
Test Negative (no smoking)	C	D (70)
Specificity = D/(D + B) × 100 = 70/(70 + 30) × 100 = 70%		

58. The answer is c. A false-negative is defined as a person who tests negative, but who is actually positive. In the above example, 2% of the positive people test negative. Therefore, the false-negative rate is 2% in this case. Sensitivity is defined as the probability that the test would be positive, given that the person has strep throat. The specificity is the probability that the test would be negative if the person does *not* have strep. The false-positive rate is defined as the percent of people who test positive, but are actually negative. The positive predictive value is the probability that a person has an illness, given that the test is positive.

	Disease Present	Disease Absent
Test Positive	A (98)	B *False Positive* (2)
Test Negative	C *False Negative* (2)	D (208)
False negative = C		

59. The answer is b. ARR and RRR are often confused. The ARR of an intervention is simply the difference between the event rate in the intervention and the control group. ARR=CER – EER. However, the RRR is the difference of the two groups expressed as a proportion of the control group. RRR = (CER – EER)/CER. As the baseline risk increases, the RRR tends to increase.

	Experimental Group (E)	Control Group (C)	Total
Events (E)	50 (EE)	50 (CE)	100
Nonevents (N)	200 (EN)	100 (CN)	300
Total Subjects (S)	250 (ES)	150 (CS)	400
Event Rate (ER)	50/250 = 0.2	50/150 = 0.33	
	EER = EE/ES	CER = CE/CS	

CER – EER = ARR: 0.33 – 0.2 = 0.13
RRR = (CER – EER)/CER = (0.33 – 0.2)/0.33 = 0.4 or 40%

60. The answer is b. The number needed to treat is the number of patients needed to treat in order to save one life. The formula is 1/ARR.

	Experimental Group (E)	**Control Group (C)**	**Total**
Events (E)	6 (EE)	8 (CE)	14
Nonevents (N)	54 (EN)	32 (CN)	86
Total Subjects (S)	60 (ES)	40 (CS)	100
Event Rate (ER)	6/60 = 0.1	8/40 = 0.2	
	EER = EE/ES	CER = CE/CS	

CER − EER = ARR: 0.2 − 0.1 = 0.1
1/ARR = NNT: 1/0.1 = 10

61. The answer is b. The incidence of a disease is the probability that a person with no prior disease will develop a new case of the disease over a specific time period. In this case, 1000 people developed diabetes. In the study, only 8000 people began with no prior disease. Therefore, the incidence is 1000/8000 or 12.5%. The prevalence is the probability of having a disease at a specific point in time, and is obtained by dividing the number of people with the disease by the number of people in the study.

62. The answer is e. The p value for any hypothesis test is the level at which we would be indifferent between accepting or rejecting the null hypothesis given the sample data at hand. It can also be thought of as the probability of obtaining a test statistic as extreme or more extreme than the actual test statistic obtained, given that the null hypothesis is true. The p-value helps us evaluate, if the observed value is likely due to chance. It does not reflect the absolute difference in the data between groups or the *correctness* of the data in the sample.

63. The answer is b. The positive predictive value refers to the probability that a positive test correctly identifies an individual who actually has the disease. Using a 4 × 4 chart:

	Disease Present	**Disease Absent**	**Total**
Test Positive	A = 300	B = 200	500
Test Negative	C = 100	D = 400	500
Total	400	600	1000
Positive Predictive Value = A/(A + B), or 300/500 = 60%			

64. The answer is d. The negative predictive value is the probability that a negative test correctly identifies an individual who does not have the disease. Using a 4 × 4 chart:

	Disease Present	Disease Absent	Total
Test Positive	A = 10	B = 0	10
Test Negative	C = 10	D = 80	90
Total	20	80	100
Negative Predictive Value = D/(C + D), or 80/90 = 89%			

Recommended Reading: Preventive Medicine

Advisory Committee on Immunization Practices (ACIP). Recommended Immunization Schedule for Adults Aged 19 or Older, United States, 2017. MMWR. 2017;66(5). Available at www.cdc.gov/mmwr/volumes/66/wr/mm6605e2.htm?s_cid=mm6605e2_w.

American Academy of Family Physicians. Summary of Recommendations for Clinical Preventive Services. July 2017. Available at https://www.aafp.org/dam/AAFP/documents/patient_care/clinical_recommendations/cps-recommendations.pdf. Accessed January 6, 2018.

Bashore TM, Granger CB, Jackson KP, Patel MR. Heart disease. In: Papadakis MA, McPhee SJ, Rabow MW (eds). *Current Medical Diagnosis & Treatment 2018*. New York, NY: McGraw-Hill.

Brunsell SC. Contraception. In: South-Paul JE, Matheny SC, Lewis EL (eds). *Current Diagnosis & Treatment Family Medicine*. 4th ed. New York, NY: McGraw-Hill.

Centers for Disease Control and Prevention. CDC-act early. Available at https://www.cdc.gov/ncbddd/actearly/pdf/checklists/all_checklists.pdf. Accessed January 14, 2018.

Centers for Disease Control and Prevention. Hib vaccine: what everyone should know. Available at https://www.cdc.gov/vaccines/vpd/hib/public/index.html. Accessed January 14, 2018.

Chapter 7. Hypothesis testing: one-sample inference. In: Rosner B (ed). *Fundamentals of Biostatistics*. 8th ed. Boston, MA: Cengage Learning.

Cheng HQ. Preoperative evaluation & perioperative management In: Papadakis MA, McPhee SJ, Rabow MW (eds). *Current Medical Diagnosis & Treatment 2018*. New York, NY: McGraw-Hill.

Conti TD, Patel M, Bhat S. Breastfeeding & infant nutrition. In: South-Paul JE, Matheny SC, Lewis EL (eds). *Current Diagnosis & Treatment Family Medicine*. 4th ed. New York, NY: McGraw-Hill.

Demian E. Preconception care. In: South-Paul JE, Matheny SC, Lewis EL (eds). *Current Diagnosis & Treatment Family Medicine.* 4th ed. New York, NY: McGraw-Hill.

Dewar JC, Dewar SB. Failure to thrive. In: South-Paul JE, Matheny SC, Lewis EL (eds). *Current Diagnosis & Treatment Family Medicine.* 4th ed. New York, NY: McGraw-Hill.

Hogge WA. Genetics for family physicians. In: South-Paul JE, Matheny SC, Lewis EL (eds). *Current Diagnosis & Treatment Family Medicine.* 4th ed. New York, NY: McGraw-Hill.

Huntington MK. Travel medicine. In: Smith MA, Shimp LA, Schrager S (eds). *Family Medicine Ambulatory Care and Prevention.* 6th ed. New York, NY: McGraw-Hill.

Marks JD. Perioperative evaluation. In: Smith MA, Shimp LA, Schrager S (eds). *Family Medicine Ambulatory Care and Prevention.* 6th ed. New York, NY: McGraw-Hill.

Mirabelli MH, Singh J, Mendoza M. The preparticipation sports evaluation. *Am Fam Physician.* 2015;92(5):371-376.

Riley M, Bluhm B. High blood pressure in children and adolescents. *Am Fam Physician.* 2012;85(7):693-700.

Rosner, B. Chapter 3. Probability. In: Rosner B (ed). *Fundamentals of Biostatistics.* 8th ed. Boston, MA: Cengage Learning.

Srinivasan S, Middleton DB. Well child care. In: South-Paul JE, Matheny SC, Lewis EL (eds). *Current Diagnosis & Treatment Family Medicine.* 4th ed. New York, NY: McGraw-Hill.

Symons AB, Mahoney MC. Neonatal hyperbilirubinemia. In: South-Paul JE, Matheny SC, Lewis EL (eds). *Current Diagnosis & Treatment Family Medicine.* 4th ed. New York, NY: McGraw-Hill.

United States Preventive Services Task Force. Available at https://www .uspreventiveservicestaskforce.org/Page/Document/Recommendation-StatementFinal/lung-cancer-screening. Accessed January 14, 2018.

Woo J. Gynecologic disorders. In: Papadakis MA, McPhee SJ, Rabow MW (eds). *Current Medical Diagnosis & Treatment 2018.* New York, NY: McGraw-Hill.

Zimmerman RK, Middleton DB. Routine childhood vaccines. In: South-Paul JE, Matheny SC, Lewis EL (eds). *Current Diagnosis & Treatment Family Medicine.* 4th ed. New York, NY: McGraw-Hill. Zuckerman JN, Faran Y. Travel medicine. In: Kellerman RD, Bope ET (eds). *Conn's Current Therapy, 2018.* Philadelphia, PA: Elsevier.

Doctor-Patient Issues

Questions

Patient-Centered Communication

65. You are seeing a patient whose reason for seeing you is listed as "sinus infection" on your schedule. In the past, this patient has had several issues to discuss at each appointment, extending the appointment time beyond what was scheduled. You have a full schedule and do not want to fall behind. Which of the following interview tactics will most likely lead to a more efficient patient visit?

a. Start by forecasting what you'd like to have happen during the interview
b. Start with an open-ended question like, "What brings you in today?"
c. Start by obtaining a list of all issues the patient wants to discuss
d. Start by indicating the time you have available for the visit
e. Start by letting the patient know that you can only discuss one issue today

66. On the way to work this morning, you passed an accident on the highway and stopped to see if your help was needed. After the emergency medical services (EMS) team arrived, you continued your commute to work. As a result, you were 30 minutes late. Your first patient is a 36-year-old patient with difficult to control hypertension who has been your patient for 5 years. When you walk in, he appears extremely angry. Which of the following statements is the most patient-centered way to approach this situation?

a. "I'm late because I had to help some people on the highway that were involved in an accident. How are you doing today?"
b. "You look very angry."
c. "I'm so sorry that I've kept you waiting and I can tell you're mad. Let's get right to the reason that you came in."
d. "Let's discuss why you're so angry right now."
e. "I can tell you're angry. I would be too if my blood pressure was so hard to control."

67. You are seeing a 34-year-old smoker in your office. She says she's thought about quitting, and although she's tried to quit unsuccessfully in the past, she's ready to consider making another attempt. Which of the following questions is the best example of using motivational interviewing with this patient?

a. "Are you really interested in quitting this time?"
b. "Has anyone close to you been able to successfully quit?"
c. "How will you make sure you're never going to smoke again?"
d. "What do you think will be hardest about trying to quit this time?"
e. "What is one step you can take to get you to your goal?"

68. You are conducting an office visit with a 54-year-old Chinese man with hypertension. He made the appointment earlier this morning because he began feeling short of breath. As you enter the room, you note that he is sitting forward and breathing heavily. Given this scenario, what interviewing technique is the most patient-centered?

a. Use open-ended questions to allow the patient to tell his story.
b. Start by obtaining a list of all issues that the patient wants to discuss during this visit.
c. Direct the interview using closed questions related to his reason for this visit.
d. Elicit the broader personal/psychosocial context of the symptoms.
e. Ask the patient about his beliefs regarding Eastern versus Western treatment options.

69. You are interviewing a 36-year-old woman who is complaining of fatigue. She says, "I'm too exhausted to help my kids with their homework!" As you gather data to help develop a differential diagnosis, which reply to her statement best exemplifies open-ended data gathering?

a. "Too exhausted?"
b. "Can you do other things with your kids?"
c. "Do you still enjoy things you used to enjoy?"
d. "Have you gained weight?"
e. "How is your sleep?"

70. A 42 year-old patient is seeing you a few weeks after the death of his brother. He has no medical history, and made the appointment "just to get checked out." When you ask about his brother's cause of death, you find out that he died after a long battle with cancer. When you ask how he's feeling about his brother's death, he says, "To be honest, I'm kind of relieved." Which of the following responses is the best example of using empathy to build a relationship with the patient?

a. "You look sad to me. Can we talk about that?"
b. "I can understand that."
c. "We all grieve differently."
d. "Are you afraid that you're at risk for cancer too?"
e. "Has anyone else in your family had cancer?"

71. An established patient made an appointment to discuss constipation. As soon as you enter and before you say anything, he begins to discuss his problem, saying that it began 5 days ago when he left on a trip out of state for his mother's funeral. Over the next several minutes, he recounts every detail of the funeral and every detail of his current problem. Which of the following would be the best way to manage this office visit?

a. Interrupt, refocus, and redirect the patient.
b. Forego developing an agenda for the visit with the patient.
c. Use open-ended questions to enhance data-gathering.
d. Ask about the emotional impact of his mother's death.
e. Gather information about his family history using closed-ended questions.

Cultural Competency and Health Disparities

72. You are treating a 61-year-old Chinese immigrant who came to see you for blurred vision. Two weeks ago, she consulted a local Chinese herbalist to help manage fatigue. The herbalist recommended ginseng, which she has been taking for around 10 days. The rest of your history and physical examination are unremarkable. Which of the following is the most culturally appropriate way to manage this situation?

a. Let her know that blurred vision can be a side effect of ginseng and ask if she is comfortable stopping the medication.
b. Let her know that blurred vision can be a side effect of the ginseng, and ask her to decrease her dosage.
c. Let her know that you understand that herbal medication plays an important role in the Chinese culture, and you'd like her to contact you prior to starting any new herbal remedies.
d. Let her know that she shouldn't use herbal remedies because they haven't been studied and can have very negative side effects.
e. Ask her to stop the ginseng and start a workup for fatigue.

73. You are caring for a patient with limited English proficiency originally from El Salvador. His chief complaint is that he's having increasingly severe headaches. He brought an English-speaking relative with him to the visit. You work in a community where there are many Spanish-speaking people, and because of that, you have learned basic medical Spanish, and have hired a medical assistant who, although American, is fluent in conversational Spanish. Which of the following is true regarding this patient visit?

a. You should engage the services of a medical translator for the visit.
b. You should engage the services of a medical interpreter for the visit.
c. You do not need assistance because the patient has an English-speaking relative with him.
d. You do not need assistance because you know enough Spanish to communicate with this patient.
e. You do not need assistance because your medical assistant can translate for you.

74. You are treating a 52-year-old female patient originally from Puerto Rico, who has been in this country for 15 years. You diagnosed her with diabetes 1 year ago, and prescribed metformin in addition to other medications in order to maximize her health. Her hemoglobin A1C has not improved, and further investigation reveals that she has not been taking her metformin. Which clinician approach is most likely to improve adherence to treatment?

a. "Talk to me about what your goals are for managing your diabetes."
b. "I can understand how hard it is to comply with the treatment recommendations."
c. "What is the biggest barrier that is preventing you from taking the medication?"
d. "Let me work with you to arrange diabetes education from someone that speaks Spanish."
e. "Given the struggles you've had with taking the pill, let's try insulin shots."

75. You are seeing a new patient to establish care. The patient is 26-year-old, identifies as Native American, and has completed an electronic review of systems as part of his previsit work. Given disease prevalence in the Native American population, which of the symptoms, if identified on a review of systems, warrants careful further evaluation?

a. Bright red blood in stool
b. Hoarseness
c. Depressed mood
d. Shortness of breath
e. Fever

76. You are caring for a refugee who is concerned about his health. Through an interpreter, you learn that he has lost weight since being in America, despite maintaining his traditional diet. In addition to a complete history and physical examination, which of the following tests would be generally advised for this patient?

a. Hepatitis B surface antibody
b. Hemoglobin
c. Transaminases
d. Erythrocyte sedimentation rate
e. Chest x-ray

Integrative Medicine

77. You diagnosed depression in a 35-year-old man, and began treatment with a selective serotonin reuptake inhibitor (SSRI). His response has been excellent, and his depression has been controlled for 2 months. At his follow-up visit, he lets you know that he has noted some erectile dysfunction. You do not want to change or adjust his antidepressant, since his response has been so good. Which of the following supplements has been used to treat the sexual dysfunction associated with the use of SSRIs?

a. Fish oils
b. Ginseng root
c. *Ginkgo biloba* leaf
d. Kava kava
e. Valerian root

78. You are caring for a 54-year-old woman who is treating her mild depression with St. John's wort. Which of the following is true regarding the mechanism of action for this botanical medicine?

a. It selectively inhibits serotonin reuptake.
b. It selectively inhibits norepinephrine reuptake.
c. It selectively inhibits dopamine reuptake.
d. It inhibits serotonin, norepinephrine, and dopamine reuptake.
e. The mechanism of action is unknown.

79. The patient in the question above is found to have hyperlipidemia that has been resistant to dietary therapy and exercise. You are considering starting a statin to help her lower her cholesterol. Which of the following is true regarding the interaction between St. John's wort and statins?

a. There is no interaction.
b. St. John's wort may lower the blood level of the statin.
c. St. John's wort may increase the blood level of the statin.
d. The statin may lower the blood level of St. John's wort.
e. The statin may raise the blood level of St. John's wort.

80. You are caring for a 36-year-old woman who is plagued by frequent viral upper respiratory infections during cold and flu season. She schedules an appointment with you and would like to discuss the possibility of using *Echinacea* to help decrease her incidence of illness. Of the following, which advice is best supported by the evidence?

a. There is no evidence to suggest that *Echinacea* will have any effect on illness incidence.
b. *Echinacea* has been shown to have a significant placebo effect, but has not been found to be effective in reducing illness incidence.
c. *Echinacea* has been shown to decrease the risk for upper respiratory infections in well-designed clinical studies.
d. The risk for using *Echinacea* outweighs the benefit for most people.
e. *Echinacea* has not been studied adequately enough for clinicians to render an opinion regarding its use.

81. You are treating a 59-year-old man with osteoarthritis of the right knee. He has been using acetaminophen daily, and is interested in adding glucosamine to his regimen. Which of the following best represents current knowledge of its mechanism of action?

a. Glucosamine serves as a substrate for synthesis of cartilage.
b. Glucosamine helps maintain articular fluid viscosity.
c. Glucosamine inhibits enzymes that break down cartilage.
d. Glucosamine stimulates cartilage repair.
e. Glucosamine is a potent anti-inflammatory.

82. You are caring for a 56-year-old man with known coronary heart disease, hypertension, hypertriglyceridemia, heart failure, and hypothyroidism. He is interested in using fish oil as a dietary supplement. Which of the following is true regarding the effect of fish oil on his health?

a. Of his conditions, fish oil will likely improve his lipid profile only.

b. Of his conditions, fish oil will likely improve his lipid profile and coronary heart disease only.

c. Of his conditions, fish oil will likely improve his lipid profile, coronary heart disease, and hypertension only.

d. Of his conditions, fish oil will likely improve his lipid profile, coronary heart disease, hypertension, and heart failure only.

e. Of his conditions, fish oil will likely improve his lipid profile, coronary heart disease, hypertension, heart failure, and thyroid disease.

83. You are caring for a 40-year-old woman with chronic low back pain without neurologic deficits. She has tried conventional therapies including anti-inflammatory medications, physical therapy, and has only seen minimal benefit. She asks you about acupuncture as a treatment modality. Based on evidence and clinical practice guidelines, which of the following statements is true regarding acupuncture in this situation?

a. Acupuncture is not recommended as a treatment option for low back pain in clinical practice guidelines.

b. Acupuncture has been shown to provide benefit when added to conventional therapies.

c. Acupuncture alone has been shown to be more effective than other active treatment modalities.

d. Acupuncture has been shown to significantly reduce disability compared to usual care and sham acupuncture in studies.

e. Acupuncture is an effective treatment for chronic low back pain, but not acute or subacute low back pain.

Palliative Care

84. After a prolonged fight with colon cancer, your 68-year-old patient decides to forego further attempts at curative treatment and focus on palliative care. He has tried nonsteroidal anti-inflammatory agents and acetaminophen for management of his pain, but this has been ineffective. Which of the following would be the best initial pain-management regimen?

a. A steroid burst to get the pain under control, and then scheduled nonsteroidal anti-inflammatory medications to maintain pain control.
b. A long-acting narcotic pain patch at the lowest dose that controls the pain.
c. A short-acting narcotic on a scheduled basis, with the possibility of additional short-acting narcotics as needed for breakthrough pain control.
d. A long-acting narcotic, with a short-acting narcotic as needed for breakthrough pain.
e. A patient-controlled analgesia device using opioids.

85. Your patient has terminal cancer with a life expectancy of less than 3 months. You are managing her chronic cancer pain with morphine sulfate. She has been stable and on the same dosage of medication for weeks, but is now requiring increasing amounts of opiates to maintain pain control. Which of the following statements is true regarding this situation?

a. The patient's disease is progressing and you should increase her medication dosage.
b. The patient's disease is progressing and you should change medications.
c. The patient is developing tolerance and you should increase her medication.
d. The patient is developing tolerance and you should maintain the dosage of medication to avoid dependence.
e. The patient is developing tolerance and you should slowly withdraw medication.

86. You are caring for a 68-year-old man with severe end-stage chronic obstructive pulmonary disease but a life expectancy longer than 6 months. One month ago, he developed a rash. The rash consisted of grouped vesicles on erythematous bases in a dermatomal pattern. You effectively treated the rash, but the patient complains of a persistent burning and itching pain in the same area as the rash. The pain is significant and keeps him from sleeping. What is the best approach for long-term pain management in this patient?

a. Nonsteroidal anti-inflammatory agents
b. Opiate analgesics
c. Steroids
d. Anticonvulsants
e. SSRIs

87. You are caring for a 65-year-old man with lung cancer. He was diagnosed 4 months ago, and is not expected to live for more than 2 months. He is experiencing dyspnea. His chest x-ray shows progression of his cancer, and his pulse oximetry shows a room air oxygen saturation of 94%. Which of the following is most likely to relieve his symptoms?

a. Oral opioids
b. Nebulized morphine
c. Steroids
d. Benzodiazepines
e. Albuterol

88. You are caring for a 68-year-old man who has had colon cancer for 3 years. Therapies have been unsuccessful, and he has chosen palliative care only. He complains of excessive fatigue, feeling tired after minimal activity, and lacking energy to perform the activities of daily living. He denies depression, and feels he is handling his diagnosis well with the support of his family and friends. His laboratory evaluation is normal, except for mild anemia. Which of the following therapies would be most likely to help his symptoms?

a. Transfusion
b. Nutritional supplementation
c. SSRIs
d. Sedative hypnotics
e. A psychostimulant, like methylphenidate

89. You are treating a 60-year-old patient with end-stage ovarian cancer. You are concerned that she may be developing depression. Which of the following would be the most reliable symptom of depression in this patient?

a. Loss of appetite
b. Fatigue
c. Insomnia
d. Sadness
e. Anhedonia

90. You are caring for a 49-year-old man with end-stage colon cancer. Despite aggressive therapy, his disease continues to progress, and he has chosen palliative care. After seeing you with symptoms of nausea and vomiting, you order imaging studies that reveal a partial obstruction, likely because of his malignancy. Which of the following therapies will be best for this patient?

a. Discontinue opiates that you are using for pain control
b. Use a 5-HT3 antagonist, like ondansetron
c. Use metoclopramide
d. Use an antihistamine
e. Use a benzodiazepine

91. You are making a home visit to a 68-year-old man with terminal cancer. His family says that his breathing seems to be labored. Upon evaluation, you know that this is the "death rattle" that often signals approaching death. Which of the following drugs would be the most useful in controlling this symptom?

a. Atropine
b. Ketorolac
c. Lorazepam
d. Haloperidol
e. Thorazine

Gay, Lesbian, Bisexual, and Transgender Issues

92. A 26-year-old sexually active, nonmonogamous gay male presents to you with urethritis and penile discharge. Which of the following represents the best test/tests to screen for in this situation?

a. Chlamydia
b. Chlamydia and gonorrhea
c. Chlamydia, gonorrhea, and HIV
d. Chlamydia, gonorrhea, HIV, and syphilis
e. Chlamydia, gonorrhea, HIV, syphilis, and herpes simplex

93. A 32-year-old gay HIV-positive man is seeing you for a routine visit. He sees an HIV specialist to manage his condition, and has had an undetectable viral load for 2 years. He is asking you about additional screening for other health concerns, and is specifically concerned about anal cancer. Which of the following is the most appropriate?

a. Anal visual inspection for condyloma yearly
b. Vaccination against human papillomavirus (HPV)
c. Anal cytologic screening
d. Anal cytologic screening and high-resolution anoscopy
e. Anal cytologic screening, high resolution anoscopy, and vaccination against HPV

94. A 30-year-old gay male asks you about preventing HIV. You discuss preexposure prophylaxis (PrEP) therapy as a potential option for him. Which of the following is true about PrEP?

a. When used daily, PrEP therapy is nearly 100% effective in preventing HIV.
b. Using PrEP daily reduces the risk of getting HIV infection by around 90%.
c. Using PrEP daily reduces the risk of getting HIV infection by around 75%.
d. Using PrEP daily reduces the risk of getting HIV infection by around 50%.
e. The risk of getting HIV infection on PrEP is about the same as the risk of getting HIV infection using postexposure prophylaxis (PEP).

95. You are seeing a 25-year-old sexually active gay man that reports having unprotected sexual activity in the last 2 weeks. At this visit, he reports fever, fatigue, and sore throat. On examination, you note adenopathy. Which of the following next steps is appropriate?

a. Watchful waiting
b. Obtain an HIV viral load test
c. Obtain an HIV antibody test
d. Obtain a complete blood count
e. Obtain a sedimentation rate

96. A 16-year-old woman comes to your office for an annual checkup for the first time without her parent present. In the encounter, she tells you that she identifies as a lesbian, and is not currently having sex with men or women. She says she is interested in "having a family someday." Which of the following is true regarding lesbians and family planning?

a. Lesbian youth are more likely to use hormonal contraceptives than their heterosexual counterparts.
b. Lesbian adults are more likely to use hormonal contraceptives than their heterosexual counterparts.
c. The rate of unintended pregnancy is higher in lesbian youth than in their heterosexual counterparts.
d. Unintended pregnancy rates are no different between lesbian adults and heterosexual adults.
e. Because she self-identifies as a lesbian, pregnancy prevention should not be discussed.

97. You are caring for a 30-year-old lesbian patient who is presenting today for routine care. She states that she has never had sex with a male partner, and tells you she has never had a Pap test. Which of the following is true?

a. Do a Pap test now and follow-up using general screening guidelines.
b. Do a Pap test now, but follow-up less often than would be required if she were heterosexual.
c. Do a Pap test now, and follow-up more often than would be required if she were heterosexual.
d. Do a Pap test now, but there is no need to repeat if again the Pap test is normal.
e. No Pap test is needed.

98. You are caring for a 32-year-old gay male. He and his husband are considering starting a family and are looking into multiple options. Their first choice would be to use a surrogate and try artificial insemination. Your patient raises a concern about the challenges the child will face if he is raised by two men. Which of the following is true of children raised by gay men?

a. Children of gay men are no different than children of heterosexual couples.
b. Female children of gay men are more likely to be lesbian than female children of heterosexual couples.
c. Male children of gay men are more likely to be gay than male children of heterosexual couples.
d. Children of gay males are more likely to struggle with their gender identity than children of heterosexual couples.
e. Children of gay men are more likely to have higher intelligence than children of heterosexual couples.

99. You are taking the complete history of a patient new to your office. The patient is dressed as a woman, but is biologically male. Further history reveals that the patient takes female hormones and is considering sexual reassignment surgery. What term most specifically describes this person?

a. Cross dresser
b. Bigender
c. Transvestite
d. Transsexual
e. Transgender

100. You are seeing a female transgender patient who has taken feminizing hormones for 5 years. At this visit, she asks about cancer screening. She has no family history of any type of cancer, and has done what she can to minimize her risks. She is specifically concerned about what types of cancer she is at risk for as a result of hormone therapy. For which of the following types of cancer is she at risk?

a. Breast cancer
b. Cervical cancer
c. Endometrial cancer
d. Colon cancer
e. Lung cancer

101. You are caring for a male-to-female (MTF) transgender patient who is considering hormone therapy and has read extensively about transdermal preparations. She is most concerned about side effects and risks. Which of the following is true regarding her morbidity and mortality, should she start hormone therapy?

a. There is no increase in morbidity or mortality.
b. There is an increase in morbidity but no change in mortality.
c. There is a decrease in morbidity but no change in mortality.
d. There is no change in morbidity but an increase in mortality.
e. There is no change in morbidity but a decrease in mortality.

102. You are seeing a female-to-male (FTM) transsexual patient for the first time. He has been taking testosterone cypionate, 50 mg subcutaneously weekly for the last year, and would like to transfer his care to you for follow-up. He is experiencing some mild acne and male-pattern baldness, which you attribute to the testosterone therapy. Which of the following options is appropriate given this scenario?

a. Stop the testosterone
b. Change the testosterone to an oral preparation
c. Change the testosterone to a topical preparation
d. Continue therapy, but monitor liver enzymes regularly
e. Continue therapy, but monitor hemoglobin regularly

103. You are caring for a MTF transgender patient who is taking feminizing hormone therapy. She is taking 17β-estradiol orally, 2 mg po bid and spironolactone, 50 mg po bid, and is not complaining of side effects. She has noted breast development (Tanner 2) and a reduction of body hair. Despite these results, she would like a more "feminine" appearance. Which of the following is the most appropriate therapeutic option?

a. No change in therapy
b. Change estrogen to transdermal
c. Change estrogen to intramuscular injection
d. Change spironolactone to 25 mg po bid
e. Stop spironolactone

Counseling for Behavior Change

104. You are caring for an unmarried 28-year-old woman. She is overweight, and you are conducting a brief intervention to help her develop an action plan for weight loss. Which of the following will be the most effective?

a. Let the patient know what has worked for you in your efforts to maintain a healthy weight.
b. Discuss the impact of successful weight loss on her overall appearance.
c. Work with her to agree to a weight loss goal, for example, losing 1 lb per week.
d. Work with her to agree to an exercise goal, for example, walking 1 mile daily.
e. Encourage her to set a start date for beginning her new dietary and exercise regimen.

105. You are addressing smoking cessation with a patient and are determining the patient's readiness to change his behaviors. During the discussion, you find that the patient is aware of the health impact of his smoking on him and his family. He understands the economic impact, and feels that if he were to quit, it would benefit him financially. He feels very addicted to cigarettes and says that he'd like to quit sometime in the future. According to the Stages of Change Model, at what stage of change is this patient?

a. Precontemplation
b. Contemplation
c. Preparation
d. Action
e. Maintenance

106. You are caring for a 41-year-old male patient with high risk for heart disease. His dietary habits are increasing his risks, and you would like to work with him to develop healthier eating habits. Assuming he is in the "precontemplation" stage, what should your action be to move him toward changing his behavior?

a. Educate him about the impact of diet on heart disease risk.
b. Outline the costs of his behaviors and contrast those to the benefits of healthy eating.
c. Show him the gap between his health goals and his current behavior.
d. Brainstorm options for healthier eating with the patient.
e. Assist him in developing a concrete action plan for behavior change.

107. You are working with a patient who recently retired from his job after 41 years. He is currently 67 years old and has hypertension and high cholesterol. His wife thinks he drinks too much, and during your visit, he admits to three alcoholic beverages per day. You have screened him for alcoholism, and he does not meet the criteria. You would like to negotiate a safe drinking amount for this patient. Which of the following best represents a safe level of alcohol intake for this patient?

a. Seven drinks per week, no more than three per occasion.
b. Fourteen drinks per week, no more than four per occasion.
c. No more than one drink per day.
d. No more than two beers or glasses of wine per day *or* no more than one alcoholic beverage per day.
e. There is no safe drinking amount for this patient.

Doctor-Patient Issues

Answers

Patient-Centered Communication

65. The answer is d. Patient-centered interviewing is built upon several premises, one of which is that patients usually bring more than one concern to their clinician. Often, the first concern mentioned is not the most important one to the patient. Sometimes, the last thing mentioned is most important, but was mentioned last because it's frightening or embarrassing for the patient. The first step in patient-centered interviewing is setting the stage for the interview by putting the patient at ease and removing communication barriers. The second stage involves obtaining the agenda. This step empowers the patient and ensures that his or her concerns are properly prioritized and addressed. If the patient is known to bring a long list of issues to each visit (as is the case in this question), indicating the time you have available for the visit is an excellent way to start, as it sets limits and helps the patient gauge what to bring up and in how much detail. Forecasting what you would like to have happen during the interview is important, but if the visit is started this way, it puts your apparent needs ahead of the patient's. Starting with a question like, "What brings you in today" is reflexive for many clinicians, but often encourages the patient to tell the entire story of the first concern on his/her list. This delays getting a full list of concerns that the patient wants to discuss, and can lead to the patient bringing up a serious concern later in the visit, increasing the likelihood of the clinician falling behind. Clinicians are often taught to obtain a list of all the things a patient wants to discuss at the start of the visit, but with patients known to bring a long list, this will lead to a negotiation with the patient about what to discuss this visit, and what to discuss at the next visit—a time consuming and sometimes dissatisfying experience for both the clinician and the patient. Beginning the visit by saying you will only discuss one issue is not recommended, as it can lead to patient dissatisfaction.

66. The answer is b. Dealing with the angry patient is challenging. A natural response to anger is defensiveness, but this can escalate the situation.

The most patient-centered approach is for the physician to first recognize and acknowledge the anger. If a physician senses that a patient is angry, but the patient has not volunteered this information, it is important to explore the anger. If the patient seems very upset, it may make him/her angrier if the provider minimizes the situation by saying something like, "you seem a little upset." It's important to choose words that seem to match the intensity of his/her feelings. Letting the patient know why you're late may make you feel better and elicit empathy from the patient, but is not patient-centered (it's clinician-centered). Apologizing for the delay and getting to the patient's needs is important, but if you don't allow the patient to express his/her thoughts, it is likely to lead to the patient harboring the anger and not being as open during the visit. Starting with a statement like, "Let's discuss why you're angry..." makes an assumption that you know what the patient is feeling. Describing how the patient looks is more patient-centered, as it allows the patient to validate that your observation is either correct or incorrect. In some instances anger is displaced, and may be truly directed at the disease process or illness. In that case, the appropriate response is empathy. However, making that assumption is not patient-centered.

67. The answer is e. Motivational interviewing is a technique conceived in the early 1980s, and is a directive, client-centered style that elicits behavior change by helping people explore and resolve ambivalence. It's an alternative to other motivational techniques often used by clinicians (including education, persuasion, or fear). The objective is not to solve the patient's problem or even develop a plan—the goal is to help the patient explore his/her own issues and let the patient develop the plan with guidance by the clinician. Using the technique, providers can help the patient identify a specific and achievable goal—but it's important for the provider to remember that it's the patient's goal that's important—not the provider's goal for the patient. The first step in motivational interviewing is asking open-ended questions that help move the patient toward a stated goal. Stating something like, "What is one behavior you can change in order to improve your health?" is a good example. In the scenario described in this question, answer e is the best example of motivational interviewing, as it helps the patient to focus on her own goal, and identifies a first step to take to achieve the goal. The first two answers are closed-ended questions that are not part of motivational interviewing. Answer c assumes that the patient's goal is to never smoke again. Answer d will help identify barriers, but is not part of motivational interviewing technique.

68. The answer is c. When interviewing patients, the patient's immediate needs always take precedence. Although patient-centered interviewing technique was developed by recognizing the limitations of clinician-centered interviewing, in specific situations, the most patient-centered thing to do is to control the interview to ensure the patient is not at immediate risk for a health emergency. Examples of these situations include times when a patient may have acute chest pain, profound shortness of breath, extreme anxiety, or is becoming overtly disruptive. In these situations, the clinician must act immediately to address the problem, and the patient needs the clinician to direct the interview. In the context of this question, it means directing the interview and using closed questions. These situations are much less common than situations in which the clinician can adopt a more overt patient-centered approach by asking open-ended questions, obtaining a list of all the issues the patient wants to discuss, reviewing the psychosocial context of the symptoms, or asking about cultural beliefs about treatment options.

69. The answer is a. When interviewing patients, clinicians can use open-ended skills and closed-ended skills to gather data. Open-ended skills can be general, or they can be used to gain more information about a specific situation. Answer "a" is an example of "echoing"—a technique where the clinician reflects what the patient has said by repeating a part of the phrase they stated to encourage them to go deeper into that aspect of their symptom or concern. Other common open-ended skills include:

- Silence: Saying nothing while continuing to be nonverbally attentive. Because people tend to be uncomfortable with silence, the patient will likely say more and fill in gaps.
- Nonverbal encouragement: leaning forward, or changing a facial expression will provide nonverbal encouragement to the patient to continue the story and add detail.
- Neutral utterances: saying things like, "I see…", "Uh-huh," or "Mmmm" will encourage the patient to talk and continue in the way that their story is progressing.
- Open-ended requests: saying things like, "tell me more about that…" or "go on…" encourages the patient to expand upon something they said earlier.
- Paraphrasing: summarizing or paraphrasing something that the patient has said encourages the patient to go deeper into that aspect of the story. It signals that he/she has been heard, and that he/she can proceed beyond that part of the story.

Closed-ended data gathering is also important, and is used to focus or clarify a patient's story. Closed-ended questions generally can be answered by yes or no, or may be answered by a brief statement or clarifier. Common closed questions can be "Did you have shortness of breath with the pain?" or "How high was your fever?"

70. The answer is b. Empathy is an excellent tool to help build the doctor-patient relationship. When a patient expresses an emotion in an interview, the clinician should respond. Remaining silent or changing the subject can lead the patient to believe that you disapprove of his/her feelings or are uncomfortable discussing feelings. You can show empathy in any number of ways, but common ways include:

- Naming: simply repeat the feeling expressed by the patient or the emotion observed
- Understanding: acknowledge that the patient's emotional reaction is reasonable
- Respecting: praising, appreciating, or acknowledging the patient's plight
- Supporting: signaling to the patient that you are prepared to help in any reasonable way that you can

In this question, although answer a names an emotion that you might observe, it does not acknowledge the emotion that the patient is expressing. By changing his expression to something you observe (sadness), it may indicate that you disapprove of "relief" and will not strengthen the relationship with the patient. Answer c is a true statement, but implies that you expected something different from the patient. Answers d and e may actually highlight the reason for the patient wanting to be "checked out," but do not acknowledge the emotion expressed, and will not enhance the patient relationship. Answer b uses understanding to acknowledge the feeling and express that it's a reasonable reaction.

71. The answer is a. The overly talkative patient can quickly overwhelm the clinician. Some talkative patients may begin without you having to say anything, and the clinician must get actively involved after no more than a minute with these types of patients or risk being left behind! If a patient recounts every detail of his/her symptoms and concerns, including issues that do not directly relate to the illness, you must respectfully and tactfully interrupt, refocus and redirect, sometimes repeatedly. It's important to control the interview and develop the agenda for the visit with the patient, even if it's difficult. Using open-ended questions will not be helpful and may enable the patient to go on even longer. While it's important to acknowledge emotion that the patient brings up, asking about the emotional impact in this situation is not going to help manage the visit. Redirecting the patient to the family history may break the cycle of over talking by forcing the patient to answer closed-ended questions, but will not help manage the time in this setting. Redirection statements like, "We need to change gears now so that I can learn more about your constipation" or "I appreciate your sharing this, but I want to be sure I address your needs in the time we have together" are appropriate ways to tactfully interrupt, refocus, and redirect the talkative patient.

Cultural Competency and Health Disparities

72. The answer is a. Health, illness, and treatment are strongly influenced by cultural contexts. Culturally and Linguistically Appropriate Services (CLAS) standards require providers to understand the important roles that cultural health practitioners have in the treatment of illness and disease. Culture influences how patients seek care, and the primary care physician may be the last person consulted for health-related issues. It is important for clinicians caring for diverse populations to be familiar with commonly consulted traditional medicine practitioners within their practice population, and respond to their use in a culturally sensitive way. Encouraging a participatory care model where the patient can negotiate preferred treatment (as in the correct answer to this question) is a culturally appropriate approach, unless the side effect or treatment regimen chosen by the patient is health threatening. Adjusting the dose would not be appropriate unless the clinician understands mechanisms of action and research behind dosing. Asking the patient to contact you prior to starting any herbal regimen may engage her as a partner, but positions you as the most important decision maker in her health, which may not be her cultural standard or belief. Asking her to stop, or telling her not to use herbals would disengage the patient.

73. The answer is b. CLAS standards assist in providing guidelines for effective communication with patients who have limited or no English proficiency. In the case described in this question, a certified interpreter is necessary. A translator converts written text into a corresponding written text in a different language. An interpreter analyzes a message and reexpresses that message accurately and objectively in another language. A certified medical interpreter has been assessed for language proficiency and knowledge of medical terminology, and includes recognizing the importance of verbal and nonverbal cues to help with context. Family members, non-native office staff, and even non-native clinicians, while convenient, have not been certified, and are therefore considered "ad hoc" interpreters. Cross-sectional error analysis was done using ad hoc interpreters, and found that the error rate for an ad hoc interpreter was 22%, and even higher than not using an interpreter at all.

74. The answer is a. Family Medicine offers many helpful strategies for initiating and maintaining a therapeutic relationship, regardless of the culture from which the clinician or patient originates. Studies have shown that eliciting the patient's goals and projecting a willingness to negotiate care options has been shown to increase adherence to treatment, therefore answer a is the best answer. While displaying empathy for the patient's challenges may be appropriate and will help the therapeutic relationship, it has not been shown to increase adherence. Eliciting barriers to compliance can be important, but just doing this does not improve adherence. Increased education, especially if it's culturally and linguistically appropriate, may be helpful in adherence, but it is not as helpful as eliciting the patient's goals for treatment. Finally, changing the regimen without engaging the patient and understanding preferences is unlikely to improve adherence.

75. The answer is c. While any of the symptoms described may warrant further evaluation and workup, Native Americans have a substantially greater prevalence of diabetes mellitus, obesity, alcoholism, and suicide than other US population groups. Therefore, the patient describing depressed mood would require the physician to further evaluate risk for suicide. Blood in stool, hoarseness, shortness of breath, and fever all are less associated with high prevalence conditions in this population.

76. The answer is b. With the exception of Southeast Asian refugees, there are not many clinical studies that evaluate the health problems of refugees upon arrival into the United States. However, we know that tuberculosis, nutritional deficiencies, intestinal parasites, chronic hepatitis B, and depression are major problems in many groups. Any of these issues may be contributing to the patient's weight loss, and should be evaluated. For most groups, the evaluation should include a hemoglobin measurement, hepatitis B surface antigen, a purified protein derivative (PPD) subcutaneous skin test for tuberculosis, and testing for ova and parasites.

Integrative Medicine

77. The answer is c. Rates of complementary and alternative medicine use have increased significantly over the past decade, and family physicians are increasingly asked to opine or even recommend supplementation for patients. Fish oils (omega-3 fatty acids) are commonly used to treat hypertriglyceridemia, prevent CHD and stroke, and have been used for many things, including depression, diabetes, and to reduce the risk of developing age-related maculopathy among other things. Ginseng root has been used to as a stress reduction agent and to improve physical performance and stamina. Kava kava and valerian root have both been used to reduce stress and as an anxiolytic or sedative. *Ginkgo biloba* leaf has been used to slow cognitive decline in patients with dementia, but is also used to improve blood circulation in patients with claudication. It has also been used to treat sexual dysfunction associated with the use of SSRIs. The standard oral dosage is 60 to 120 mg of extract twice daily.

78. The answer is d. Throughout history, plants have been used for medicinal purposes. In the United States, botanicals are used by one in five Americans at an annual total cost of more than $4 billion. St. John's wort is a perennial plant native to Europe that has been transferred to and grown in North America. It is one of the most studied botanicals. There have been more than 60 randomized controlled clinical trials, systematic reviews, and meta-analyses that have been done to establish its evidence base. A 2015 meta-analysis of 66 studies involving more than 15,000 patients found that St. John's wort is as effective for the treatment of depression as other drug classes with significantly fewer dropouts due to side effects. The mechanism of action for St. John's wort is that it inhibits serotonin, norepinephrine, and dopamine reuptake in the central nervous system (CNS), and may modulate autonomic system reactivity. Overall, it is very well-tolerated.

79. The answer is b. Many people believe that botanical medicines are natural and therefore safe. While it is true that the vast majority of medicinal botanicals are safe, a few have significant toxicity (for example, ephedra or ma huang, which has been banned in the United States due to case reports of severe and fatal reactions when used for weight management or to increase energy). Other botanicals have drug interactions that family physicians should be aware of. St. John's wort is known to potently induce the cytochrome P450 system (specifically the isozyme CYP3A4), and may lower the blood levels of medications that are metabolized by this system. These medications include alprazolam, ethinyl estradiol, warfarin, cyclosporine, indinavir, and statins.

80. The answer is c. *Echinacea* originated in Eastern North America and its plants were used extensively by Native Americans. Their use continues to be popular today, with preparations made from roots, stems, leaves, flowers, or combinations of parts. There have been dozens of studies using *Echinacea* preparations for the prevention and treatment of upper respiratory tract infections. A 2014 Cochrane review evaluated 12 studies for the prevention of colds and found that although none of the trials individually showed a reduction in colds, when the data were pooled, there was a 10% to 20% risk reduction in the treatment group. A meta-analysis in 2015 included six clinical studies with a total of 2458 participants and found a relative risk of 0.65 for upper respiratory tract infection in the experimental group. In 2016, there was a large double-blind, randomized, placebo-controlled prevention trial in which 755 healthy people were followed while either taking *Echinacea* or placebo. Those in the *Echinacea* arm experienced 58% fewer days of cold symptoms. There are few risks in using *Echinacea*, and although some trials show a placebo effect, there are well-designed studies that support its use.

81. The answer is a. Glucosamine and chondroitin have been used extensively for osteoarthritis in Europe and in the United States. Glucosamine is an amino-monosaccharide that serves as a substrate for the synthesis of cartilage. It may have anti-inflammatory activity, but it is not a potent anti-inflammatory agent. Chondroitin is a glycosaminoglycan that helps to maintain articular fluid viscosity, inhibit enzymes that break down cartilage, and stimulate cartilage repair. Despite more than 30 years of clinical research, glucosamine and chondroitin use remain controversial. Even the most recent trials, reviews, and meta-analyses report mixed results with some reporting no benefit, while others support their use and highlight potential disease-modifying activity. Fortunately, even with the lack of clear guidance from existing literature, both glucosamine and chondroitin are well-tolerated, safe, and have fewer side effects than non-steroidal anti-inflammatory drugs (NSAIDs).

82. The answer is d. Fish oil has been studied for decades after discovering that certain populations in Greenland had low rates of heart disease despite consuming a diet high in saturated fats. The protection was thought to be because of the consumption of omega-3 fatty acids through their diet which was high in fish. The benefits of fish oil include reductions in triglyceride levels, inflammation, blood pressure, blood clotting, and atherosclerotic plaque formation. Dozens of clinical trials have looked at the benefit of fish oil in reducing serum triglycerides, and a meta-analysis of 21 studies confirmed the benefit. There appears to be a linear dose-response relationship, and a dose of 4 g/day can lower triglyceride levels by up to 40%. With regard to coronary heart disease, large-scale observational studies and randomized controlled trials that have included hundreds of thousands of patients show that fish oil is effective for secondary and possibly primary prevention of CHD. Three different meta-analyses and a systematic review concluded that high dose fish oil supplementation can lower blood pressure. Although the results were statistically significant, the blood pressure improvement is relatively small. Clinical and epidemiologic trials have shown that fish oil is beneficial for heart failure, and this was confirmed by a meta-analysis. Results showed that treatment led to a significant reduction of all-cause mortality and improvement in left ventricular end-diastolic volume. Studies have not identified a significant effect on hypothyroidism.

83. The answer is b. Acupuncture as a treatment method has been around for thousands of years, and despite being well-studied, its mechanism of action is not well-understood. As more patients become interested in integrative medicine, primary care physicians should be aware of the broad benefits of therapies like acupuncture. Treatment typically involves inserting 4 to 15 needles at selected points, then stimulating the needles either manually or with electricity. In the past 30 years of literature, significant complications are rare. More than 1000 reviews of the clinical use of acupuncture have been published since the 1970s. It has been shown to be most effective in treating pain, nausea, and vomiting. Regarding low back pain, more than 50 trials using acupuncture as a treatment modality were reviewed by the American Pain Society and the American College of Physicians (ACP) to develop clinical practice guidelines. The ACP recommends its use as an option for acute, subacute, and chronic low back pain. In most studies, acupuncture alone has not been shown to be more effective compared to other active treatments, but provides additional benefit when added to conventional therapies. In addition, a 2012 multicenter randomized controlled trial showed that acupuncture reduced levels of disability compared to usual care, but not significantly more than sham acupuncture in acute low back pain.

Palliative Care

84. The answer is c. The World Health Organization published guidelines for pain control in 1996. These guidelines have been well-studied and lead to effective pain control in most situations. In general, failing nonopioid pain control should lead to the use of opioid analgesics. Steroids have limited, if any, use in chronic cancer pain. Fentanyl patches, even at the lowest dose, may be excessive in opiate naïve patients, and should never be used alone. Most start with immediate-release morphine sulfate to determine a baseline need. This can be converted to sustained release quickly, and titrated based on pain control. Patient-controlled analgesia devices have an important role, but require intravenous or subcutaneous administration, and should not be used first-line, unless pain is extreme.

85. The answer is a. Managing chronic cancer pain with opiates is often concerning for physicians. Physicians may fear addiction or be concerned about causing harm. It is important to remember that there is no specific limit to opioid dose, and medications should be titrated to pain control or development of significant side effects. Fear of addiction should not hinder the use of opiates in this situation. Addiction is a rare occurrence in patients with terminal illness, especially in patients without a history of drug abuse. In patients on previously steady doses, dose escalation generally means the disease is progressing rather than tolerance. Tolerance, like addiction, is rarely seen in these patients.

86. The answer is d. Neuropathic pain, like that described from shingles in this question, frequently requires opioids in the short term, but often requires the use of other medications for long-term relief. Commonly used medications include tricyclic antidepressants, anticonvulsants (valproic acid, carbamazepine, and gabapentin are the most common), and antihistamines. The data on using SSRIs are unconvincing.

87. The answer is a. Dyspnea, like pain, is a subjective sensation. It can be present in the absence of hypoxia. Opioids can relieve breathlessness associated with advanced cancer by an unclear mechanism. Nebulized morphine is not more effective than placebo. Steroids and albuterol are useful for dyspnea caused by bronchospasm, but that is unlikely in this case. Anxiolytics, like benzodiazepines and buspirone, may help if anxiety is a significant component, but that is usually expressed by patients as a feeling of "choking" or "suffocation."

88. The answer is e. Excessive fatigue seen with end-stage cancer may result from direct tumor effects, paraneoplastic neuropathy, or tumor involvement of the CNS. It is often an effect of therapy. When no specific cause is apparent, as in this question, therapy is difficult. Transfusion is unlikely to be beneficial given his hemoglobin level. There is no evidence that the patient has a nutritional deficit, and supplementation may not be helpful. Although fatigue is frequently seen as a symptom of depression and may respond to SSRI therapy, in this case it is unlikely. Sleeping pills would not help unless insomnia is the cause. A short course of steroids or a psychostimulant can increase energy and improve mood.

89. The answer is e. It is commonly assumed that all patients with cancer are, and should be, depressed. Physicians often do not recognize depression because they feel they would be depressed in the same situation. While neurovegetative symptoms (loss of appetite, difficulty with concentration, fatigue, or insomnia) are a compelling indication of depression in the physically healthy patient, they may be less reliable for the diagnosis of depression in patients with advanced cancer. Loss of appetite may be due to therapy, and fatigue may be due to sleep loss from untreated pain. Sadness may be appropriate, given the diagnosis. Anhedonia is a useful, if not the most useful symptom to monitor. Hopelessness, guilt, and a wish to die are also predictive.

90. The answer is c. Palliative care treatment for nausea and vomiting should be geared toward the cause. If nausea and vomiting are symptoms of malignant gastrointestinal partial obstruction, the use of metoclopramide, with dexamethasone and a low-fiber diet, can provide significant relief for several weeks. Discontinuing opiates may exacerbate pain and increase discomfort. Antiemetics, including 5-HT3 antagonists, are generally used for chemotherapy and radiation induced nausea and vomiting. Benzodiazepines are commonly used for anticipatory nausea associated with chemotherapy. Antihistamines like meclizine and diphenhydramine are not as effective in this case but are very effective if the nausea and vomiting are related to vestibular dysfunction.

91. The answer is a. Atropine can decrease secretions and help the "death rattle." Other medications that may be useful include scopolamine, glycopyrrolate, mycosamine, or morphine. Ketorolac may help pain, lorazepam may help restlessness, and haloperidol and thorazine may help agitation and hallucinations, both of which are also symptoms of impending death.

Gay, Lesbian, Bisexual, and Transgender Issues

92. The answer is d. Many sexually active gay men are at increased risk for sexually transmitted infections (STIs). Suspicion or diagnosis of one STI should routinely lead to testing for concomitant HIV and syphilis. In this case, his discharge is likely to be either gonorrhea or chlamydia, and additional testing should be completed for HIV and syphilis. Herpes simplex testing is not indicated in the absence of vesicular genital lesions.

93. The answer is d. The risk of anal squamous cell carcinoma in gay men is significant, and anal HPV DNA was detected in more than 90% of HIV-positive men in one study. High-resolution anoscopy and cytologic screening of all gay men with HIV is supported by current knowledge. Vaccination against HPV can prevent genital warts, but the vaccination is currently indicated in boys and men 9 to 26 years old. If the patient in this case had visible anal condyloma, screening would be indicated regardless of HIV status.

94. The answer is b. PrEP is a way to help prevent HIV by taking medication every day. The recommended medication is a combination of two antiretroviral drugs, tenofovir and emtricitabine (brand name Truvada). Studies have shown that the risk of getting HIV infection was up to 92% lower for participants in studies who took PrEP consistently as compared with those that did not take the medications. PEP is generally recommended for someone that feels they have had a significant exposure to HIV, and must be started within 72 hours of exposure. When administered correctly, PEP is also effective in preventing HIV, but should not be a substitute to other proven HIV prevention methods (including PrEP, using condoms with every sexual encounter, and using sterile needles).

95. The answer is b. When someone at risk for HIV presents with nonspecific symptoms compatible with acute viral infection, acute HIV infection should be in the differential. These symptoms are generally indistinguishable from common viral infections. Although not valuable as screening tests, HIV viral load tests (polymerase chain reaction tests) become positive 1 to 2 weeks prior to routine antibody-based HIV tests and may be useful in diagnosis. Obtaining nonspecific tests like a complete blood count (CBC) or sedimentation rate would not be helpful in differentiating HIV infection from other common viral infections.

96. The answer is c. Family planning, including discussion of unintended pregnancy, is important to discuss with lesbian patients. The majority of lesbians have been sexually active with men at some point in their lives, and as many as 30% of women that self-identify as lesbians are currently sexually active with men. Fewer lesbian youth use hormonal contraception than their heterosexual counterparts, and that seems to continue into adulthood. The unintended pregnancy rate in female lesbian youth is higher than that of comparison heterosexual female youth, and that risk continues into adulthood, perhaps because of decreased use of hormonal contraceptives.

97. The answer is a. Cervical cancer may be less prevalent in women who have never had heterosexual vaginal intercourse; however, even in women reporting that they have never had sex with a man, up to 20% were found to have HPV DNA. Also, many physicians assume self-reported lesbians to have never had sex with a man, when some studies have reported that a majority of lesbians have reported having sex with a male in the past. Therefore, physicians should follow Pap smear screening guidelines in place for all women regardless of the woman's reported sexuality.

98. The answer is a. Existing evidence suggests that gay men and lesbians have parenting skills comparable to heterosexual parents. When compared with children from heterosexual couples, children of gay couples seem to be no different with regard to several variables, including their sexual or gender identity and their intelligence.

99. The answer is d. Transgender is an umbrella term describing a group of people who cross culturally defined gender categories. Cross dressers wear the clothes of the other gender, but may not completely identify with that gender. Bigender individuals identify with both genders. Transvestites dress as another gender, but have not considered surgery. Transsexuals wish to change their sex, and have considered or undertaken surgery.

100. The answer is a. In transgender patients, it's important to screen based on current anatomy and consider the use of hormones that might impact cancer risks. MTF transgender patients are at risk for both prostate and breast cancers. They are at average risk for colon and lung cancer, and since she would have no uterus or cervix, would not be at risk for those cancers. FTM transgender patients often require screening for breast, uterine, cervical, endometrial, and ovarian cancers.

101. The answer is a. Extensive experience with hormonal therapies in transgender patients indicates that hormonal therapy does not cause increased morbidity or mortality.

102. The answer is e. Testosterone can be injected or applied topically. The typical introductory dosage is 20 mg injected (either subcutaneously or intramuscularly), with various initial dosages for creams, gels, or patches, depending on the preparation. A typical maintenance dosage is around 50 mg/week, if injected. Clinical endpoints include development of facial hair, deepening of the voice, and induction of amenorrhea by 6 months. Concerns about hepatotoxicity surrounded the use of oral methyltestosterone, but there is no evidence to support a concern of hepatotoxicity in transsexual men using parenteral testosterone. Common side effects include male-pattern baldness and acne, both of which can be treated as they would in any patient, without needing to change the testosterone preparation. Testosterone and other androgens have an erythropoietic effect and can cause polycythemia. Therefore, hemoglobin and hematocrit should be monitored, and the preparation should be changed if elevated.

103. The answer is a. The goal of feminizing hormone therapy is the development of female secondary sex characteristics and the minimization of male secondary sex characteristics. The maximum Tanner stage expected should be around Tanner 2 or 3. Given that the patient described above has achieved the expected clinical endpoint, no change should be considered in her therapy; however, it's important to monitor kidney function and potassium levels periodically. To achieve a more feminine appearance, other cosmetic options can be considered rather than changing hormone therapy.

Counseling for Behavior Change

104. The answer is d. The components of an effective brief intervention for lifestyle change should have the following components:

- It should be patient-focused (framed around the patient's needs and interests).
- It should be health-connected (review the projected impact of the intervention on the patient's physical or emotional health).
- It should be behavior-oriented (focused on what the patient can "do" differently).
- It should be realistic.
- It should be controllable (framed in terms of what the patient can reasonably control, for example, exercise daily rather than a specific amount of weight loss).
- It should be measurable.
- It should be practical.

Answer a is not patient-focused. Answer b is not health-connected, it is appearance-connected. Answer c is not as controllable as answer d. Answer e is incorrect, as once an intervention is agreed upon, the caregiver should encourage the patient to begin to make changes immediately.

105. The answer is b. The Stages of Change Model can be applied to virtually any change in lifestyle or behavior. It outlines the current stage of change, what it represents for the patient, and the provider's task. The stages are outlined below:

Stage of Change	Description of Patient
Precontemplation	No intention to change, may be unaware of the problem
Contemplation	Aware of the problem, but unwilling to make a change; may feel stuck, or say he/she will do it in the future
Preparation	Planning to make a change, usually within 1 month
Action	Involved in implementing or making a change
Maintenance	Has sustained change for some time, usually around 6 months
Addressing relapse or relapse prevention	Patient behavior starts to slip, falls back to old behaviors

In this question, the patient best fits in the contemplation stage.

106. The answer is a. All of the actions listed in the answers would be appropriate at some stage of change, but in the precontemplation stage, education is the provider action that will best move the patient toward the next step in making a change. The following table outlines the recommended provider actions at each stage of change.

Stage of Change	Provider Task
Precontemplation	Education about the health area
Contemplation	Cost-benefit analysis; develop discrepancy between patient goals and current behavior
Preparation	Brainstorm options; assist in developing a concrete action plan
Action	Encourage tracking/monitoring actions; validate patient and provide feedback; discuss and elicit social support
Maintenance	Check progress; troubleshoot slips/concerns of the patient; reinforce successes and build patient confidence
Addressing relapse or relapse prevention	Judge choices, not the patient; focus on past success; identify new supports that reinforce healthy behavior

107. The answer is c. Managing alcohol use is challenging. If a person is alcoholic or has a history of substance abuse, there is no safe drinking amount. However, if patients do not have this history, it is important to know how much alcohol use is considered "too much." General guidelines for non-pregnant women are no more than seven drinks per week, and no more than three per any one occasion. For men, the guidelines are no more than 14 drinks per week and no more than four per any one occasion. For patients older than age 65, it is recommended that they ingest no more than one drink per day. There is not a difference between the recommended amounts of beer, wine, or alcohol—one beer is equivalent to one glass of wine or one alcoholic beverage.

Recommended Reading: Doctor-Patient Issues

Barrows K. Chapter e4. Integrative medicine. In: Papadakis MA, McPhee SJ, Rabow MW (eds). *Current Medical Diagnosis & Treatment.* New York, NY: McGraw-Hill; 2018.

Bullock KA, Graves DL. Cultural & linguistic competence. In: South-Paul JE, Matheny SC, Lewis EL (eds). *Current Diagnosis & Treatment Family Medicine.* 4th ed. New York, NY: McGraw-Hill.

Chan M. Popular herbs and nutritional supplements. In: Bope ET, Kellerman RD (eds). *Conn's Current Therapy.* Philadelphia, PA. Elsevier; 2017.

Chapter 1. The medical interview. In: Fortin AH, Dwamena FC, Frankel RM, Smith RC (eds). *Smith's Patient-Centered Interviewing: An Evidence-Based Method.* 3rd ed. New York, NY: McGraw-Hill.

Chapter 2. Data-gathering and relationship-building skills. In: Fortin AH, Dwamena FC, Frankel RM, Smith RC (eds). *Smith's Patient-Centered Interviewing: An Evidence-Based Method.* 3rd ed. New York, NY: McGraw-Hill.

Chapter 3. The beginning of the interview. In: Fortin AH, Dwamena FC, Frankel RM, Smith RC (eds). *Smith's Patient-Centered Interviewing: An Evidence-Based Method.* 3rd ed. New York, NY: McGraw-Hill.

Chapter 7. Adapting the interview to different situations and other practical issues. In: Fortin AH, Dwamena FC, Frankel RM, Smith RC (eds). *Smith's Patient-Centered Interviewing: An Evidence-Based Method.* 3rd ed. New York, NY: McGraw-Hill.

Mallin R, Hood-Watson K. Alcohol and drug abuse. In: Smith MA, Shimp LA, Schrager S (eds). *Family Medicine Ambulatory Care and Prevention.* 6th ed. New York, NY: McGraw-Hill.

Obedin-Maliver J, Robertson PA, Ard KL, Mayer KH, Deutsch MB. Lesbian, gay, bisexual & transgender health. In: Papadakis MA, McPhee SJ, Rabow MW (eds). *Current Medical Diagnosis & Treatment.* New York, NY: McGraw-Hill; 2018.

Pre-exposure Prophylaxis (PrEP) for HIV Prevention. May, 2015. Available at https://www.cdc.gov/hiv/pdf/PrEP_fact_sheet_final.pdf. Accessed January 1, 2018.

Reitschuler-Cross EB, Arnold RM. Hospice & palliative medicine. In: South-Paul JE, Matheny SC, Lewis EL (eds). *Current Diagnosis & Treatment Family Medicine.* 4th ed. New York, NY: McGraw-Hill.

South-Paul JE, Lewis EL. Health & healthcare disparities. In: South-Paul JE, Matheny SC, Lewis EL (eds). *Current Diagnosis & Treatment Family Medicine.* 4th ed. New York, NY: McGraw-Hill.

Wolfe SR. Caring for lesbian, gay, bisexual, & transgender patients. In: South-Paul JE, Matheny SC, Lewis EL (eds). *Current Diagnosis & Treatment Family Medicine.* 4th ed. New York, NY: McGraw-Hill.

Acute Complaints

Questions

Acute Complaints—Cardiovascular

108. You are evaluating a 40-year-old male patient in the office who is complaining of chest pain. His father had a myocardial infarction at age 42, and the patient is quite concerned. Which characteristic, if included in the history, decreases the likelihood that his chest pain is cardiac in origin?

a. The pain is worse with inspiration.
b. The pain radiates to his right arm.
c. The pain radiates to his left arm.
d. The pain is associated with nausea.
e. The pain is associated with sweatiness.

109. You are evaluating a 61-year-old man in the office who is complaining of chest pain. Given his history and risk factors, you are concerned about myocardial ischemia, and order an electrocardiogram (ECG). Which of the following ECG features, if present, would most markedly increase the likelihood of an acute myocardial infarction?

a. Any ST-segment elevation greater than or equal to 1 mm
b. Any ST-segment depression
c. Any Q wave
d. Any conduction defect
e. A new conduction defect

110. A 43-year-old woman with a history of well-controlled hypertension and diabetes presents to your office complaining of intermittent chest pain for the last 3 months. The most recent episode was 1 week ago, after climbing four flights of stairs at work. The pain was relieved with rest. An ECG in your office is shown below. She is currently asymptomatic. Which of the following is the most appropriate next step?

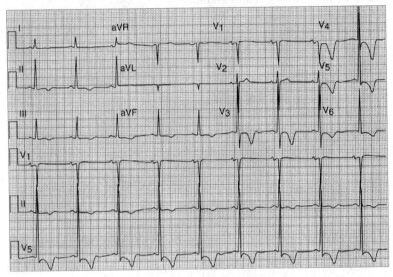

(Reproduced, with permission, from Ferry D. Basic Electrocardiography in Ten Days. New York, NY: McGraw-Hill; 2001: 35.)

a. Reassure the patient and have her return if symptoms continue.
b. Reassure the patient, but increase her medication to ensure tight control of her blood pressure and glucose levels.
c. Admit the patient to the hospital for serial enzymes.
d. Obtain a treadmill stress ECG.
e. Obtain a treadmill stress echocardiogram.

111. You are evaluating a 75-year-old woman with diabetes and hyper-lipidemia who is complaining of chest pain. She reports having occasional chest pain with exertion for years, but yesterday she reported chest pain while walking up steps, then she passed out. On examination, she is afebrile with mildly elevated blood pressure. Cardiac auscultation demonstrates a harsh, rasping crescendo-decrescendo systolic murmur heard best at the second intercostal space at the right upper sternal border. Her carotid pulse is small and rises slowly. Which of the following is the most likely diagnosis?

a. Pulmonary embolism (PE)
b. Aortic dissection
c. Left ventricular hypertrophy (LVH)
d. Aortic stenosis
e. Mitral valve prolapse

112. You are caring for a 38-year-old male patient who reports episodic chest pain. He reports that the pain feels like "tightness," is located right behind his sternum, lasts less than 3 minutes, and is relieved with rest. He takes no medications, has no family history of coronary disease, and has never smoked. His ECG in the office is normal. Which of the following tests should be done to determine whether or not his chest pain is due to ischemia?

a. Exercise ECG
b. Resting echocardiogram
c. Stress echocardiography
d. Radionuclide angiography
e. Electron-beam computed tomography (CT)

113. You are evaluating a 33-year-old woman complaining of palpitations. Which of the following characteristics, if present, increase the likelihood that the symptoms are cardiac in etiology?

a. The fact that the patient is female
b. The fact that the patient has a sister with similar symptoms
c. Her description of the symptoms as an "irregular heartbeat"
d. The fact that her father has a history of heart disease
e. The fact that the episodes last less than 1 minute

114. The patient in the question above reports random and episodic feelings of palpitations. You complete a detailed history and physical examination and do not find an obvious cause or precipitating factor. Her 12-lead ECG, thyroid-stimulating hormone (TSH), hemoglobin/hematocrit, and electrolytes are all normal. Which of the following is the best next step?

a. Ambulatory ECG for 2 weeks
b. Ambulatory ECG for 4 weeks
c. Electrophysiology consultation
d. Echocardiogram
e. Observation and reassurance

115. You are seeing a hypertensive 56-year-old woman who is complaining of a "fluttering in her chest." She is otherwise well, and denies shortness of breath, light-headedness, pedal edema, or other symptoms when her "fluttering" occurs. On examination, her pulse rate is rapid and irregular. She has no other complaints and the rest of her physical examination is normal. Which of the following is her most likely diagnosis?

a. Atrial fibrillation
b. Paroxysmal supraventricular tachycardia (PSVT)
c. Stable ventricular tachycardia
d. Stimulant abuse
e. Hyperthyroidism

116. You are seeing a 32-year-old otherwise healthy woman who is complaining of palpitations. She describes the sensation as a "flip flop" in her chest. They only last an instant and are not associated with light-headedness or other symptoms. She denies other symptoms. Which of the following is the most likely etiology of her complaint?

a. Atrial fibrillation
b. PSVT
c. Ventricular premature beats
d. Stimulant abuse
e. Hyperthyroidism

117. You are seeing a 19-year-old African-American student who reports that he can "feel his heartbeat." It happens with exercise and is associated with some light-headedness and shortness of breath. On examination, his heart has a regular rate and rhythm, but you hear a holosystolic murmur along his left sternal border. It increases with Valsalva maneuver. Which of the following is the most likely cause of his symptoms?

a. Mitral valve prolapse
b. Hypertrophic obstructive cardiomyopathy
c. Dilated cardiomyopathy
d. Atrial fibrillation
e. Congestive heart failure (CHF)

118. You are evaluating a 23-year-old swimmer who is complaining of episodes of symptomatic rapid heart beating. Twice during swim practice, he has developed a sensation that his heart is racing. When he measures his heart rate, he finds it to be between 160 and 220 beats/min. The first episode lasted approximately 4 minutes and the second lasted more than 10 minutes. He denies light-headedness or other symptoms during the events. Limited laboratory evaluation is normal, and ECG shows a normal QRS duration. Which of the following is the next step in the evaluation?

a. Reassure and continue observation
b. Ambulatory ECG monitoring
c. Consultation with an electrophysiologist
d. Stress testing
e. Echocardiography

119. The patient in the question above completed the appropriate testing and all was normal, but his symptoms persist. The patient has tried mechanical measures, including Valsalva, coughing, holding breath, and cold water without success. What is the preferred next step to prevent his symptoms?

a. Cardioversion
b. Catheter ablation
c. Use of a β-blocker
d. Use of a class Ic anti-arrhythmic (flecainide, propafenone)
e. Use of a class III anti-arrhythmic (sotalol, amiodarone)

120. You are seeing a man complaining of symptomatic palpitations. His ECG is shown below:

Which of the following is the likely diagnosis?

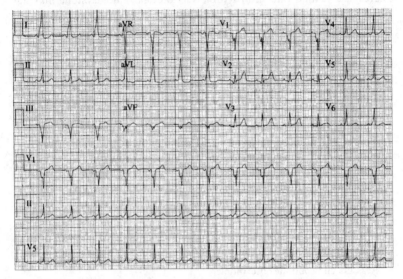

(*Reproduced, with permission, from Ferry D. Basic Electrocardiography in Ten Days. New York, NY: McGraw-Hill; 2001: 177.*)

a. Sinus tachycardia
b. Supraventricular tachycardia
c. Wolff-Parkinson-White syndrome
d. Ventricular tachycardia
e. Premature atrial contractions

121. You are evaluating a 42-year-old previously healthy man who has presented to the emergency department with a complaint of chest pain. He reports substernal sharp pain that radiates to the back and shoulders, is worse with deep breathing or lying flat. For the past week, he has felt fatigued with increasing dyspnea when lying down as well as a mild cough. The patient's ECG is shown below.

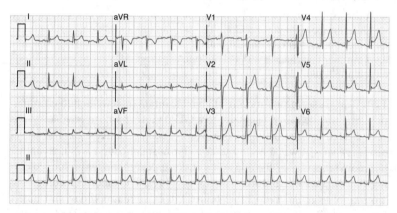

(Reproduced with permission from Kasper DL, Fauci AS, Hauser SL, Longo DL, Jameson JL, Loscalzo J. Harrison's Principles of Internal Medicine, *19th Ed. New York, NY: McGraw-Hill Education; 2015: Figure 269e-13, p. 269-e7.)*

What is the most likely diagnosis?

a. PE
b. Acute myocardial infarction
c. Acute pericarditis
d. Acute myocarditis
e. Acute community-acquired pneumonia

122. You are discharging a 35-year-old female patient who was recently diagnosed with acute viral pericarditis. The patient will follow-up with you in the office later this week, but she is very anxious about her symptoms returning. Which of the following is the most effective in preventing recurrence of viral pericarditis?

a. Restricted activity for 3 months
b. No treatment has been shown to prevent recurrence
c. Aspirin or nonsteroidal anti-inflammatory drugs (NSAIDs)
d. Oral corticosteroids
e. Colchicine

123. You are seeing a healthy 12-month-old male infant in the office for a well-child examination. He was delivered vaginally to a G2P1 mother and the pregnancy and delivery were uneventful. His examination at delivery and previous well checks have been normal. Today, you auscultate a cardiac murmur on examination; previous examinations have been documented as normal. Which of the following murmur characteristics would favor a benign etiology for the murmur (an "innocent murmur")?

a. A pansystolic murmur
b. The presence of a systolic click
c. A murmur associated with an S_4 gallop
d. A murmur that changes with the position of patient
e. A diastolic murmur

124. You are seeing a 1-month-old female infant for a well-child examination. She was delivered vaginally to a G1P0 mother whose pregnancy was complicated by preexisting poorly controlled type 2 diabetes. The baby's discharge weight was 6 lbs; 8 ounces. Her hospital course was uneventful, but mom reports poor feeding and a dusky appearance after prolonged crying. The infant's weight today is 6 lbs, 4 ounces. The infant is feeding ½ to 1 ounce of formula every 2 to 3 hours. On examination today, you note a harsh grade III/VI continuous "machinery" type murmur in the left infraclavicular fossa and pulmonic area with an associated thrill. Faint wheezes are auscultated bilaterally in the lungs and hepatomegaly is present. Which of the following is the most likely cause?

a. Atrial septal defect
b. Patent ductus arteriosus (PDA)
c. Aortic stenosis
d. Still's murmur
e. Transposition of the great vessels

Acute Complaints—Dermatologic and Breast

125. You are seeing a 25-year-old male patient with a rash. It began as pink spots on his extremities including on his palms and soles, but the lesions have begun to coalesce and become purple in color. He recently returned from a hiking trip in the mountains. Which of the following is the most likely cause?

a. Lyme disease
b. Rocky Mountain spotted fever
c. Tularemia
d. Brown recluse spider bite
e. Black widow spider bite

126. You are caring for a person who presents with severe symptoms. He started with fatigue, myalgias, arthralgias, headache, and low-grade fever several weeks ago. He also noted a "rash" on his upper back near the right scapula that looked "like a bull's eye." That rash has since resolved. Currently, he complains of musculoskeletal pain and attacks of joint pain and swelling for the past week, and today he reports pleuritic chest pain. On examination, he has lymphadenopathy, tenderness in his joints, and right axillary adenopathy. You also notice a friction rub. What is the best treatment for this condition?

a. Doxycycline for 10 to 14 days
b. Amoxicillin for 10 to 14 days
c. Tetracycline for 2 to 3 days after the patient becomes afebrile
d. Streptomycin intramuscularly for 1 week
e. Ceftriaxone intravenously for 2 to 3 weeks

127. You are seeing a patient who is complaining of an itching scalp. There are erythematous papules on her scalp especially behind the ears, and you note small black bulbs at the bases of several hair follicles. Which of the following is the preferred treatment option for this condition?

a. Extermination of the home
b. Permethrin 1%
c. Permethrin 5%
d. Lindane 1%
e. Oral ivermectin (Stromectol)

128. A 16-year-old camp counselor sees you to evaluate a severely pruritic rash. You note pruritic erythematous papules in between his fingers, on his wrists, and around his waist. For which of the following is this distribution characteristic?

a. Flea bites
b. Bedbugs
c. Body lice
d. Scabies
e. Chigger bites

129. A 34-year-old woman presents to your office with a complaint of 4 days of fever, itchy rash, "pink eye," and aching in her joints. She has no prior medical history and has not traveled recently, but she does note that her husband has just returned home from a business trip to Brazil. On examination, you note a temperature of 101.3°F and a diffuse maculopapular rash. There is no erythema or swelling of the joints or soft tissues. Which of the following conditions is most likely?

a. Disseminated gonococcal disease
b. Dengue fever
c. Zika virus
d. Chikungunya fever
e. Yellow fever

130. You are seeing a 21-year-old patient with pruritic, erythematous papules in clusters on his ankles and legs. He noticed the rash the day after he stayed in a hotel on his way back from a Spring Break vacation in Florida. Based on this history and description, which is the most likely culprit?

a. Flea bites
b. "Hot tub" folliculitis
c. Spider bites
d. Scabies
e. Lice

131. A 20-year-old man presents to you 30 minutes after being stung by a bee on his right thigh. He was stung by a bee twice last year. The first sting caused a 3-cm × 3-cm area of erythema, induration, and pain around the sting site. The second sting caused a similar 5-cm × 7-cm area. When you examine him, he has an expanding 2-cm × 2-cm area of erythema, induration, and pain around the sting site on his thigh. He reports pruritis, fatigue, and some nausea, but denies dyspnea. Which of the following is true?

a. This is a typical local reaction, and should spontaneously resolve within hours.
b. This is a large local reaction, and the patient has minimal risk for the development of anaphylaxis upon subsequent exposure.
c. This is a large local reaction, and the patient is at significant risk for the development of anaphylaxis upon subsequent exposure.
d. This is considered a toxic systemic reaction, and increases his risk for anaphylaxis if he is exposed in the future.
e. This is considered a mild anaphylactic reaction.

132. A 15-year-old adolescent boy comes to your office complaining of bilateral breast enlargement. He is otherwise healthy and on no medications. On examination, there is mildly tender palpable breast tissue bilaterally. The rest of his physical examination, including his testicular examination, is normal. Which of the following is true?

a. No further workup is necessary.
b. Serum liver studies will help to elucidate the cause.
c. Thyroid function assessment will help to elucidate the cause.
d. Serum estradiol, testosterone, and luteinizing hormone levels are needed to elucidate the cause.
e. His serum chorionic gonadotropin level is likely to be elevated.

133. A 22-year-old woman is seeing her physician with complaints of breast pain. It is associated with her menstrual cycle and is described as a bilateral "heaviness" that radiates to the axillae and arms. Examination reveals groups of small breast nodules in the upper outer quadrants of each breast. They are freely mobile and slightly tender. Which of the following statements is most accurate?

a. The patient has bilateral fibroadenomas, and reassurance is all that is necessary.
b. The patient has bilateral fibroadenomas, and a mammogram is necessary for further evaluation.
c. The patient has bilateral fibrocystic changes, and reassurance is all that is necessary.
d. The patient has bilateral fibrocystic changes, and a mammogram is necessary for further evaluation.
e. The patient has bilateral mastitis and antibiotic therapy is needed.

134. A 35-year-old woman presents to you concerned about a breast mass. Examination reveals no skin changes, diffusely nodular breasts bilaterally with a more dominant, firm, and nontender fixed nodule on the left side. The nodule is approximately 7 mm in size, in the upper outer quadrant of the left breast. Her mammogram is negative. Which of the following statements is true?

a. The patient should be reassured and resume routine care.
b. The mass should be closely followed with repeat mammogram in 3 to 6 months.
c. The patient should undergo testing for breast cancer genetic mutations, and base further workup on the results.
d. The patient should be referred for an ultrasound (US) and possible biopsy.
e. If clear amber fluid is aspirated from the mass, it is likely benign, and no further workup is necessary.

135. You are seeing a 36-year-old woman with a complaint of nipple discharge. Which of the following characteristics of the discharge is most suspicious for breast cancer?

a. Spontaneous discharge (not related to physical manipulation)
b. Green discharge
c. Bilateral discharge
d. Discharge associated with menses
e. Bloody discharge

136. You are working in the emergency department (ED) and evaluating a 21-year-old man with an erythematous, tender, and edematous hand. He reports helping a neighbor get her cat out of a tree around 10 hours ago, and was bitten on the hand. On examination, you note erythema with some purulent discharge around a fairly deep wound with a jagged laceration. You irrigate the wound thoroughly and do not see tendon involvement. Which of the following is the most likely infecting organism?

a. *Clostridium perfringens*
b. *Staphylococcus aureus*
c. *Streptococcus pyogenes*
d. *Pasteurella multocida*
e. *Haemophilus influenzae*

137. In the case described above, what is the best treatment option?

a. Hospitalization
b. Treat with amoxicillin/clavulanic acid as an outpatient for 5 days
c. Treat with amoxicillin/clavulanic acid as an outpatient for 10 days
d. Treat with amoxicillin/clavulanic acid and perform primary closure of the wound
e. Treat with amoxicillin/clavulanic acid along with clindamycin, and perform primary closure of the wound

138. You are seeing a 14-year-old high school wrestler for a skin condition. About a week ago, he noted a patch of erythematous skin on his right thigh. The patch has enlarged since he first noted it, and the central part of the lesion seems to be clearing. He reports that it is mildly pruritic. You scrape the lesion and evaluate the shavings under the microscope using potassium hydroxide (KOH). The slide is shown below. Which of the following is the most likely diagnosis?

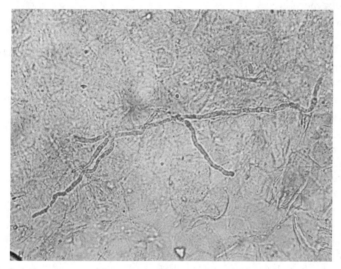

(*Reproduced, with permission, from Usatine RP, Smith MA, Chumley H, Mayeaux EJ Jr, Tysinger J.* The Color Atlas of Family Medicine. *New York, NY: McGraw-Hill; 2009: 542.*)

a. Tinea corporis
b. Tinea cruris
c. Pityriasis rosea
d. Nummular eczema
e. Impetigo

139. You are caring for a teenager who complains of acne. It is most apparent on his forehead and his cheeks. It is causing a great deal of stress in his life and impacting his self-confidence. Of the following, which is most likely a contributing factor to his condition?

a. Leaning his face on his hands while sitting at his desk at school
b. Eating fast food
c. Not washing his hair often enough
d. Eating chocolate
e. Not eating enough vegetables

140. You are caring for a 20-year-old male patient who is concerned about facial acne. He has had moderate symptoms since his teenage years, but has not ever tried a formalized treatment regimen. He is otherwise healthy and developmentally normal. Which of the following tests or set of tests is best to help guide treatment of his disorder?

a. Free testosterone.
b. Dehydroepiandrosterone sulfate (DHEAS).
c. Free testosterone and DHEAS.
d. Free testosterone, DHEAS, follicle-stimulating hormone, and luteinizing hormone.
e. No laboratory examinations are required.

141. You are caring for a 13-year-old girl with acne. She is becoming increasingly concerned about her appearance and is worried about getting teased at school because of her skin. After assessment, you diagnose her with moderate acne. Of the following treatment regimens, which would be best for her at this time?

a. Topical antibiotics
b. Benzoyl peroxide gel
c. Topical antibiotics and benzoyl peroxide gel
d. Topical antibiotics, benzoyl peroxide gel, and topical retinoids
e. Oral antibiotics, benzoyl peroxide gel, and topical retinoids

142. You are caring for a 16-year-old girl with moderate acne. Her current regimen includes topical retinoids, benzoyl peroxide gel, and oral minocycline, but after 6 months on this regimen, she has not had improvement. You are considering treatment with oral isotretinoin (Accutane). In addition to ensuring that pregnancy is prevented during her therapy, which of the following must occur during her therapy?

a. She must avoid Tylenol use.
b. She must stop wearing her contacts.
c. She must have transaminases checked regularly.
d. She must be screened for depression every 3 months.
e. She must not use topical glucocorticoids.

143. You are caring for a 45-year-old woman who reports a 2- to 3-year history of episodic flushing of her cheeks, nose, and forehead. Over the last several months, this has been more constant, and she has developed papules and some pustules on her cheeks. Her picture is shown below:

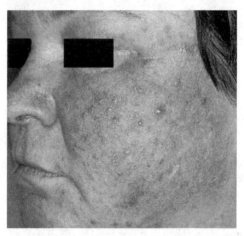

(Reproduced with permission from Wolff K, Johnson RA, Saavedra AP, Roh EK. Fitzpatrick's Color Atlas and Synopsis of Clinical Dermatology, 8th Ed. New York, NY: McGraw-Hill Education; 2017: Figure 1-9, p. 10.)

Which of the following is the most effective treatment for this condition?

a. Topical metronidazole cream
b. Topical sodium sulfacetamide
c. Topical antibiotics
d. Topical steroids
e. Oral antibiotics

144. You are seeing a 17-year-old woman for a rash. She was helping her father rake leaves in their yard this past weekend, and now, 4 days later, complains of a severely pruritic rash. It is on her legs, arms, and face. A picture of her leg is below.

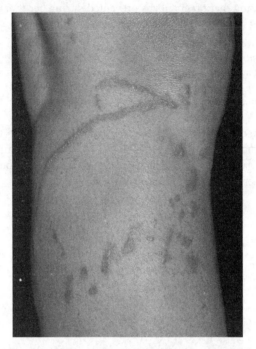

(Reproduced with permission from Wolff K, Johnson RA, Saavedra AP, Roh EK. Fitzpatrick's Color Atlas and Synopsis of Clinical Dermatology, 8th Ed. New York, NY: McGraw-Hill Education; 2017: Figure 2-8, p. 30.)

She reports that she hasn't slept in the last couple of days because the itching is keeping her awake. Which of the following is the most effective treatment?

a. Topical glucocorticoid ointment
b. Topical glucocorticoid gel
c. Low-dose oral prednisone for 1 to 2 weeks
d. High-dose oral prednisone tapered over 2 weeks
e. Oral tacrolimus

145. A 55-year-old male patient comes to you with concerns about a nodule underneath his right eye. The nodule is shown below. He reports that it "popped up" a couple of weeks ago and has been growing ever since. Which of the following is the most likely diagnosis?

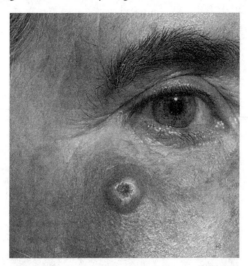

(Reproduced with permission from Wolff K, Johnson RA, Saavedra AP, Roh EK. Fitzpatrick's Color Atlas and Synopsis of Clinical Dermatology, *8th Ed. New York, NY: McGraw-Hill Education; 2017: Figure 11-17A, p. 236.)*

a. Verruca vulgaris
b. Molluscum contagiosum
c. Keratoacanthoma
d. Nodular basal cell carcinoma (BCC)
e. Squamous cell carcinoma

146. You are caring for a 28-year-old man with a rash. The rash has been present for 3 to 4 years and has remained fairly stable. He describes the rash as a single patch that is mildly itchy. On examination, you identify an erythematous scaly patch on his right elbow. You also note pitting and subungual hyperkeratosis of the fingernails. Which of the following is the best therapeutic choice for his rash?

a. Topical fluorinated glucocorticoids
b. Topical pimecrolimus (Elidel)
c. Oral penicillin
d. Oral retinoids (Accutane)
e. Oral methotrexate

147. You are talking with a 24-year-old man who reports an outbreak of a mildly pruritic rash. The rash initially began with a large pink patch on his chest, to the right of his sternum. About a week later, he noted a more generalized eruption. The rash is shown below. Which of the following treatments is indicated?

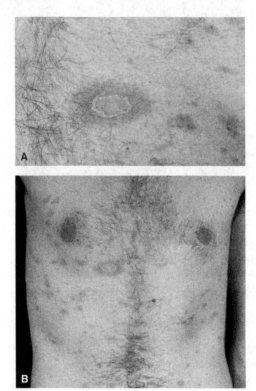

(Reproduced with permission from Wolff K, Johnson RA, Saavedra AP, Roh EK. Fitzpatrick's Color Atlas and Synopsis of Clinical Dermatology, 8th Ed. New York, NY: McGraw-Hill Education; 2017: Figure 3-19, p. 66.)

a. Antihistamines
b. Antibiotics
c. Antivirals
d. Antifungals
e. Cyclosporine

148. You are seeing a young child whose mother brings him in with a rash. It developed on his upper lip underneath his nose. He has recently had cold symptoms with a runny nose. On examination, you note erythematous scattered discreet lesions on his upper lip, chin, and around his nares. Many have a golden-yellow crust. Which of the following is the most likely cause of this rash?

a. Contact dermatitis
b. Infection with *S aureus*
c. Infection with an *Enterococcus* species
d. Infection with *H influenzae*
e. Infection with a *Pseudomonas* species

149. After returning from a ski trip in the mountains, your 35-year-old patient developed a rash. He has multiple erythematous papules and pustules over his legs, arms, and chest. They are not pruritic and do not seem to be spreading. He denies any new soaps, lotions, foods, or medications. He did spend time in a hot tub on the trip. Which of the following treatments is the best first-line therapy for this patient?

a. Reassurance and follow-up if no improvement
b. Topical steroid medication
c. Systemic steroid medication
d. Topical antibiotics with activity against *Streptococcus* and *Staphylococcus* species
e. Oral antibiotics with activity against *Pseudomonas* species

150. You are seeing a 26-year-old woman with a lesion on her lip. It began with a burning at the site of the lesion, then an eruption of vesicles. She describes outbreaks of this rash many times in the past. The rash is shown below. Which of the following is true of the treatment for this infection?

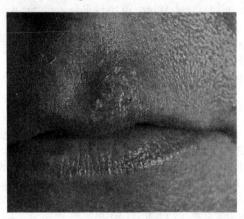

(Reproduced with permission from Wolff K, Johnson RA, Saavedra AP, Roh EK. Fitzpatrick's Color Atlas and Synopsis of Clinical Dermatology, 8th Ed. New York, NY: McGraw-Hill Education; 2017: Figure 27-35B, p. 684.)

a. Oral antiviral agents are more effective treating recurrences than they are treating primary infections.
b. Oral therapy begun within 2 days of onset is the best treatment for recurrent outbreaks.
c. Chronic suppression with daily therapy is beneficial for oral herpes.
d. Acyclovir resistance makes it a poor choice for therapy.
e. Docosanol cream (Abreva) is ineffective.

151. An otherwise healthy 61-year-old male patient complains of a burning sensation on the back of his right shoulder for 24 hours, and subsequent development of a rash. On examination, you note grouped vesicles on an erythematous base in a dermatomal pattern that does not cross the midline. Which of the following is true about this condition?

a. The varicella (chicken pox) vaccine has led to an increase in cases of this rash in the general population.
b. Compared with no treatment, antiviral therapy has been shown to decrease the incidence of postherpetic neuralgia 6 months after treatment.
c. Treatment with corticosteroids will not reduce the prevalence of postherpetic neuralgia.
d. Narcotics are rarely necessary for this condition.
e. Antiviral resistance is common.

152. You are seeing a 5-year-old otherwise healthy girl whose mother brings her in for evaluation. The mother reports that last week, she had 3 days of upper respiratory tract symptoms and associated headache, sore throat, abdominal pain, and some loose bowel movements. That resolved a few days ago, but today she developed a facial rash which was concerning to the mother. A picture of the rash is shown below:

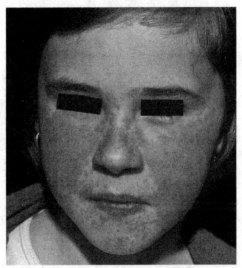

(Reproduced with permission from Wolff K, Johnson RA, Saavedra AP, Roh EK. Fitzpatrick's Color Atlas and Synopsis of Clinical Dermatology, 8th Ed. New York, NY: McGraw-Hill Education; 2017: Figure 27-27A, p. 684.)

Which of the following is the most likely cause of her symptoms?

a. An enterovirus
b. A parvovirus
c. A parainfluenza virus
d. A varicella virus
e. Cytomegalovirus

153. The patient described in the question above is treated appropriately and recovers as expected. Which of the following is true of the weeks following the acute symptoms?

a. The patient should be tested for anemia.
b. The patient is contagious as long as the rash persists.
c. The rash may recur in association with bathing.
d. The patient should continue antivirals as long as the rash persists.
e. Serum should be tested for immunoglobulin G (IgG) to ensure future immunity.

154. You are seeing a young man who is complaining of patchy hair loss. He denies pulling the hair and complains that his scalp is itchy and flakey. His scalp is shown below. Which of the following is the treatment of choice for this condition?

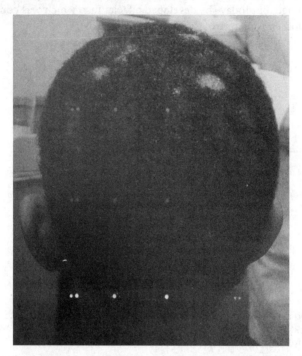

(Reproduced with permission from Usatine RP, Smith MA, Mayeaux EJ Jr, Chumley H, and Tysinger J. The Color Atlas of Family Medicine, 1st ed. New York, NY: McGraw-Hill Education; 2009: Figure 131-1, p. 549.)

a. Selenium sulfide lotion, applied daily for 4 to 8 weeks
b. Ketoconazole (Nizoral) shampoo, applied daily for 4 to 8 weeks
c. Clotrimazole (Lotrimin) cream, twice daily for 4 to 8 weeks
d. Griseofulvin tablets, daily for 4 to 8 weeks
e. Fluconazole (Diflucan) tablets, daily for 4 to 8 weeks

155. You are caring for a 35-year-old woman who works in a veterinary hospital. She noted an itchy rash on her calf approximately 3 to 4 weeks ago. It started as a small pink circular lesion, but is spreading, and has not responded to over-the-counter antifungal ointments. The rash is shown below.

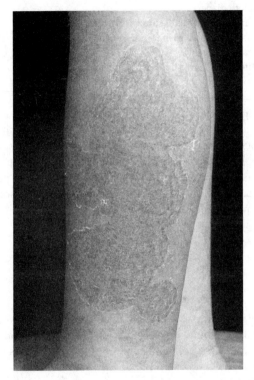

(Reproduced with permission from Wolff K, Johnson RA, Saavedra AP, Roh EK. Fitzpatrick's Color Atlas and Synopsis of Clinical Dermatology, 8th Ed. New York, NY: McGraw-Hill Education; 2017: Figure 26-38, p. 626.)

Which of the following therapies is likely to be most effective?

a. Topical clotrimazole (Lotrimin)
b. Topical ketoconazole (Nizoral)
c. Topical terbinafine (Lamisil)
d. Oral griseofulvin
e. Oral griseofulvin with oral steroids

156. You are caring for a 5-month-old infant whose mother complains that he has a diaper rash. Examination of his diaper area reveals erythematous patches with skin erosion and satellite lesions. He also has a white coating on his buccal mucosa. Which of the following interventions is most likely to cure his rash?

a. Change to cloth diapers
b. Frequent gentle cleaning with commercially available wipes
c. Application of a barrier preparation (such as zinc oxide, petroleum jelly, or vitamin A & D ointment)
d. Topical antifungal creams such as clotrimazole
e. Combination antifungal cream and oral nystatin

157. A 7-year-old girl's mother brought her in to have you evaluate her rash. The child describes significant itching for 3 days, and it seems to be worsening. She shares these symptoms with several friends, all of whom are now complaining of an itchy rash after having had a sleep over 3 weeks ago. On examination, your patient has slightly erythematous papules in her interdigital spaces, wrists, ankles, and waist. You diagnose scabies. Which of the following treatments is most effective?

a. Permethrin 5% cream (Elimite)
b. Oral ivermectin
c. Benzyl benzoate
d. Lindane cream
e. 10% sulfur

158. You are caring for a 25-year-old man who presents to you for evaluation of a new lesion found on his groin. On examination, you find a single small umbilicated flesh-colored papule, 4 mm in size, in his pubic region. Which of the following is true?

a. A family history of skin cancer is likely in this person.
b. The patient is probably immunocompromised.
c. This is likely to be a sexually transmitted infection.
d. This can be spread through aerosolized droplets.
e. Treatment for this condition must be surgical.

159. You are caring for a 72-year-old woman who reports a mole on the right side of her nose that has been increasing in size. She says it has been there for at least 4 years, but is enlarging and more noticeable. On examination, you see a nodule with raised lighter edges, telangiectasias, and a slightly ulcerated center. Given this history and these clinical features, what is the most likely diagnosis?

a. Intradermal nevus
b. Molluscum contagiosum
c. Basal cell carcinoma
d. Squamous cell carcinoma
e. Seborrheic keratosis

Acute Complaints—Gastrointestinal

160. You are evaluating a 41-year-old man in your office who reports abdominal pain. He says the pain began suddenly and is located in the right lower quadrant. He describes the pain as "gnawing" and it seems to get worse after eating. He has vomited twice since the pain began. Which historical feature would lead you toward an emergent evaluation?

a. The pain's location in the right lower quadrant
b. The fact that the pain began suddenly
c. The description of the pain
d. The fact that it is worse after eating
e. The fact that it is associated with emesis

161. A 42-year-old woman presents to your office complaining of the recent onset of abdominal pain. She describes pain that starts in the midepigastric region, radiating to the back. It is associated with nausea and vomiting. You suspect pancreatitis. If that is true, what is the most likely underlying cause of the condition?

a. Idiopathic
b. Overeating
c. NSAID use
d. Biliary tract disease
e. Congenital anomaly

162. Based on the previous question, which of the following imaging modalities is most suitable for diagnosis in this patient?

a. Abdominal x-rays
b. Abdominal US
c. Abdominal magnetic resonance imaging (MRI)
d. Abdominal CT
e. Esophagogastroduodenoscopy (EGD)

163. An 80-year-old man presents with mild, crampy, bilateral lower quadrant pain, decreased appetite, and low-grade fever for about 48 hours. Which of the following is the most likely diagnosis?

a. Small-bowel obstruction
b. Appendicitis
c. Constipation
d. Irritable bowel syndrome (IBS)
e. Pancreatitis

164. A 62-year-old woman is complaining of gnawing abdominal pain in the center of her upper abdomen associated with a sensation of hunger and darker stool over the last 3 weeks. She had an intentional 20 pound weight loss last year, but recently her weight has been stable. Her only medical history includes osteoarthritis of the knees. Which of the following is the most likely cause of her illness?

a. Alcoholism
b. NSAID abuse
c. *Helicobacter pylori* infection
d. Gallstones
e. Gastroparesis

165. A 26-year-old man complains of heartburn. He also complains of regurgitation, belching, and occasional dry cough. His symptoms are worse when he is lying down. He denies melena, weight loss, or dysphagia. What is the appropriate next step, if you suspect gastroesophageal reflux disease (GERD) in this patient?

a. Treat with H_2-receptor antagonists or a proton-pump inhibitor, and evaluate the response
b. Obtain a barium swallow
c. Obtain a CT scan of the abdomen with oral and intravenous (IV) contrast
d. Obtain an US of the abdomen
e. Perform an EGD

166. You are seeing a 75-year-old patient with complaints of heartburn, regurgitation, and belching. You suspect GERD. Which symptom, if present, would necessitate a referral for an upper endoscopy?

a. Pain radiating to the back
b. Dysphagia
c. Chronic use of NSAIDs for coexisting arthritis
d. Bloating
e. Nausea

167. A 44-year-old woman is admitted to the hospital for acute right upper quadrant pain consistent with biliary colic. Her symptoms have been present for 4 hours, and she also has fever and a positive Murphy sign. She has a history of asymptomatic gallstones, identified incidentally several years ago. Her laboratory evaluation is as follows:

White blood cell (WBC):	17.5 K/μL (H) with a left shift
Aspartate aminotransferase (AST):	88 U/L (H)
Alanine aminotransferase (ALT):	110 U/L (H)
Alkaline phosphatase:	330 U/L (H)
Bilirubin (total):	3.2 mg/dL (H)

What would the next test of choice be?

a. US of the abdomen
b. CT scan of the abdomen
c. MRI of the abdomen
d. Endoscopic retrograde cholangiopancreatography (ERCP)
e. Cholescintigraphy

168. A 63-year-old previously healthy female patient presents to the office complaining of 2 to 3 days of achy abdominal pain, nausea with two episodes of emesis, anorexia, and a low-grade fever. She denies any hematemesis or hematochezia, in fact, she has not had a bowel movement in several days. On examination, she is afebrile, appears in no acute distress, mucous membranes are moist, abdomen is soft, nondistended, and without rebound or guarding. However, she does have significant tenderness to palpation of the left lower quadrant. Her complete blood count (CBC) reveals a mildly elevated WBC without a left shift and normal RBC. Which of the following is the best initial treatment for this patient?

a. IV antibiotics and oral hydration
b. Oral antibiotics and oral hydration
c. Further evaluation with colonoscopy
d. Clear, liquid diet with close follow-up in 24 to 48 hours
e. Emergent surgical consultation

169. You are seeing a 53-year-old man who was hospitalized for pancreatitis. His admission laboratory studies include a WBC count of 18,000/mm³, glucose of 153 mg/dL, lactate dehydrogenase (LDH) of 254 IU/L, and AST of 165 U/L. According to Ranson criteria, which of these factors suggest a poor prognosis in this patient?

a. Age
b. WBC count
c. Glucose
d. LDH
e. AST

170. A 17-year-old previously healthy man presents to your office with a chief complaint of nausea and increasing, constant abdominal pain for the past 3 days. He denies diarrhea, fever, or respiratory symptoms. No one else at home or school has been sick with similar symptoms. His knees and ankles have been aching badly as well and he has noticed some hematuria that started today along with a bumpy, purple rash on his buttocks and posterior legs. Which of the following conditions is most likely?

a. Poststreptococcal glomerulonephritis
b. Reiter's syndrome
c. Henoch-Schönlein purpura
d. Renal lithiasis
e. Disseminated gonococcal disease

171. You are seeing a 46-year-old man who reports 3 months of discomfort centered around his upper abdomen. It is associated with heartburn, frequent belching, bloating, and occasional nausea. What is the most likely result that will be found after workup for these symptoms?

a. Peptic ulcer disease (PUD).
b. GERD.
c. Gastric cancer.
d. Gastroparesis.
e. No cause is likely to be identified.

172. You are caring for a healthy 41-year-old man on no medication who is complaining of difficulty with defecation. He reports a recent onset of having fewer bowel movements per week that include difficult passage of stool. He denies hematochezia, melena, or weight loss. He has no family history of colon cancer or inflammatory bowel disease. His physical examination and fecal occult blood test in the office are negative. What initial laboratory testing is indicated in the workup of his condition?

a. No blood tests are needed.
b. TSH only.
c. TSH and electrolytes only.
d. TSH, electrolytes, and ionized calcium only.
e. TSH, electrolytes, ionized calcium, and CBC.

173. The patient above is no better despite appropriate workup. He has tried to increase fluid intake and dietary fiber with no change in his complaint. What is the most appropriate next step?

a. Stimulant laxatives
b. Osmotic laxatives
c. Chloride secreting agents
d. Opioid receptor antagonists
e. Referral to gastroenterology

174. You are seeing a 28-year-old woman who is complaining of constipation. She reports that her symptoms have been present since she can remember, and no dietary changes have seemed to benefit her. She has never tried pharmacologic therapy in the past. Which of the following would be the best first-line therapy for her?

a. Psyllium (Metamucil)
b. Magnesium hydroxide (milk of magnesia)
c. Bisacodyl (Dulcolax)
d. Saline enemas
e. Lubiprostone (Amitiza)

175. You are caring for a 46-year-old male patient who reports new onset constipation. The frequency of his bowel movements has gone from once every day to once every 3 days, and he describes a feeling of bloating that improves after defecation. His weight on this visit is 12 pounds less than at his last visit 4 months ago. He denies hematochezia or melena, and his fecal occult blood test in the office is negative. What is the most appropriate next step?

a. A trial of increased fiber and fluid intake
b. A trial of stimulant laxatives
c. A trial of osmotic laxatives
d. A trial of chloride secreting agents
e. A referral to gastroenterology

176. You are caring for a 27-year-old man who is generally healthy. He reports a several month history of a change in his bowel habits. He reports increased stool frequency with "diarrhea" several times per week. He states that his mother suffered with inflammatory bowel disease, and he's very concerned that he has developed the same condition. Which of the following signs or symptoms by itself would lead you to think that his symptoms are related to irritable bowel syndrome (IBS)?

a. Abdominal pain relieved by defecation
b. Blood in the stool
c. Unintentional weight loss
d. Anemia
e. An abdominal mass

177. You are seeing a 34-year-old man who is complaining of diarrhea. It's been an intermittent problem or some time, but seems to be worsening. He describes intermittent bouts of low-grade fever, occasional right lower quadrant pain, some bloody diarrhea, and weight loss. Endoscopic findings are consistent with a diagnosis of mild to moderate Crohn disease. Which of the following medications is best for treating the acute symptoms?

a. Mesalamine
b. Metronidazole
c. Budesonide
d. Azathioprine
e. Methotrexate

178. The above patient's course has been one of intermittent exacerbations and remissions. His most recent evaluation indicates that he now has moderate to severe Crohn disease. Based on the best current data, which of the following statements is true regarding treatment with anti-tumor necrosis factor (anti-TNF) therapies like infliximab?

a. Anti-TNF agents should be used as "step-up" therapy after patients have failed corticosteroids and azathioprine.
b. Single drug therapy with an anti-TNF agent should be initiated early in the course of the disease.
c. Anti-TNF agents should be used in combination with an immunomodulatory agent for most patients.
d. Anti-TNF agents should only be used in post-surgical patients to maintain remission.
e. Side effects from anti-TNF agents limit their use to only the most severe cases.

179. You are seeing a 42-year-old man for diarrhea. After hearing his reports of recurrent bloody diarrhea, you order a colonoscopy, the results of which show mild to moderate ulcerative colitis. Which of the following is the most appropriate initial treatment plan?

a. A 5-ASA agent (for example, mesalamine) alone
b. A corticosteroid alone
c. A 5-ASA agent and a corticosteroid in combination
d. A 5-ASA agent and an immune modulating agent (for example, azathioprine) in combination
e. A 5-ASA agent and an anti-TNF agent (for example, infliximab) in combination

180. You are seeing a 6-month-old boy whose mother reports that he has had diarrhea for almost 2 weeks. He has had four to six bowel movements a day, with a loose to liquid consistency. His mother stays at home with him and the child is not in day care. His symptoms began after his young cousins visited for Christmas. Which of the following is the most likely cause of his diarrhea?

a. Rotavirus
b. Norwalk virus
c. Giardiasis
d. *Salmonella*
e. Enterotoxigenic *Escherichia coli*

181. A 26-year-old man returned from a vacation in Mexico 1 day ago. He spent the last 2 days of his trip with loose, more frequent bowel movements that are continuing. He has not had nausea, vomiting, bloody stool, or fever. His examination does not reveal dehydration, and is otherwise normal, except for mildly diffuse lower abdominal pain. Which of the following is an appropriate treatment option for his condition?

a. Erythromycin
b. Doxycycline
c. Loperamide
d. Opioid agents
e. Anticholinergic agents

182. The patient described in the above question is no better after 7 days and returns to your office for an evaluation. He reports that he has had up to 10 watery stools per day. He reports no appetite, and denies nausea, fever, or bloody stools. What is the best therapy to try at this time?

a. Loperamide
b. Loperamide and ciprofloxacin
c. Azithromycin
d. Loperamide and azithromycin
e. Rifaximin

183. You are seeing a 13-month-old Caucasian boy. His growth chart is shown below. His past medical history and physical examination are otherwise unremarkable, and he is meeting his developmental milestones. Which of the following is most likely to reveal the cause of his growth pattern?

a. Thorough dietary history
b. Serum albumin levels
c. Serum prealbumin levels
d. Assessment of the TSH
e. Serum IgA levels

Birth to 36 months: Boys
Length-for-age and Weight-for-age percentiles

NAME _____

RECORD # _____

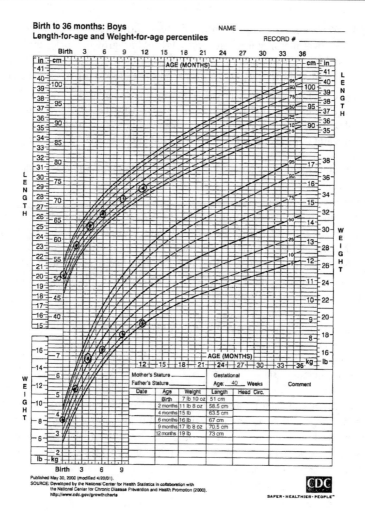

Age	Weight	Length	Head Circ.
Birth	7 lb 10 oz	51 cm	
2 months	11 lb 8 oz	58.5 cm	
4 months	15 lb	63.5 cm	
6 months	16 lb	67 cm	
9 months	17 lb 8 oz	70.5 cm	
12 months	19 lb	73 cm	

Mother's Stature _____
Father's Stature _____

Gestational
Age: __40__ Weeks

Comment

Published May 30, 2000 (modified 4/20/01).
SOURCE: Developed by the National Center for Health Statistics in collaboration with
the National Center for Chronic Disease Prevention and Health Promotion (2000).
http://www.cdc.gov/growthcharts

CDC
SAFER · HEALTHIER · PEOPLE™

184. You are seeing a 15-month-old child and note that her weight has dropped two major percentile brackets on her growth curve and have remained low. You evaluate the child's median weight for age and find it to be 71%. Which of the following is the most appropriate statement in this case?

a. The child is in no immediate danger. Follow-up as scheduled.
b. The child is mildly undernourished and may be safely observed over time.
c. The child is moderately undernourished and requires close observation.
d. The child warrants immediate evaluation and intervention with close outpatient follow-up.
e. The child has severe malnutrition and should be hospitalized for evaluation and nutritional support.

185. You are evaluating a 9-month-old Caucasian girl for poor weight gain. She has gone from the 75th percentile to the 10th percentile in height and weight. She has had recurrent respiratory infections and diarrhea, but cultures obtained have been negative. Her mother's health is excellent, and the child's birth history was unremarkable. Which of the following will be the most useful test in this setting?

a. Mantoux test for tuberculosis
b. Assessment for human immunodeficiency virus (HIV)
c. Stool for ova and parasites
d. Sweat chloride test
e. Renal function tests

186. You are evaluating an infant for poor weight gain. History from his mother reveals that he has frequent "wet burps" after eating. He coughs during and after eating, and his mother has heard him "wheeze" on occasion. He has not had diarrhea. Which of the following tests, if any, would be best to reveal the diagnosis?

a. No testing is necessary.
b. Esophageal pH probe.
c. Stool hemoccult.
d. Lactose tolerance test.
e. Abdominal US.

187. You are seeing a 15-month-old boy for a well-child check. His parents have no concerns and his developmental history is normal. His growth chart is shown. Which of the following is the most likely observation?

a. Familial short stature
b. Failure to thrive (FTT)
c. Hypothyroidism
d. A normal breast-fed infant
e. Constitutional growth delay

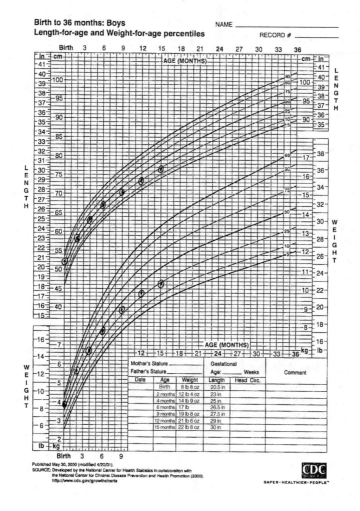

Birth to 36 months: Boys
Length-for-age and Weight-for-age percentiles

Date	Age	Weight	Length	Head Circ.
	Birth	8 lb 8 oz	20.5 in	
	2 months	12 lb 4 oz	23 in	
	4 months	14 lb 9 oz	25 in	
	6 months	17 lb	26.5 in	
	9 months	19 lb 8 oz	27.5 in	
	12 months	21 lb 6 oz	29 in	
	15 months	22 lb 8 oz	30 in	

Published May 30, 2000 (modified 4/20/01).
SOURCE: Developed by the National Center for Health Statistics in collaboration with
the National Center for Chronic Disease Prevention and Health Promotion (2000).
http://www.cdc.gov/growthcharts

188. You have been following a 15-month-old male infant. At 9 months, his height was at the 25th percentile while his weight was at the 5th percentile. At his 12-month visit, his weight and height are unchanged, so you asked his family to bring in a detailed dietary history and counseled them on a healthy diet. At his 15-month visit, his weight is up slightly, and his vital signs are as follows:

Blood pressure: 62/32 mm Hg (low)
Heart rate: 72 beats/min
Respiratory rate: 16 breaths/min
Temperature: 98.8°F

Which of the following is the best therapeutic option for this child?

a. Nutritional instruction to take two times the normal caloric intake
b. Iron supplementation with increased calorie intake
c. Zinc with increased caloric intake
d. Referral to social services for neglect
e. Hospital admission

189. A mother brings her son in to see you emergently. He is almost 2 years old, and began to have significant abdominal pain, vomiting, and bloody stool today. He is currently hemodynamically stable, in obvious pain, and on examination you notice a palpable firm tube-like mass in his left lower quadrant. He has never had an episode like this before. You suspect intussusception. Which of the following is the best next step for treating this condition?

a. Watchful waiting
b. Upper endoscopy
c. Lower endoscopy
d. A barium enema
e. A surgical referral

190. A 34-year-old man reports a 1-day history of hematemesis. He feels well, but does describe occasional abdominal discomfort. He denies alcohol use. On examination, his abdomen is slightly tender without peritoneal signs. His stool is not bloody, but his fecal test for occult blood is positive. Which of the following is the most appropriate next step?

a. Gastric lavage
b. Barium study
c. Endoscopy
d. Red cell scan
e. Angiography

191. You are evaluating a 21-year-old normally healthy college student who presents to the ED after a night of heavy drinking to celebrate his 21st birthday. His friends report that he has had multiple episodes of retching and vomiting and they brought him in after they noticed streaks of bright red blood in the emesis. After fluid hydration and antiemetics, the patient is resting comfortably and is hemodynamically stable. Stool guaiac testing is negative and the abdomen is soft and nontender. What is the most likely cause of the bleeding?

a. PUD
b. Acute gastritis
c. Mallory-Weiss tear
d. Esophageal varices
e. Aortoenteric fistula

192. A 56-year-old man is found to have asymptomatic diverticulosis on screening colonoscopy. He is concerned about his risk for gastrointestinal (GI) bleeding from the diverticula. Which of the following statements is the most accurate regarding his concern?

a. Severe diverticular bleeding is relatively common, occurring in up to 50% of patients with diverticulosis.
b. Diverticular bleeding is usually triggered by the ingestion of nuts, berries, seeds, popcorn, or other relatively indigestible material.
c. Diverticular bleeding resolves spontaneously in the vast majority of cases.
d. In patients with diverticular bleeding, colonoscopy should be avoided.
e. If colonoscopy fails to localize the source of active bleeding, a subtotal colectomy is needed to ensure no future bleeding.

193. You are evaluating a 26-year-old man with rectal pain for 48 hours. The pain was initially associated with bright red blood on the toilet paper after a bowel movement. Over the last day, his pain has worsened. On examination, he has an exquisitely tender purple nodule distal to the dentate line. Which of the following is the best treatment for his condition?

a. Hydrocortisone suppositories
b. Rubber-band ligation
c. Sclerotherapy
d. Incision and drainage
e. Excision

194. You are evaluating a 30-year-old male patient in the office with hematochezia. He has had chronic constipation, and reports bright red blood from his rectum associated with extremely painful bowel movements. After defecation, he complains of a dull ache and a feeling of "spasm" in the anal canal. The pain resolves within a few hours. On external examination, no abnormalities are noted. Which of the following is his most likely diagnosis?

a. Anal fissure
b. Thrombosed external hemorrhoid
c. Internal hemorrhoid
d. Thrombosed internal hemorrhoid
e. Perianal abscess

195. A 45-year-old woman comes to your office after her husband noticed that her "skin turned yellow." She reported "flu symptoms" a couple of weeks ago, with weakness, loss of appetite, nausea, and abdominal pain for 2 days. She has felt better since, but noted the skin discoloration yesterday. On examination, her skin tone, conjunctivae, and mucous membranes are yellow-tinged. Serologies indicate acute hepatitis A infection. Which of the following is true about this infection?

a. She is most infectious while she is jaundiced.
b. Most infected adults are asymptomatic.
c. This infection never results in chronic hepatitis.
d. Relapses are common.
e. Fecal shedding of the virus continues until liver enzymes have normalized.

196. You are examining a newborn whose mother has a positive screen for hepatitis B surface antigen (HBsAg). Which of the following is true regarding this situation?

a. When acquired early in life, the large majority of those infected with hepatitis B will have chronic disease.
b. If the child has a normal immune system, his likelihood of developing chronic disease is small.
c. A higher percentage of adults infected with hepatitis B will develop chronic disease as compared with children.
d. A high percentage of children acutely infected will develop fulminant liver disease.
e. When hepatitis B is transmitted perinatally, the child generally develops the typical symptoms of acute hepatitis.

197. You are following a patient after an acute hepatitis B infection. His serologies are shown below:

- HBsAg: Positive
- HBeAg: Positive
- IgM anti-HBc: Negative
- IgG anti-HBc: Positive
- Anti-HBs: Negative
- Anti-HBe: Negative

Which of the following terms best describes his disease status?

a. Acute infection, early phase
b. Acute infection, recovery phase
c. Chronic infection, replicating virus
d. Chronic infection, nonreplicating virus
e. Previous exposure with immunity

198. You check serologies on a patient exposed to hepatitis B. His serologies are shown below:

- HBsAg: Negative
- HBeAg: Negative
- IgM anti-HBc: Negative
- IgG anti-HBc: Negative
- Anti-HBs: Positive
- Anti-HBe: Negative

Which of the following terms best describes his disease status?

a. Acute infection, early phase
b. Acute infection, window phase
c. Acute infection, recovery phase
d. Previous exposure with immunity
e. Vaccination

199. You are following a patient after an acute hepatitis B infection. His serologies are shown below:

- HBsAg: Positive
- HBeAg: Positive
- IgM anti-HBc: Positive
- IgG anti-HBc: Negative
- Anti-HBs: Negative
- Anti-HBe: Negative

Which of the following terms best describes his disease status?

a. Acute infection, early phase
b. Acute infection, recovery phase
c. Chronic infection, replicating virus
d. Chronic infection, nonreplicating virus
e. Previous exposure with immunity

200. You are evaluating a 5-year-old girl whose mother brought her in to evaluate jaundice. Laboratory evaluation reveals a conjugated hyperbilirubinemia. Which of the following is the most likely cause of her problem?

a. G6PD deficiency
b. Gilbert disease
c. Crigler-Najjar syndrome
d. Wilson disease
e. Viral hepatitis

201. You are caring for a 65-year-old man with new-onset jaundice. Laboratory evaluation reveals conjugated hyperbilirubinemia. Statistically speaking, which of the following is the most likely cause of his condition?

a. Hemolytic anemia
b. Viral hepatitis
c. Extrahepatic obstruction
d. Metastatic disease
e. Heart failure

202. You are evaluating a 45-year-old woman with significant jaundice. Her alkaline phosphatase is seven times normal, and her transaminases are twice normal. You perform a US of her right upper quadrant, and it is negative for obstruction and shows no bile duct dilation. You still suspect obstruction. Which of the following should be the next step in the workup?

a. CT of the abdomen
b. ERCP
c. Percutaneous transhepatic cholangiography (PTC)
d. Magnetic resonance cholangiopancreatography (MRCP)
e. Nuclear scintigraphy of the biliary tree (HIDA)

203. A 62-year-old woman is seeing you because of nausea and vomiting. She has a 15-year history of type 2 diabetes mellitus. She describes her symptoms as being worse after eating, and on occasion she will vomit food that appears to be undigested. Her weight is stable and she does not appear dehydrated. On examination, she has abdominal distension and diffuse tenderness. Which of the following is the best treatment for her condition?

a. An anticholinergic medication, like scopolamine (Transderm Scop)
b. An antihistamine, like promethazine (Phenergan)
c. A benzamide, like metoclopramide (Reglan)
d. A cannabinoid, like dronabinol (Marinol)
e. A phenothiazine, like chlorpromazine (Thorazine)

204. You are evaluating a 63-year-old man who complains of abdominal pain, distension, nausea, and vomiting. It began rather suddenly this morning, though he has had mild diffuse pain for several days. His past history is significant for a recent partial sigmoid resection for diverticulosis and an appendectomy at 23 years of age. On examination, he is afebrile, his mucous membranes are dry, but he has no orthostatic symptoms. His abdomen is distended and diffusely tender, and his bowel sounds are high-pitched. Which of the following is the most likely cause of his nausea and vomiting?

a. Gastroenteritis
b. Ileus
c. Obstruction
d. Diverticulosis
e. Diverticulitis

205. You are seeing a 14-year-old girl who asked her mother to take her to the doctor for nausea and vomiting. She was diagnosed as having viral gastroenteritis in the emergency department more than 6 weeks ago, but since that time has had difficulty keeping food down. She states that whenever she eats, she gets nauseated and vomits within 10 to 30 minutes. She has been using antiemetics to control her symptoms, but they do not work consistently. She has always done well in school, and denies social stressors since she was adopted at the age of 8. Prior to that, she was in an abusive home. Her medical history is otherwise unremarkable. On examination, she is well-nourished, interactive, and in no distress with no signs of dehydration. Her weight is 147 lb (5 lb less than at her well examination 6 months ago) and her height is 5 ft. Which of the following is the most likely cause of her symptoms?

a. Chronic gastroenteritis
b. Psychogenic vomiting
c. Anorexia nervosa
d. Bulimia nervosa
e. Central nervous system malignancy

206. You are seeing a 6-year-old boy with nausea and vomiting. His symptoms began acutely last evening, starting with malaise, headache, low-grade fever, body aches, and diarrhea. On examination, he has dry mucous membranes, but no orthostatic symptoms. He has slight tachycardia, but the rest of his vital signs are normal. Examination reveals diffuse mild abdominal pain without rebound or involuntary guarding. Which of the following is the most appropriate next step?

a. Abdominal x-ray.
b. Abdominal CT without contrast.
c. Abdominal CT with contrast.
d. Abdominal US.
e. No testing is necessary.

207. In the patient described in the question above, which of the following is the best treatment for his condition?

a. Nothing by mouth until his symptoms improve
b. Oral rehydration with clear liquids, advancing the diet as tolerated
c. IV rehydration, advancing to oral as tolerated
d. Antiemetics, given intravenously or intramuscularly
e. Trimethoprim-sulfamethoxazole therapy

208. You are seeing a 44-year-old woman with hypertension controlled with lisinopril, who presents with severe nausea and vomiting. She reports having months of occasional right upper quadrant pain, usually after eating out with her husband, that resolves within a couple of hours. Over the last 24 hours, her symptoms have been severe, and she is unable to eat or drink without vomiting. Her pain is significant, radiates to her back, and is better when she leans forward. On laboratory evaluation, her amylase and ALT are elevated. Which of the following would be the best approach to avoid recurrent problems after her acute symptoms subside?

a. Discontinue lisinopril
b. Avoid calcium in the diet
c. Work with the patient to remain sober
d. Remove the patient's gallbladder
e. Use medication to lower the patient's triglyceride level

209. A new mother brings her infant son to see you to discuss his vomiting. He is 4 weeks old and is exclusively breast-fed. He vomits with every meal. On examination, his abdomen is distended with normal bowel sounds, and he appears dehydrated. He has lost 4 oz since his visit with you 2 weeks ago. Which of the following is the most likely diagnosis?

a. Allergy to breast milk
b. GERD
c. Hypertrophic pyloric stenosis
d. Intussusception
e. Small-bowel obstruction

210. A 42-year-old woman is seeing you to evaluate nausea and vomiting. It happens about 60 minutes after eating a big meal and is associated with pain in the epigastric area. Which of the following tests is most likely to be abnormal in this case?

a. Amylase and lipase level assessment
b. Hemoccult testing of the stool
c. Abdominal x-rays
d. Right upper quadrant US
e. Upper endoscopy

Acute Complaints—Urogenital

211. You are caring for a 24-year-old generally healthy woman. She is sexually active and currently in a monogamous relationship. You recently completed her annual examination. Her Pap smear reports "atypical squamous cells of undetermined significance" (ASC-US). Which of the following is the most appropriate next step?

a. Repeat cytology immediately
b. Treat the patient with metronidazole and repeat cytology when the course of antibiotics is finished
c. Order reflex Human Papillomavirus (HPV) testing
d. Repeat cytology in 1 year
e. Perform colposcopy

212. You are caring for a 33-year-old woman without medical concerns. She is married and monogamous, and on oral contraceptives. Her Pap test Reports normal cytology but insufficient transformational zone cells. Her HPV status is negative. Which of the following is the most appropriate next step?

a. Repeat cytology immediately
b. Repeat cytology in 4 to 6 months
c. Repeat cytology in 1 year
d. Repeat cytology in 3 years
e. Co-testing in 5 years

213. You are reviewing the results of a recent Pap test you performed on a 23-year-old female patient. Last year, her cytology was low-grade squamous intraepithelial lesion (LSIL). You recommended repeat cytology at 12 months and this was performed last week. The new results are atypical squamous cells of undetermined significance (ASC-US). What is the next best step?

a. Repeat cytology in 1 year
b. Resume routine screening with cytology alone in 3 years
c. Resume routine screening with cytology alone in 5 years
d. Order reflex HPV testing
e. Proceed to colposcopy

214. You are caring for a 58-year-old postmenopausal woman who is not on estrogen replacement therapy. You perform her Pap test, and the results are reported as "atypical squamous cells of undetermined significance: Cannot Exclude High-Grade SIL (ASC-H)." HPV testing was not performed. Which of the following is the most appropriate next step?

a. Repeat the cytology immediately
b. Repeat the cytology in 1 year
c. Perform HPV testing
d. Proceed to colposcopy
e. Treat with a 4-week course of vaginal estrogen cream and repeat Pap testing

215. You are caring for a 35-year-old female patient. She had her well-woman examination last week and you performed co-testing (cytology and HPV testing) as per current guidelines. Her co-testing results showed normal cytology, endocervical/transition zone cells present, and HPV 16 or 18 positive. What do you recommend as the next step for this patient?

a. Repeat the cytology immediately
b. Repeat the cytology in 1 year
c. Repeat the co-testing in 1 year
d. Perform colposcopy
e. Continue with routine screening with co-testing in 5 years

216. You are caring for a 36-year-old generally healthy woman. She is sexually active and currently in a monogamous relationship with her husband, using oral contraceptives. You recently completed her annual examination. Her cytology report show "atypical glandular cells (AGC)," but does not specify if those cells are endocervical or endometrial in origin. Her HPV status is negative. She has not had any abnormal vaginal bleeding. Which of the following is the most appropriate next step?

a. Continue routine screening.
b. Repeat cytology in 1 year.
c. Perform colposcopy and endometrial biopsy.
d. Perform colposcopy.
e. Perform endometrial biopsy.

217. You recently saw a 32-year-old patient for an initial prenatal visit. She reports she was finishing grad school and had not had a Pap test in more than 5 years, so you performed co-testing as part of the initial prenatal examination. The pathology results indicate "low-grade squamous intraepithelial lesion (LSIL) and HPV other positive." What do you recommend as the preferred course of action for this patient?

a. Repeat co-testing in 1 year
b. Repeat cytology alone in 1 year
c. Perform colposcopy without endocervical sampling
d. Perform colposcopy with endocervical sampling
e. Defer further workup until 6 weeks postpartum

218. An 23-year-old woman is seeing you for back pain, frequency, and dysuria. She reports being treated for acute cystitis in the past on two other occasions. She denies vaginal discharge. What is the most appropriate and cost-effective next step?

a. Empiric 3-day treatment for urinary tract infection (UTI)
b. Treating with a 7 to 10 day course of antibiotics
c. Clean catch urinalysis with treatment depending on results
d. Send urine for culture
e. Testing for a sexually transmitted infection

219. You are evaluating a 25-year-old woman who reports frequent UTIs since getting married last year. In the last 12 months, she has had five documented infections that have responded well to antibiotic therapy. She has tried voiding after intercourse, she discontinued her use of a diaphragm, and tried acidification of her urine using oral ascorbic acid, but none of those measures decreased the incidence of infections. At this point, which of the following would be an acceptable prophylactic measure?

a. An antibiotic prescription for the usual 3-day regimen with refills, to be used when symptoms occur
b. Single-dose antibiotic therapy once daily at bedtime for 12 months
c. Single-dose antibiotic therapy once daily at bedtime for 2 years
d. Single-dose antibiotic therapy after sexual intercourse
e. Antibiotics for 3 days after sexual intercourse

220. A 36-year-old woman comes to your office complaining of recurrent dysuria. This is her fourth episode in the past 10 months. Initially, her symptoms were classic for a UTI, and she was treated empirically without testing. For the second episode, her urinalysis was positive for blood only. Her culture was negative, as was evaluation for nephrolithiasis. The third episode was similar, also with a negative culture. All episodes have resolved with a standard course of antibiotic therapy. Which of the following is the most appropriate next step?

a. Evaluate for somatization disorder
b. Consider cystoscopy
c. Consider potassium iodide sensitivity testing
d. Consider a 14-day regimen of antibiotics
e. Use daily antibiotic therapy for prophylaxis

221. A screening urinalysis in a female patient reveals asymptomatic bacteriuria. In which of the following patients would treatment be indicated?

a. A sexually active teenager
b. A pregnant 26-year-old woman
c. A 45-year-old woman with uncontrolled hypertension
d. A menopausal woman
e. An otherwise healthy 80-year-old woman

222. You receive a telephone call from an otherwise healthy 33-year-old woman on a Saturday night while you are on call. She complains of dysuria, frequency, and urgency. She reports a history of two other UTIs in the past 3 years, and denies fever, vaginal discharge, back pain, or visible blood in her urine. She denies allergies to medications. Which of the following is the appropriate next step?

a. Call in a prescription for trimethoprim-sulfamethoxazole
b. Call in a prescription for ciprofloxacin
c. Prescribe empiric antibiotics today, and have the patient follow-up on Monday in your office for a urinalysis
d. Prescribe empiric antibiotic today, but have the patient collect a home urine sample and bring it into the office on Monday for culture
e. Prescribe symptom relief today and follow-up Monday in your office for a urinalysis

223. You are seeing a 34-year-old man with urinary symptoms. He reports frequency, urgency, and moderate back pain. He is febrile and acutely ill. He has no penile discharge. His urinalysis shows marked pyuria. He has never had an episode like this before, and has no known urinary tract abnormalities. Which of the following is the most likely diagnosis?

a. Gonococcal urethritis
b. Nongonococcal urethritis
c. Acute bacterial cystitis
d. Pyelonephritis
e. Acute prostatitis

224. You are seeing a 7-year-old girl whose parents brought her in to have her bed-wetting evaluated. She has been toilet trained during the day since the age of 4, but still wets the bed at night. Her father wet the bed until the age of 8 years. Her physical examination reveals no abnormalities and her urinalysis is normal. Which of the following is the appropriate next step?

a. Reassurance with no testing or treatment
b. Obtain a post-void residual using US
c. Obtain a blood count and serum chemistry
d. Obtain a renal US
e. Obtain a voiding cystourethrogram (VCUG)

225. You are evaluating a 5-year-old boy. His mother has brought him in because he wets the bed. He has never been dry at night and his parents are starting to get concerned. You obtain a thorough voiding history, and find the child to be completely normal on physical examination. He is otherwise developmentally normal. His urinalysis is normal and his post-void residual is also normal. What should be the next step in the workup of this patient?

a. Observation
b. X-rays of the lumbar and sacral spine
c. Renal US
d. VCUG
e. Both renal US and VUCG

226. The patient in the question above is now 8 years old and has had no improvement. He has never been consistently dry through the night, and his physical examination continues to be normal. Which of the following has been shown to be the most effective intervention for this condition?

a. Frequent nighttime wakening to encourage voiding
b. Use of an alarm that wakes the child when he wets at night
c. Use of desmopressin (synthetic DDAVP)
d. Use of tricyclic antidepressant medications (for example, imipramine)
e. Use of an anticholinergic antispasmodic (for example, oxybutynin)

227. You are caring for a 7-year-old boy with enuresis. His physical examination and initial testing are all normal. His parents want to try lifestyle modifications to improve the situation. Which of the following is NOT an effective lifestyle intervention for this child?

a. Discontinue pull ups
b. Include child in clean up if he wets the bed at night
c. Use positive reinforcement like stickers for dry nights
d. Set an alarm for 3 hours after he goes to bed, and wake him up to urinate at that time
e. Discontinue fluids after 5 pm

228. The child described in the question above has tried the lifestyle modifications for 6 months with only slight improvement. His mother is not interested in pharmacologic therapies, but would like to discuss using a moisture-sensitive alarm. Which of the following is true regarding the use of these alarms for nocturnal enuresis?

a. The goal of this alarm is to wake the child just after the initiation of urination.
b. The success rate is greater for boys than for girls.
c. The success rate is less than 50%.
d. If the process will be successful, it only takes 3 to 4 weeks on average.
e. The alarms are easier for families because the child takes responsibility for the treatment.

229. You are evaluating a 56-year-old generally healthy man who is seeing you after finding blood in his urine. He denies pain, dysuria, frequency, or urgency. He is a smoker, and has worked for years in the printing industry. Which of the following is the most likely cause of his hematuria?

a. Acute prostatitis
b. Chronic prostatitis
c. Cystitis
d. Urinary stones
e. Bladder carcinoma

230. A 16-year-old girl comes to your office complaining of blood in her urine. She also complains of dysuria and frequency; she is not currently menstruating but has normal cycles. She denies sexual activity. Urinalysis reveals grossly pink urine; urine dipstick is positive for blood but negative for leukocytes or nitrites. Which of the following is the most appropriate next step?

a. Pelvic US
b. Urine cytology
c. Speculum examination and bimanual examination
d. Empiric treatment for cystitis
e. Urine culture and sensitivity

231. A 30-year-old man was found to have hematuria on routine urinalysis. He had no symptoms and is otherwise healthy. His urinalysis is negative for casts and protein, but is positive for moderate blood. His urine culture is negative. IV pyelogram and serum creatinine are both normal and you send urine cytology just to be safe. It is also normal. Which of the following is the most appropriate in this case?

a. Reassurance and periodic monitoring
b. Renal US
c. Cystoscopy
d. Antistreptolysin O (ASO) titer
e. Renal biopsy

232. During a routine physical examination, you notice isolated hematuria in a 49-year-old male patient. The patient is a former smoker, but has no current medical problems. He denies urinary symptoms or other sources of bleeding. You ask the patient to return in a month for a repeat urinalysis and this also confirms isolated hematuria. What is the best imaging study to evaluate this patient's hematuria?

a. Intravenous pyelogram (IVP)
b. Renal US
c. Contrast-enhanced abdominal CT
d. Non-contrast abdominal CT
e. Plain x-ray (KUB) of the abdomen

233. You are evaluating a 74-year-old woman for the recent onset of incontinence. She has diabetes, controlled by diet but with recently increasing sugars, and hypertension, controlled with a combination of lisinopril/hydrochlorothiazide. She has complained of constipation recently and has not had a bowel movement for 3 days. Microscopic analysis of her urine is positive for bacteria, but she does not report dysuria, urgency, or frequency. Which of the historical features mentioned is inconsequential in the workup of her incontinence?

a. Hyperglycemia
b. Diuretic use
c. Constipation
d. Bacteriuria
e. Postmenopausal state

234. A 44-year-old mother of two reports leakage of a small amount of urine with sneezing. Recently, it began to occur with exercise. She denies recent life stressors. Which of the following best describes the type of incontinence she is experiencing?

a. Functional incontinence
b. Senile incontinence
c. Urge incontinence
d. Stress incontinence
e. Overflow incontinence

235. You are seeing a 74-year-old man who is complaining that he is leaking urine. You have ruled out secondary causes and choose to measure his "post-void" residual. It is 250 mL. Which of the following is true?

a. Post-void residual measurement has no place in the workup of incontinence.
b. This amount is below what is expected, and leads one to suspect urge incontinence.
c. This amount is about average, and is not helpful in determining this patient's type of incontinence.
d. This amount is more than average, but is not helpful in determining this patient's type of incontinence.
e. This amount is more than average, and would lead one to suspect overflow incontinence.

236. You are treating a 40-year-old woman for incontinence. She would prefer not to use medications, and would like to try pelvic floor strengthening (Kegel) exercises. Which of the following types of incontinence has shown the best response to pelvic floor strengthening exercises?

a. Functional incontinence
b. Stress incontinence
c. Urge incontinence
d. Overflow incontinence
e. Mixed incontinence

237. One of your patients has tried and failed behavioral therapy for incontinence. He describes a strong urge to urinate, followed by involuntary loss of urine. Which of the following would be the best medication for him to use?

a. Oxybutynin (Ditropan)
b. Pseudoephedrine (Sudafed)
c. Trimethoprim-sulfamethoxazole (Bactrim, Septra)
d. Finasteride (Proscar)
e. Terazosin (Hytrin)

238. You are treating a 45-year-old man for hypertension. Since beginning therapy, he complains of urinary leakage and urgency. Which antihypertensive class is most likely to cause this?

a. Thiazide diuretics
b. ACE inhibitors
c. β-Blockers
d. Calcium channel blockers
e. α-Blockers

239. An obese 29-year-old woman is complaining of polyuria. Her workup, including serum glucose, is negative. She is not taking any prescription medications. Which of the following, if present in her history, is the most likely cause?

a. Marijuana abuse
b. Over-the-counter diet pill use
c. Over-the-counter decongestant use
d. Over-the-counter sleeping pill use
e. Caffeine overuse

240. You are evaluating a 14-year-old female patient whose mother brought her in for evaluation. Despite the fact that all of her friends have started menstruating, the daughter has not. On examination, she has no breast development, no axillary or pubic hair, and her pelvic examination reveals normal-appearing anatomy. She has not lost weight recently and is not excessively thin. Which of the following is the most likely cause of her primary amenorrhea?

a. Gonadal dysgenesis
b. Hypothalamic failure
c. Pituitary failure
d. Polycystic ovarian syndrome
e. Constitutional delay of puberty

241. You are seeing a 17-year-old patient who began menstruating at age 14, and has been relatively regular since age 15. She made an appointment to be seen today because she stopped having periods 2 months ago. She denies sexual activity. Which of the following is the most likely cause of her secondary amenorrhea?

a. Polycystic ovarian syndrome
b. Functional hypothalamic amenorrhea
c. Pregnancy
d. Hypothyroidism
e. Hyperprolactinemia

242. A 16-year-old woman comes to your office complaining of unpredictable menstrual periods. She began her periods at age 14 and they have never been predictable. She denies sexual activity in her lifetime, has no systemic illness, uses no medications regularly, and her physical examination is normal. Which of the following is her most likely diagnosis?

a. Pregnancy
b. Ovulatory bleeding
c. Anovulatory bleeding
d. Uterine leiomyoma
e. Endometrial polyposis

243. A healthy 60-year-old woman is seeing you to evaluate vaginal bleeding. She has not had a menstrual period for approximately 7 years, but 3 months ago noted occasional pink spotting. Since then, it has increased in amount and has become almost continuous. She is currently sexually active with her husband. On examination, she appears well, her pelvic examination is normal, and screens for sexually transmitted infections are negative. Which of the following should be your next step?

a. Pelvic US to evaluate for fibroids
b. Pelvic CT scan to evaluate for pelvic tumor
c. Laparoscopy to evaluate for endometriosis
d. Endometrial biopsy
e. Begin hormone-replacement therapy to regulate bleeding

244. You are considering treatment for a 19-year-old female patient with primary dysmenorrhea. Which of the following should be your first-line therapy?

a. Use of NSAIDs during menses
b. Use of NSAIDs daily
c. Use of opiates during menses
d. Use of a selective serotonin reuptake inhibitor (SSRI) daily
e. Use of combined oral contraceptive pills daily

245. You are evaluating a 32-year-old woman complaining of amenorrhea. She has mild hypertension, hypothyroidism, GERD, and depression. On evaluation, her prolactin level was found to be 89 ng/mL (H). Which of the following medications would be the most likely to cause the elevated prolactin level?

a. Proton pump inhibitors
b. SSRIs
c. Thiazide diuretics
d. ACE inhibitors
e. Thyroid hormone replacement

246. You are evaluating a 16-year-old girl who has never menstruated. She has normal secondary sexual characteristics and her laboratory evaluation is negative. She has no withdrawal bleeding after a progestin challenge and you choose to perform an estrogen-progestin challenge. She has no withdrawal bleeding after that challenge as well. Which of the following is the most likely reason for her amenorrhea?

a. Outflow tract obstruction or anatomic defect
b. Hypergonadotropic amenorrhea
c. Hypogonadotropic amenorrhea
d. Polycystic ovarian syndrome
e. Pituitary adenoma

247. You are caring for a 23-year-old woman complaining of pelvic pain. She reports one-sided pain that she describes as "pressure." On further questioning, she reports that it is diffuse and dull, but occasionally sharp. Menses have been normal. She denies fever. Based on this history alone, which of the following is the most likely cause of the pain?

a. Pelvic inflammatory disease (PID)
b. Ectopic pregnancy
c. Ovarian cyst
d. Uterine leiomyoma
e. Appendicitis

248. You are caring for a 21-year-old woman complaining of pelvic pain. She reports a gradual onset of bilateral pain associated with fever, vaginal discharge, and mild dysuria. Her pelvic examination demonstrates uterine, adnexal, and cervical motion tenderness, and her pregnancy test is negative. Which of the following is the best treatment option?

a. Ceftriaxone 250 mg intramuscular (IM) in a single dose
b. Oral doxycycline 100 mg twice a day for 14 days
c. Metronidazole 500 mg twice a day for 14 days
d. Ceftriaxone 250 mg IM in a single dose plus oral doxycycline 100 mg twice a day for 14 days plus oral metronidazole 500 mg twice a day for 14 days
e. Inpatient admission for parenteral antibiotics

249. You are caring for a 27-year-old woman complaining of pelvic pain. She denies vaginal bleeding and does not remember the date of her last menstrual period. She reports localized pain on the left side that has increased in severity over the last 2 days. She also reports nausea and breast tenderness. On examination, you note a tender adnexal mass on the left. Which of the following is the most likely cause?

a. PID
b. Ectopic pregnancy
c. Ovarian cyst
d. Uterine leiomyoma
e. Appendicitis

250. You are evaluating a 30-year-old woman with chronic pelvic pain. She reports cyclic pain, generally during the premenstrual period and during her menses. She has been trying to conceive for 15 months without success. Her pelvic examination is normal, and her pregnancy test is negative. Given her history, which of the following treatments should you consider?

a. Oral contraceptives
b. An antispasmodic
c. An intrauterine device
d. Laparoscopic ablation
e. Adhesiolysis

251. You are evaluating a 13-year-old girl with pelvic pain. She denies being sexually active and you do not suspect abuse. On pelvic examination, you confirm that she has never been sexually active, see no discharge, and find no cervical motion tenderness, but feel an ovarian mass on the right side. Which of the following is the most appropriate next step in this situation?

a. Reassurance and use of NSAIDs for pain control
b. Reassurance and repeat pelvic examination in 6 to 8 weeks
c. Transvaginal pelvic US
d. CT scanning of the abdomen and pelvis
e. MRI evaluation of the pelvis

252. You are caring for a married, 31-year-old man who complains of severe pain in his left testicle. He describes a gradual onset of pain, with mild dysuria. He denies fever. On examination, his cremasteric reflex is present, and you identify a swollen and tender epididymis. You diagnose epididymitis. Which of the following is the most likely cause?

a. *Neisseria gonorrhoeae*
b. *E coli*
c. *Ureaplasma*
d. *Mycoplasma*
e. *Enterobacter*

253. You are seeing a 14-year-old boy who was brought emergently to your office after developing severe testicular pain while weight lifting 3 hours ago. He had a sudden onset of severe pain without fever, and has had associated nausea and vomiting. On examination, his cremasteric reflex is absent, and when the patient is in the supine position, elevation of the testis increases the pain. Which of the following is the most likely diagnosis?

a. Epididymitis
b. Testicular torsion
c. Inguinal hernia
d. Orchitis
e. Testicular cancer

254. You are performing an examination on a premature newborn delivered hours ago. During the examination, you note that the patient has only one descended testicle. When is the most appropriate time to obtain a urologic consultation, assuming there is no resolution?

a. Immediately
b. Before the age of 3 months
c. Before the age of 6 months
d. At 1 year of age
e. At 2 years of age

255. You are evaluating a 20-year-old woman complaining of vaginal discharge. She reports vaginal itch and white discharge. She has no history of vaginal infections in the past and has never been sexually active. Examination shows a white discharge with vulvar erythema. A KOH preparation of the discharge demonstrates spores and pseudohyphae. Which of the following will relieve the patient's symptom of itch faster?

a. Topical azole cream
b. A single dose of oral fluconazole
c. Topical metronidazole
d. Oral clindamycin
e. Doxycycline

256. You are seeing a 17-year-old girl who reports intense vaginal itching and urinary frequency. She has been sexually active for 6 months. On examination, you note frothy yellow-green discharge with bright red vaginal mucosa and red macules on the cervix. What is the saline preparation of the discharge most likely to show?

a. Sheets of epithelial cells "studded" with bacteria
b. "Moth-eaten" epithelial cells
c. Motile triangular organisms with long tails
d. Few WBCs
e. Hyphae

257. Your patient describes a recent vaginal discharge. She reports more discharge than usual and an unusual odor after intercourse with her husband. A KOH preparation of the discharge produces a fishy odor, and a saline preparation shows classic "clue" cells. Which of the following is the treatment of choice for her condition?

a. Metronidazole
b. Doxycycline
c. Clotrimazole
d. Imiquimod
e. Acyclovir

Acute Complaints—Hematologic and Other Causes of Fatigue

258. You are caring for a patient who reports fatigue. A laboratory analysis reveals a microcytic anemia with a hemoglobin level of 9.9 g/dL. The red cell distribution width (RDW) is elevated. Which of the following is the best treatment plan?

a. Start erythropoietin
b. Treat with vitamin B$_{12}$ injections weekly for 1 month and then monthly
c. Treat with ferrous sulfate 325 mg twice daily
d. Treat with elemental iron 325 mg once daily
e. Consider a bone marrow biopsy

259. A 60-year-old man is being evaluated for fatigue, weakness, and exercise intolerance. Laboratory assessment reveals:

Hemoglobin:	9.1 mg/dL (low)
Serum iron:	46 µg/dL (low)
Ferritin:	9 ng/mL (low)
Total iron binding capacity (TIBC):	626 µg/dL (high)
Mean corpuscular volume (MCV):	76 fL (low)

What is the most common cause of this condition?

a. Blood loss
b. Poor nutrition
c. Inadequate absorption of iron
d. Chronic disease
e. Folic acid deficiency

260. You are performing a presurgical clearance evaluation on a 44-year-old otherwise healthy African-American man who is undergoing a laparoscopic cholecystectomy. His CBC is shown below:

Hemoglobin:	10.6 g/dL (low)
MCV:	54 fL (low)
Red blood cell (RBC) count:	6.3 M/µL (high)
RDW:	14.1 (normal)

What is the most appropriate step prior to surgery?

a. Oral iron replacement for 4 weeks, then recheck before surgery
b. Parenteral iron replacement for 4 weeks, then recheck before surgery
c. Transfusion
d. Hemoglobin electrophoresis
e. Erythropoietin

261. You are evaluating a 26-year-old woman with fatigue. She also complains of light-headedness and paresthesias in her hands and feet. On examination, her vital signs are normal, but you note pallor and glossitis. Laboratory evaluation reveals a hemoglobin of 9.8 g/dL (L) and an MCV of 102 fL (H). Which of the following would be the most likely to treat her condition?

a. Diet rich in green leafy vegetables
b. Diet rich in iron
c. Vitamin B_{12} supplementation
d. Folic acid supplementation
e. Iron supplementation

262. A 68-year-old man complains of fatigue. He has a history of hypertension, well-controlled with hydrochlorothiazide. He has recently lost 30 lb on a high-protein, low-carbohydrate diet. He drinks 2 to 3 beers daily, and smokes 10 cigarettes daily. Laboratory evaluation reveals a macrocytic anemia and vitamin B_{12} deficiency. Which of the following is the most likely cause?

a. Side effects of hydrochlorothiazide
b. High-protein diet
c. Low-carbohydrate diet
d. Alcohol intake
e. Inadequate vitamin B_{12} absorption

263. A 3-year-old African-American boy is brought in by his parents with inconsolable crying. He reports extreme pain in his hands and upper extremities. Laboratory evaluation reveals a hemoglobin of 8.2 mg/dL. His peripheral blood smear is shown as follows:

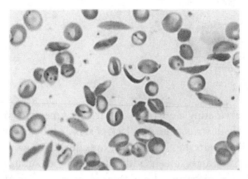

(Reproduced with permission from Lichtman MA, Shafer MS, Felgar RE, Wang N. Lichtman's Atlas of Hematology. Access Medicine. New York, NY: McGraw-Hill. accessmedicine.com.)

Which of the following measures would be the most likely to reduce these events in the future?

a. Chronic use of analgesics
b. Adequate hydration
c. Immunization against streptococcal pneumonia
d. Monthly transfusions
e. Daily penicillin prophylaxis until the age of 5 years

264. A 19-year-old male patient presented to your office with a 3-day history of fatigue, sore throat, and low-grade fevers. On examination, his temperature was 100.3°F, and you noted an exudative pharyngitis with anterior and posterior cervical adenopathy. You sent a throat culture and started him on amoxicillin prophylactically. Two days later, he presents for follow-up with continued symptoms and a diffuse, symmetrical erythematous maculopapular rash. Which of the following is the most likely cause of his symptoms?

a. Scarlet fever
b. Allergic reaction to amoxicillin
c. Viral exanthem
d. Mononucleosis
e. Rubella

265. A 33-year-old woman presents to your office to discuss fatigue. She describes a "lack of energy" and "tiredness," but denies weakness or hypersomnolence. Her symptoms have been present for around 4 months, and have not progressively worsened. Which of the following is the next step in the workup?

a. Screen for depression
b. Screen for sleep apnea
c. Screen for anemia
d. Screen for hypothyroidism
e. Screen for pregnancy

266. You are evaluating a 56-year-old African-American man complaining of fatigue. He describes this as a lack of stamina, but he has motivation to do things. Sleep refreshes him, but he tires quickly at work. His physical examination is unremarkable. In addition to a blood count, sedimentation rate, urinalysis, chemistry panel, and thyroid testing, which of the following should be included in your initial workup to help ascertain the diagnosis?

a. Chest x-ray
b. ECG
c. HIV test
d. Prostate cancer screen
e. Drug screen

Acute Complaints—Musculoskeletal

267. You are seeing an 18-year-old boy who reports acute pain in the left posterior heel. His symptoms occurred while he was playing intramural basketball for his college dorm's team. On examination, he has swelling and ecchymosis over the posterior left heel. He is unable to walk normally, and has a positive Thompson test. What is the most likely diagnosis?

a. Lisfranc injury
b. Tarsal navicular bone fracture
c. Planar fascia rupture
d. Achilles tendon rupture
e. Calcaneus fracture

268. You are seeing a 45-year-old woman who reports increasingly severe right foot pain for 2 weeks. She has been trying to lose weight, and has recently started a walking regimen. She describes a sharp pain in the inferior heel when weight bearing after a period of rest. With continued movement, the pain improves, but becomes more dull and achy. She has tried anti-inflammatory agents with only temporary relief. Of the following, which is the best next step?

a. Right foot x-ray
b. Arch support
c. Physical therapy
d. Referral to a foot specialist
e. Steroid injection over the site of pain

269. You are caring for a 61-year-old man complaining of neck pain for several weeks. He denies injury or illness. The pain is aggravated by movement, worse after activities, and there is a dull ache in the interscapular region. His examination reveals a limited range of motion, no tenderness to palpation, no radiation, and no neurologic signs. Which of the following is the most likely diagnosis?

a. Osteoarthritis
b. Chronic mechanical neck pain
c. Cervical nerve root irritation
d. Whiplash
e. Cervical dystonia

270. You are seeing a 66-year-old man complaining of right-sided neck pain and stiffness. He complains that his right hand has become "numb." On examination, you confirm paresthesia of his fingers that continues up to the back of his arm, and his pain worsens when he turns his head to the right. Which of the following studies, if any, should be your next step in the workup?

a. Cervical spine radiographs.
b. CT scan of his neck.
c. MRI of his neck.
d. Electromyography (EMG).
e. No testing is necessary.

271. You are seeing a 67-year-old man who is following up in your office 2 days after being involved in a motor vehicle collision. He was the restrained driver and was going 45 mi/h when he ran into a car that was stopped in front of him. Thankfully, he denies head injury or loss of consciousness. He was ambulatory after the event and only had slight neck pain, but was taken to the emergency department for evaluation. They released him that evening without any imaging studies. On follow-up with you, he denies neck pain or numbness and tingling in his extremities. His range of motion is appropriate for his age. What testing, if any, should be done at this time?

a. No testing is needed.
b. He should have C-spine radiographs.
c. He should have a CT scan of the neck.
d. He should have an MRI of the neck.
e. He should have an EMG.

272. You perform a Spurling test on a 36-year-old woman complaining of neck pain. The test causes neck discomfort only. What is the most likely diagnosis for this patient?

a. Herniated disk
b. Spinal stenosis
c. Osteoarthritis
d. Mechanical neck pain
e. Cervical dystonia

273. You are caring for a 16-year-old gymnast who is complaining of neck pain. Although she is very active, she denies significant trauma precipitating the pain. She has tried nonsteroidal anti-inflammatory agents, ice, rest, and physical therapy with no results. She denies radiculopathy, fever, chills, weight loss, or other significant symptoms. Her medical and social histories are unremarkable, other than the fact that she reports trying marijuana once at a friend's house. In addition to the fact that she isn't getting better with treatment, which item described in her history represents a "red flag" for a serious underlying condition or disease?

a. Her age
b. The fact that she is a gymnast
c. Lack of traumatic cause
d. Admitted drug abuse
e. Lack of radiculopathy

274. You are seeing a 16-year-old high school football player to discuss a recent injury. Last night, during football practice, he dislocated his shoulder. His trainer took him to an urgent care where an x-ray confirmed the diagnosis. They relocated his shoulder and put him in a sling. This is the first time he has dislocated his shoulder. Which of the following represents the most appropriate next steps?

a. If his range of motion is normal, allow him to return to play without restriction.
b. Immobilization until an MRI can be obtained.
c. Referral for physical therapy as soon as possible.
d. Immobilization for 2 to 3 weeks, then begin physical therapy.
e. Immediate surgical referral.

275. A 49-year-old man presents to your office complaining of right shoulder pain for the past 6 months. He denies prior injury and works as a mason. His pain is worse at night when he is trying to sleep and with overhead motions at work. He denies neck pain, numbness/tingling, or loss of strength. You suspect rotator cuff tendonitis. Which of the following examinations is most likely to be positive (or abnormal) in this patient?

a. Spurling maneuver (axial compression of the cervical spine)
b. Cross-arm maneuver (passively moving the extended arm toward the opposite shoulder)
c. Hawkins test (flexing the shoulder while it is in a passive internally rotated position)
d. Sulcus test (looking for a gap at the acromion with a caudal load)
e. O'Brien test (internal rotation and adduction of the arm while in active forward flexion)

276. A 55-year-old female patient has been having increasing left shoulder pain for the past month. Past medical history includes obesity and type 2 diabetes. She has no prior history of shoulder or neck problems. On physical examination, you note exquisite tenderness diffusely around the shoulder with movement and reduced passive and active motions in all planes. Upper extremity strength is within normal limits. Plain x-rays of the left shoulder are unremarkable. What should be your next course of action to improve this condition?

a. Corticosteroid injection in the subacromial space
b. Referral to physical therapy
c. Corticosteroid injection in the glenohumeral joint
d. MRI of the left shoulder
e. Referral to orthopedic surgery

277. A 30-year-old male cyclist comes to your office complaining of knee pain. He describes lateral knee pain when he goes for a long bike ride that does not improve with activity. On examination, he has tenderness over the lateral aspect of the knee just above the joint line. Which of the following is the mostly likely diagnosis?

a. Iliotibial (IT) band syndrome
b. Patellofemoral pain syndrome
c. Medial collateral ligament sprain
d. Anterior cruciate ligament (ACL) sprain
e. Medial meniscal tear

278. A patient comes to see you after a skiing accident 6 days ago. She reports twisting her left knee during a fall, feeling a "pop," and noting significant immediate swelling. She was able to bear weight immediately, but did not ski for the rest of the trip. Her pain is now improved, and she is ambulating, but she says the knee feels unstable. On examination, she has a tense effusion in her left knee and is unable to extend her knee fully. Which of the following is the most likely cause of her symptoms?

a. Patellofemoral pain syndrome
b. ACL tear
c. Posterior cruciate ligament (PCL) tear
d. Meniscal injury
e. Medial collateral ligament sprain

279. After diagnosis, the patient described above is ready for her treatment plan. She hopes to return to a high level of activity, and knee stability is necessary for her. Which of the following is best?

a. Immediate surgical referral
b. Surgical referral after 1 to 2 weeks to allow improvement of range of motion and strength
c. Surgical referral after 3 to 4 weeks to allow swelling to improve
d. 6 to 8 weeks of physical therapy to see if surgery can be avoided
e. Return to play after effusion clears

280. You are caring for a 20-year-old male patient with knee pain. He is a runner and reports bilateral anterior knee pain. He is unable to localize the pain to a specific region. The pain is worse with stairs and he has been unable to run because of the pain. When he sits for prolonged periods of time, the knees start to ache. Strengthening of which of the following muscles will lead to improvement of this problem?

a. Hip abductors
b. Hip adductors
c. Quadriceps
d. Hamstrings
e. Internal rotators

281. You are seeing a 14-year-old girl who hurt her ankle while dancing yesterday. She reports that her ankle "twisted in" causing immediate pain and the inability to bear weight. In the office, she has bruising and tenderness over the anterior talofibular ligament (ATFL) with acute swelling. She is unable to bear weight due to the pain. Which of the following is the most appropriate next step?

a. Obtain x-rays of her ankle
b. Encourage early mobilization
c. Prescribe rest, ice, compression, and elevation
d. Use an NSAID to help with the pain and inflammation
e. Begin physical therapy

282. One of your patients had a significant finger injury when playing basketball. He described having a forced flexion injury of an actively extended distal interphalangeal (DIP) joint. That action disrupted the extensor mechanism at the insertion into the distal phalanx. As a result, he was unable to actively extend his DIP joint. You diagnosed him with "mallet finger" and advised continuous extension splinting of the DIP joint for 6 weeks. After 4 weeks, the patient took off his splint to "give his finger some air," and is able to flex his finger appropriately. Which of the following statements is true in this case?

a. The patient can keep the splint off, as he is functionally healed.
b. The patient should keep the splint on for an additional 2 weeks as initially recommended.
c. The patient should keep the splint on for an additional 4 weeks, but only at night and during activity.
d. The patient should keep the splint on for an additional 6 weeks.
e. Surgical referral is indicated.

283. A 35-year-old female patient presents to your office complaining of acute low back pain. She reports she was folding laundry last night and felt a sharp pain in her left lower back which quickly progressed to a severe pain with movement. She is unable to stand up straight today without excruciating pain. She has no past medical history and takes no chronic medications. On examination today, she has no bony tenderness to palpation, positive left paraspinal muscle spasm, reduced active range of motion, negative straight leg raise test, and normal muscle strength and neurologic examination. What is the best course of action for this patient?

a. Bed rest for 2 to 3 days
b. X-ray of the lumbar spine
c. Referral to physical therapy
d. Maintain normal activity and start an NSAID
e. Start a daily NSAID and muscle relaxant

284. A 15-year-old baseball player presents to your office with a 3-week history of progressively worsening low back pain. His mother reports that he has been taking ibuprofen daily and has not been able to practice for the last week due to the pain. He has no past medical history, denies fevers/chills, nocturnal pain, weight loss, or changes in his appetite or bowels. Pain is worse with activity and better with rest. On physical examination, he has full lumbar spine range of motion but has pain with extension. Stork testing is positive. There is some pain to palpation along the spinous processes at the level of the iliac crests. Lower extremity strength testing is 5/5 bilaterally, and patellar and ankle reflexes are 2/4 bilaterally. What is the best imaging tool to confirm this patient's diagnosis?

a. CT of the lumbar spine.
b. Anteroposterior (AP)/lateral/oblique plain radiographs of the lumbar spine.
c. SPECT bone scan of the lumbar spine.
d. MRI of the lumbar spine.
e. No imaging is indicated for this condition.

Acute Complaints—Neurological

285. A 33-year-old woman is seeing you with a chief complaint of "dizziness." Upon further characterization, she describes a "spinning" sensation and a sense of "falling forward." Based on this description, which of the following terms should be used to characterize her complaint?

a. Vertigo
b. Orthostasis
c. Presyncope
d. Dysequilibrium
e. Light-headedness

286. The patient described in the above question reports that this is not the first time she's had this symptom. She says that the symptoms are often precipitated when she rolls over in bed. Symptoms occur a few seconds after a change in head movement, and last a few minutes per spell. This time, her symptoms have been occurring for 3 days. Which of the following would you recommend as first-line treatment?

a. Oral meclizine
b. Oral diazepam
c. Oral valproic acid
d. Intratympanic corticosteroid injections
e. Physical therapy directed at the condition

287. A 42-year-old woman is seeing you to follow-up with a new complaint of "dizziness." She reports that symptoms first began several months ago. At that time, she reported a subjective hearing loss and a ringing in her left ear only. Symptoms were mild, and her physical examination was normal, so you elected to follow her. Since that time, her symptoms have progressed to include dizziness and some facial numbness. Which of the following is her most likely diagnosis?

a. Vestibular neuronitis
b. Benign positional vertigo
c. Acoustic neuroma
d. Meniere disease
e. Cerebellar tumor

288. In the evaluation of a 55-year-old man complaining of dizziness, you perform the Dix-Hallpike (Nylen-Barany) maneuver several times. You had the patient sit on the edge of the examining table and lie down suddenly with the head hanging 45 degrees backward and turned to either side. With this maneuver, the vertigo was reproduced immediately and symptoms did not lessen regardless of repetition. The direction of the nystagmus changed with changing the direction that the head is turned, and the symptoms were of mild intensity. Which of the following is the most likely cause of the vertigo?

a. Stroke
b. Vestibular neuronitis
c. Benign positional vertigo
d. Meniere disease
e. Acoustic neuroma

289. You are caring for a 26-year-old man with vertigo. You have diagnosed him with a peripheral vestibular disorder, and are considering treatment options. Which of the following would be the first-line therapy?

a. NSAIDs
b. Antihistamines
c. Antiemetics
d. Antibiotics
e. Benzodiazepines

290. You are talking with a 24-year-old woman complaining of a headache. She reports that before she has the headache, she experiences visual symptoms associated with slight nausea. When the headache occurs later, it is throbbing, pulsating, and unilateral. During the headache, she experiences light sensitivity. Sleep improves the symptoms. Her symptoms are disrupting her daily life, and you decide to try prophylactic therapy. Which of the following prophylactic agents has established efficacy data to support its use?

a. Propranolol
b. Amitriptyline
c. Fluoxetine
d. Gabapentin
e. Clonazepam

291. One of your patients has been on β-blocker therapy for migraine prophylaxis. Her symptoms are not controlled and she is interested in trying another prophylactic medication. Which class of antidepressants has the strongest evidence base for prophylactic use in migraines?

a. Tricyclic antidepressants
b. SSRIs
c. Monoamine oxidase inhibitors (MAOIs)
d. Selective norepinephrine reuptake inhibitors
e. Bupropion

292. You are caring for a patient who is complaining of a headache. Which of the following, if present, represents a "red flag" and necessitates a workup?

a. Headache that presents after the age of 50 years
b. Headache with a consistent location
c. Frequent, severe headaches
d. Visual disturbances with the headache
e. Severe nausea with the headache

293. You are seeing a 27-year-old male migraine sufferer. His attacks happen approximately monthly, and he would like to discuss abortive therapy. Which of the following options is the best initially prescribed option?

a. Acetaminophen
b. NSAIDs
c. A triptan
d. Ergotamines
e. Narcotics

294. You are seeing a 34-year-old woman for a follow-up of her headaches. She has been having these headaches for the past 5 months and describes them as starting at the base of her neck and wrapping around her head. The pain is constant, bilateral, and typically lasts the whole day if she does not take an NSAID. She denies any photophobia or nausea/vomiting. She has been taking ibuprofen, with relief of her pain, at least three times a week and would like to talk about a prophylactic medication. Which of the following would be the most efficacious for her condition?

a. Botulinum A toxin injections
b. Amitriptyline
c. Topiramate
d. Sumatriptan
e. Butalbital

295. A 38-year-old man comes to the office to discuss his headache symptoms. He describes the headaches as severe and intense, "like an ice pick in my eye!" The headaches begin suddenly, are unilateral, last up to 2 hours, and are associated with a runny nose and watery eye on the affected side. He gets several attacks over a couple of months, but is symptom-free for months in between flare-ups. Which of the following is the best approach for prophylactic management of the attacks?

a. SSRIs
b. Triptans
c. NSAIDs
d. Calcium channel blockers
e. Ergotamine

296. You are talking with a 33-year-old woman who is complaining of headaches. She has had these headaches for 5 months, and they are increasing in frequency. She reports that the headaches may last anywhere from an hour to several days. They are now occurring about 5 to 10 times a month, without relationship to her menstrual cycle. She describes the headache as bilateral, and the pain is described as a pressure around her forehead. She denies nausea, is not sensitive to sound, but is sensitive to light during an attack. On examination, she has no obvious neurologic deficit. Which of the following is the best approach to take at this point?

a. Prescribe a triptan for abortive therapy
b. Prescribe NSAIDs and follow-up if no improvement
c. Order blood work to rule out secondary cause
d. Order a CT of the brain
e. Order an MRI of the brain

297. You are caring for a 45-year-old obese man who is complaining of poor sleep. He reports that he can fall asleep relatively quickly, but wakes up hours later unable to return to sleep for the rest of the night. He has stopped using caffeine, but this has not improved his symptoms. His medications include propranolol, hydrochlorothiazide, and naproxen as needed. He is a smoker, and drinks two to three glasses of wine nightly after work. Which of the following is the most likely reason for his sleep problems?

a. Obesity
b. Propranolol
c. Hydrochlorothiazide
d. Naproxen
e. Alcohol

298. You are caring for a patient who complains of transient insomnia. His problems are associated with stressful times at work, and he generally inhibits his activities approximately three to four times per month. When he is impacted, he generally can fall asleep easily, but has difficulty maintaining sleep. He wakes up at around 2:30 AM and finds it difficult to get back to sleep before he needs to wake up at 5:30 AM. He has eliminated caffeine and has maintained effective sleep hygiene. Which of the following medications would work best to maintain sleep in this patient?

a. Zolpidem (Ambien)
b. Eszopiclone (Lunesta)
c. Zaleplon (Sonata)
d. Diphenhydramine (Benadryl)
e. Melatonin

299. You are seeing a 78-year-old man who was brought to the office by his daughter. The daughter says her father is becoming increasingly forgetful. His medical history is significant for a 20-year history of type 2 diabetes and well-controlled hypertension. On examination, he is mildly hypertensive with otherwise normal vital signs. He is oriented to time, place, and person, but is unable to complete "serial sevens" on a mini-mental status examination. Which of the historical features make this diagnosis more consistent with dementia as opposed to delirium?

a. His history of hypertension
b. His history of diabetes
c. His current level of orientation
d. His inability to complete serial sevens
e. The recent onset of his symptoms

300. You are caring for a 72-year-old hospitalized man who is currently 1 day out from a carotid endarterectomy. You are called to the floor at 3 AM because the patient removed his peripheral IV and is demanding to go home. Reviewing his chart, you see that he has a history of hypertension and hyperlipidemia, both of which are well controlled with medication. He is working part time as an auto mechanic and lives at home with his wife. On evaluation, he is agitated but responds to questions, is oriented to person only, and denies chest pain, palpitations, shortness of breath, dizziness, or other problems. Which of the following characteristics points to delirium instead of dementia in this case?

a. The acute onset of his symptoms
b. The fact that he is disoriented to time and place
c. His history of hypertension
d. The fact that he is responsive to questions
e. The fact that this happened in the early morning hours

301. The patient described in the above question did not respond to reassurance and reorientation. An appropriate review of his medications and an acute evaluation at the bedside including laboratory testing is unrevealing as to the cause of his symptoms. You are fearing that the patient is going to harm himself if left untreated. Which of the following medications would be best to help treat his delirium?

a. Alprazolam (Xanax)
b. Zolpidem (Ambien)
c. Diphenhydramine (Benadryl)
d. Amitriptyline (Elavil)
e. Haloperidol (Haldol)

302. You are in the ER caring for a 47-year-old man who was brought in by his wife. She states that he complained of a headache and started to become irritable. She then noticed that he started acting confused. His past medical history is unremarkable, without evidence of drug or alcohol use. On examination, you find his blood pressure to be 210/130 mm Hg, his pulse to be 97 beats/min, and his respirations to be 20 breaths/min. His temperature is 98.4°F. Strength, sensation, and gait are normal. He has no tremor. Which of the following would you expect to find on ophthalmologic examination?

a. Pinpoint pupils
b. Dilated pupils
c. Papilledema
d. Sixth cranial nerve palsy
e. Anisocoria of 1 mm

303. You are evaluating a person in the emergency department who is displaying an acute fluctuating state of confusion. He is irritable, restless, and hypervigilant. Withdrawal from which of the following substances is most likely to cause this state?

a. Levothyroxine
b. Fluoxetine
c. Oxycodone/acetaminophen
d. Alcohol
e. Amphetamine

304. You are seeing a 26-year-old male patient complaining of a red eye who says, "I think I have pink eye." He reports redness, irritation, tearing, watery discharge, and fairly intense eye pain. Which of his reported symptoms is more suggestive of something other than conjunctivitis?

a. Redness
b. Irritation
c. Tearing
d. Discharge
e. Pain

305. You are seeing a 20-year-old college student who reports that her left eye became pink over the last 24 hours. She is otherwise healthy and takes no medications except oral contraceptives. She reports redness, irritation, tearing, discharge, and itching. Which of her symptoms are more specific for an allergic etiology for her condition?

a. Single eye involvement
b. Irritation
c. Tearing
d. Discharge
e. Itching

306. You are caring for a 3-year-old boy who goes to daycare while his parents are at work. His mother brought him to see you because the daycare will not take him back until he's had a doctor evaluate his eye symptoms. He developed an acute redness of the left eye, associated with runny nose, cough, and increased irritability. On examination, his eye is red and watery. The discharge is clear, and he has mild eyelid edema. Which of the following is the most common cause for his condition?

a. Coxsackie virus
b. Parainfluenza virus
c. Adenovirus
d. Rhinovirus
e. Herpesvirus

307. You are seeing a 32-year-old nurse who was treated in an urgent care for bacterial conjunctivitis. Despite the appropriate use of ciprofloxacin ophthalmic solution over the last 4 days, her purulent discharge and erythema have not improved. What should be the next step in treatment of this patient?

a. Ciprofloxacin ointment
b. Polymyxin-trimethoprim ophthalmic solution
c. Oral ciprofloxacin
d. Oral sulfamethoxazole-trimethoprim
e. Immediate ophthalmologic referral

308. You are seeing a 4-year-old boy whose mother brought him in to be assessed. He's been irritable and feverish for 3 days, with runny nose, slight cough, and ear pain. Today, he woke up with bilateral eye redness and discharge. After evaluation and examination, you diagnose otitis media and bilateral conjunctivitis. You are treating his otitis media with high-dose amoxicillin therapy. Which of the following is true regarding treatment of his conjunctivitis?

a. No additional treatment is necessary.
b. Treatment with a topical antibiotic ophthalmologic solution is indicated.
c. Treatment with a topical antibiotic ophthalmologic ointment is indicated.
d. Treatment with a topical antiviral ophthalmologic solution is indicated.
e. Treatment with a topical corticosteroid is indicated.

309. You are caring for a 21-year-old college junior who comes to see you for a red eye. He noticed the problem after waking up this morning, and it caused him significant concern. He denies eye pain, loss of vision, discharge, or trauma. He has never had an episode like this before. He reports that he was very ill yesterday with nausea and intense vomiting for several hours, but is feeling better today. On examination, you note a localized and sharply circumscribed bright red patch on his left eye. Which of the following statements is true?

a. Trauma is the likely cause.
b. Underlying hypertension is the likely cause.
c. An unrecognized bleeding disorder is the likely cause.
d. Increased intrathoracic pressure is the likely cause.
e. Referral to an ophthalmologist is indicated.

310. You are seeing a 59-year-old man who reports that he "passed out" a day ago. He had a witnessed rapid loss of consciousness followed by complete rapid recovery without intervention. This is his first episode. Which of the following tests is always indicated in the workup?

a. CBC
b. TSH assessment
c. ECG
d. Echocardiogram
e. Tilt table testing

311. A 21-year-old generally healthy college student is seeing you in your office after having "passed out" playing basketball. This has never happened before. He has no significant past medical history and takes no medications. On examination, you note a harsh crescendo-decrescendo systolic murmur, heard best at the apex and radiating to the axilla. Which of the following tests is most likely to reveal the etiology of his syncopal episode?

a. Echocardiogram
b. Holter monitoring
c. ECG
d. Stress testing
e. Tilt table testing

312. You are caring for a 49-year-old type 2 diabetic woman who presents to you after passing out. The event occurred 1 day ago, while she was walking up steps to her seat at a movie theatre. She reports that she felt breathless, became hot and sweaty, and the next thing she remembers, she was waking up on the floor. Her diabetes has been fairly well-controlled with metformin, and her last glycosylated hemoglobin 1 month ago was 7.9%. Her examination is benign, as is her ECG. Which of the following tests would be most likely to reveal the cause of her syncope?

a. Serum glucose assessment
b. Hemoglobin A_{1C}
c. Echocardiogram
d. Stress testing
e. Twenty-four hour Holter monitoring

313. You are evaluating a 28-year-old woman who has had several episodes of passing out. In general, the events are unpredictable, and are not preceded by any prodrome. Her examination has been consistently normal. Initial workup, including a pregnancy test, hematocrit, serum glucose, orthostatic blood pressures, and ECG were normal. She underwent 24-hour Holter monitoring and long-term ambulatory loop ECG evaluation, both of which were negative. Which of the following is the most appropriate next test?

a. Psychiatric evaluation
b. Carotid Doppler
c. MRI of the brain
d. Stress testing
e. Tilt table testing

314. You are asked to see a 67-year-old alcoholic for an evaluation. You notice that he demonstrates a wide-based unsteady gate. He also demonstrates proprioceptive defects. Which of the following terms best describes this condition?

a. Ataxia
b. Chorea
c. Dystonia
d. Generalized myoclonus
e. Focal myoclonus

315. You are caring for a 45-year-old man who comes to see you with a chief complaint that "my hands are shaking." He noted it around 4 months ago, and although it is not progressing, he is worrying about it. He describes bilateral hand involvement, and he notices it most when he tries to pour liquid into a glass or drink from a glass or can. He denies caffeine and drug use, is on no other medications and has no other medical problems. Interestingly, he notes that when he drinks alcohol, the tremor improves significantly. Based on these characteristics, which of the following tests should you order to help diagnose the tremor?

a. A chemistry profile
b. A CT scan of the head
c. An MRI of the head
d. An EMG
e. No testing is necessary

316. You are in your office seeing a patient when your medical assistant asks you to come to the lobby immediately. You find a patient of yours, a 4-year-old child, on the floor having what appears to be tonic-clonic convulsions. Her mother is present and witnessed the event. The event began around 1 minute prior. The child stops the movement and starts to arouse after about 3 minutes. You take her back to an examination room, and although she seems sleepy, is neurologically normal. Her appointment was initially for a suspected ear infection. On examination, the patient has a temperature of 102°F, but her other vital signs are normal. There is no sign of stiff neck, and no evidence of otitis media. The child has no history of seizures, and no family history of epilepsy. After administering acetaminophen, which of the following is the best next step in the workup of this patient?

a. Recommend laboratory testing with routine chemistry tests and a blood count
b. Recommend a CT scan of the head
c. Recommend MRI of the head
d. Recommend EEG
e. Recommend no further workup

Acute Complaints—Respiratory Tract

317. A 33-year-old healthy nonsmoking man presents to you for evaluation of his cough. He says the cough has been present for about 8 weeks. After a few days, he went to an urgent care where he received antitussives and a bronchodilator. Those did not help, and he returned 2 weeks later and was given a course of azithromycin. His cough has persisted. He complains of an associated sore throat, but no fever. He reports worsening nighttime symptoms, and drinking coffee seems to precipitate the cough. Which of the following treatments is most likely to help??

a. A proton pump inhibitor
b. An antihistamine
c. An angiotensin-converting enzyme (ACE)-inhibitor
d. A steroid inhaler
e. Levofloxacin

318. You are treating a 52-year-old woman with a 40-pack-year history of smoking. She reports a productive cough that has been present for the last 3 to 4 months, beginning in the fall. She remembers having the same symptoms last year in the fall, and attributed it to a "cold that she just couldn't kick." She does not have fevers, reports mild dyspnea when walking up stairs, and denies hemoptysis. Which of the following is the most likely diagnosis?

a. Irritation of airways from cigarette smoke
b. Chronic bronchitis
c. Postnasal drainage due to seasonal allergies
d. Lung cancer
e. Asthma

319. Four weeks ago, you treated a 22-year-old woman for acute bronchitis with supportive care. Although she feels much better, the cough has persisted. She has used bronchodilators, antihistamines, and antitussives without relief. Of the choices listed below, which of the following is the best course of treatment at this time?

a. A 10-day course of amoxicillin
b. A 5-day course of azithromycin
c. A steroid nasal spray
d. An NSAID
e. An inhaled steroid

320. You are seeing an otherwise healthy 18-year-old man who has had an acute cough for 2 weeks. It started like a typical "cold," but has persisted. Over the last 3 days, he reports dyspnea and some wheezing. On examination, his temperature is 38.3°C, but his other vital signs are normal. Chest auscultation reveals crackles in the left lower lobe. What is the appropriate next step?

a. Supportive therapy without antibiotics
b. Treatment with a bronchodilator
c. A 10-day course of amoxicillin
d. A 5-day course of azithromycin
e. A posteroranterior (PA) and lateral chest film

321. In the patient described above, which of the following pathogens is the most likely culprit in this case?

a. *Chlamydia pneumoniae*
b. *Mycoplasma pneumoniae*
c. *H influenzae*
d. *Legionella*
e. Respiratory syncytial virus

322. You are evaluating a 57-year-old farmer who is complaining of dyspnea. His history includes being hospitalized for bronchiolitis as a young child leading to childhood asthma, and a history of pneumonia 2 years ago, for which he was also hospitalized. He has a 36-pack-year history of smoking. Which of the following increase his risk for having restrictive lung disease as the cause of his dyspnea?

a. A history of childhood bronchiolitis
b. A history of asthma
c. A smoking history
d. A recent history of pneumonia
e. His occupation as a farmer

323. You are seeing a 60-year-old patient in the ambulatory setting who is complaining of new onset shortness of breath. He looks to be in moderate distress, with a respiratory rate of 22 breaths/min and a pulse rate of 108/min. Then patient does not have a history of asthma, and has never smoked as an adult. You hand the patient a peak flow meter, and obtain a peak expiratory flow rate (PEFR). The PEFR is 100 L/min. What should you do next?

a. Administer oxygen and have the patient transported to the hospital
b. Provide a nebulized bronchodilator in the office and reassess the PEFR in 10 minutes
c. Provide a prescription for a bronchodilator and an oral steroid taper, and reassess the next day
d. Obtain a D-dimer and follow-up based on the results
e. Obtain an ECG in the office

324. You are seeing a 55-year-old smoker in the ambulatory setting. He is complaining of new onset shortness of breath. He looks to be in mild to moderate distress with a respiratory rate of 20 breaths/min and a pulse of 110/min. The patient is on an ACE-inhibitor for hypertension. His pulmonary examination is normal other than his respiratory rate, and his cardiac examination is normal except for tachycardia. The rest of his examination is unremarkable. You obtain an in-office PEFR and find it to be 450 L/min. What should you do next?

a. Administer oxygen and have the patient transported to the hospital
b. Provide a nebulized bronchodilator in the office and reassess the PEFR in 10 minutes
c. Provide a prescription for a bronchodilator and an oral steroid taper and reassess the next day
d. Obtain a D-dimer and follow up based on results
e. Obtain an ECG in the office

325. You are evaluating a 69-year-old woman with a history of asthma and ischemic cardiomyopathy who is complaining of dyspnea. You are not sure if her symptoms are related to asthma or CHF, and you order a B-type natriuretic peptide to help in her evaluation. The level is found to be 76 pg/mL (normal is 0-100 pg/mL). Which of the following is most correct regarding the interpretation of this laboratory value?

a. It is unlikely that her symptoms are related to CHF.
b. The probability that her symptoms are related to CHF is low.
c. The probability that her symptoms are related to CHF is moderate.
d. The probability that her symptoms are related to CHF is high.
e. The probability that her symptoms are related to CHF is indeterminate.

326. You are seeing a sedentary, obese 41-year-old woman who presents to you with acute shortness of breath. She has tachycardia, but no other abnormal examination findings. You order a D-dimer and it comes back low at 326 ng/mL. Which of the following is the most appropriate option?

a. Order a spiral CT of the chest.
b. Order a ventilation-perfusion (V/Q) scan.
c. Order Doppler-flow studies of her lower extremities.
d. Order a pulmonary angiogram.
e. Reassure the patient that her symptoms are not suspicious for a pulmonary embolus.

327. You are seeing a 25-year-old patient complaining of a left-sided earache. She describes the pain as deep, and it worsens with eating. Her ear examination is normal, but she has tenderness and crepitus during palpation of the left temporomandibular joint. Which of the following would be the most appropriate next step?

a. Antibiotic therapy
b. Treatment with NSAIDs
c. Dental referral
d. MRI of the temporomandibular joint
e. Obtaining an erythrocyte sedimentation rate (ESR)

328. The mother of a 9-month-old infant brings him in for irritability. The child has been fussy and has not been sleeping well for 2 days. His highest temperature has been 100°F, and he has had a clear runny nose and cough. On examination, the child is crying and irritable. Which physical examination finding, by itself, is insufficient to diagnose acute otitis media?

a. Opaque tympanic membrane
b. Bulging tympanic membrane
c. Impaired tympanic membrane mobility
d. Erythematous tympanic membrane
e. Purulent discharge in the ear canal

329. You are seeing a 4-year-old male child 2 weeks after being diagnosed with left acute otitis media. He completed his therapy, and is afebrile, acting well, and apparently back to normal. On examination, he has a persistent effusion in the left ear. There is no erythema, purulence, or hearing loss. Which of the following is the most appropriate next step?

a. Reassurance and reevaluation in 2 to 4 weeks
b. Ten-day course of a second-line antibiotic
c. Regular use of a decongestant and reevaluation in 2 weeks
d. Regular use of an antihistamine and reevaluation in 2 weeks
e. Referral to an otolaryngologist

330. You are seeing a 6-year-old patient whose mother brought him in for severe ear pain and fever. On examination, he is febrile with a temperature of 102.5°F, and his right tympanic membrane is shown below:

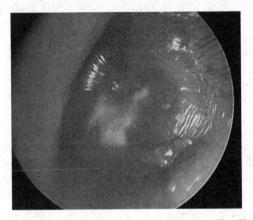

(Reproduced with permission from Brunicardi FC, Andersen DK, Billiar TR, Dunn DL, Hunter JG, Matthews JB, and Pollock RE. Schwartz's Principles of Surgery. 10th ed. Figure 18-1. Available at: www.accessmedicine.com. Copyright © McGraw-Hill Education. All rights reserved.)

Which of the following would be the best initial treatment?

a. A weight-adjusted dose of Tylenol
b. A weight-adjusted course of amoxicillin
c. A weight-adjusted course of amoxicillin-clavulanate
d. A weight-adjusted 3-day course of azithromycin
e. A weight-adjusted 5-day course of azithromycin

331. You are seeing a 16-year-old student complaining of ear pain. His pain has been present for 2 days. He denies fever and has no symptoms of upper respiratory infection. On examination, his ear canal is tender, erythematous, and swollen. His tympanic membrane is obscured by discharge and debris. Which of the following is the treatment of choice for this patient?

a. Flushing of the ear canal with hydrogen peroxide
b. Acetic acid washes
c. Topical antibiotics
d. Systemic antibiotics
e. Oral steroids

332. You are seeing a 15-year-old patient complaining of sore throat. She complains of 3 days of symptoms that have included hoarseness and cough. She denies any medication allergies. On examination, she is afebrile, has erythematous tonsils and cervical adenopathy. Which of the following would be the best next step?

a. Symptomatic care
b. Antiviral therapy
c. Treatment with penicillin (Pen VK)
d. Perform a rapid antigen detection test (RADT)
e. Perform a throat culture

333. A 7-year-old boy comes to see you for a sore throat. He reports fevers, chills, myalgias, and pain on swallowing. On examination, you note anterior adenopathy, erythematous tonsils, and edema of his uvula. He has no drug allergies. Which of the following would be the best next step?

a. Symptomatic care
b. Antiviral therapy
c. Penicillin (Pen VK)
d. RADT
e. Throat culture

334. You are evaluating an 17-year-old man with a sore throat. It has been present for 3 days and began with chills. He now has fever (to 103°F), aches, and fatigue. On examination, he has enlarged tonsils, exudative pharyngitis, soft palate petechiae, and anterior and posterior cervical adenopathy. Which of the following would most likely be found, if testing occurs?

a. Erythrocytosis
b. Neutropenia
c. Atypical lymphocytes
d. A positive heterophile antibody test
e. A positive culture for group A β-hemolytic streptococcus (GABHS)

335. An 11-year-old patient has a history of recurrent pharyngitis with repeatedly positive streptococcal RADTs. You test him when he is asymptomatic and find that the test continues to be positive. Assuming that the patient has no allergies, what would be the best treatment for him?

a. No antibiotics are required.
b. Penicillin (Pen VK).
c. Amoxicillin (Amoxil), using high dosages.
d. Azithromycin (Zithromax).
e. Clindamycin (Cleocin).

336. You are caring for a 15-year-old who came in for evaluation of his sore throat. He has been ill for 24 hours. In addition to the sore throat, he has a fever, but no cough. On physical examination, his temperature is 101°F, tender anterior cervical adenopathy, and tonsillar exudate. His RADT is positive. He denies allergies to medication. Which of the following is the appropriate next step?

a. Reassurance and observation
b. Perform a throat culture
c. Treat with oral penicillin (Pen VK)
d. Treat with oral azithromycin (Zithromax)
e. Treat with cephalexin (Keflex)

337. You are caring for a 32-year-old female smoker with a history of allergic rhinitis who presents to discuss upper respiratory symptoms. She reports congestion, facial pressure, nasal discharge, tooth pain, and headache. Her symptoms have been present for 5 days and they have not improved with decongestants. Sinus palpation causes significant pain. Which of the following is true regarding the criteria for diagnosing acute bacterial rhinosinusitis in this adult?

a. Pain with sinus palpation is one of the minor criterion.
b. Purulent nasal drainage is one of the minor criterion.
c. Facial pain is one of the minor criterion.
d. Tooth pain is one of the major criterion.
e. There are no agreed upon criteria for the diagnosis of acute bacterial rhinosinusitis in an adult.

338. You are seeing a 21-year-old college student who complains of congestion, headache, sinus pressure, and tooth pain for more than 2 weeks. She is otherwise healthy, but feels like she's "having trouble shaking this cold." She has used over-the-counter decongestants with limited relief. A CT scan of her sinuses demonstrates acute sinusitis. Which of the following is the most common organism causing her symptoms?

a. *Moraxella catarrhalis*
b. *S aureus*
c. Group A β-hemolytic streptococcal species
d. *Streptococcus pneumoniae*
e. A polymicrobial mixture of many organisms

339. You are caring for a 42-year-old woman with a 10 days of congestion, purulent nasal discharge, headache, and tooth pain. Based on clinical grounds, you diagnose her with uncomplicated rhinosinusitis. According to studies, which of the following statements regarding treatment of this condition is true?

a. Treatment with amoxicillin is superior to placebo.
b. Treatment with erythromycin is superior to placebo.
c. Treatment with ciprofloxacin is superior to placebo.
d. Treatment with trimethoprim-sulfamethoxazole is superior to placebo.
e. No significant difference has been demonstrated between any antibiotic and placebo.

340. You are caring for a patient with recurrent bouts of acute sinusitis. She has had multiple courses of analgesics, decongestants, and occasional rounds of antibiotics. Among other remedies, she has tried nasal steroids without relief from her acute symptoms. Which of the following statement is true regarding imaging in this case?

a. No imaging will be helpful in this case.
b. Sinus films may be helpful in this case.
c. CT of the sinuses is only helpful for chronic sinusitis.
d. MRI is the most sensitive in the evaluation of sinusitis.
e. US is recommended based on cost and sensitivity in this case.

341. You are caring for an 18-month-old infant, whose mother brings him in for "wheezing." She reports that he has had a runny nose and a slight cough for 2 days, along with a low-grade fever. On examination, he does not appear to be in respiratory distress, but his lung examination does reveal bilateral wheezing. Which of the following is the most likely diagnosis?

a. Acute viral respiratory tract infection
b. Pneumonia
c. Bronchiolitis
d. Aspiration
e. Asthma

342. You are seeing a 23-year-old man for shortness of breath. He has no history of asthma or wheezing and is otherwise healthy. His lung examination does reveal significant wheezing bilaterally. Which of the following tests is necessary?

a. Observation and treatment
b. Chest x-ray
c. Peak flow testing
d. Pulmonary function tests
e. CBC

343. You are evaluating an 18-week-old child whose mother brings him in for "wheezing." She says that it has occurred several times in the last few weeks, and it is usually worse after he eats. She says that the child does spit up more than his older sibling did. On examination, you note that he is not in any distress. His weight is a few ounces down from his visit 3 weeks ago. He is interactive and seems otherwise normal. Given this history, what is the test most likely to determine the cause of his wheezing?

a. Chest x-ray
b. Pulmonary function testing
c. Upper GI barium swallow
d. Upper endoscopy
e. Twenty-four hour pH probe

Acute Complaints

Answers

Acute Complaints—Cardiovascular

108. The answer is a. When someone presents to the office complaining of chest pain, the history is invaluable in helping determine if the pain is due to a life-threatening cause (myocardial infarction, PE, aortic dissection, and tension pneumothorax, to name a few). The likelihood ratios for the clinical features associated with acute myocardial infarction follow:

- Chest pain radiating to the left arm: 2.3
- Chest pain radiating to the right arm: 2.9
- Chest pain associated with nausea or vomiting: 1.9
- Chest pain associated with diaphoresis: 2.0
- Pleuritic chest pain: 0.2

Sharp or stabbing pain (rather than dull, aching, a feeling of pressure, tightness, or squeezing) and positional chest pain also decrease the likelihood that the pain is ischemic.

109. The answer is a. Unless a competing diagnosis can be confirmed, an ECG is warranted in the initial evaluation of most patients with acute chest pain. The likelihood ratios for ECG features associated with acute myocardial infarction are listed below.

- Any ST-segment elevation: 11.2
- Any ST-segment depression: 3.2
- Any Q wave: 3.9
- Any conduction defect: 2.7
- New conduction defect: 6.3

ST-segment elevation is the ECG finding that is the strongest predictor of acute myocardial infarction. However, it is important to remember that up to 20% of patients with acute coronary syndrome can have a normal ECG.

110. The answer is e. The ECG shown has no acute changes, but is suggestive of LVH. Her symptoms are quite suggestive of angina. Since she is currently asymptomatic and her ECG shows nothing acute, transfer to the hospital is unwarranted. The best approach would include patient education for warning signs, and some sort of stress testing. For women in her age group, stress ECGs are often false positive, so a stress test with imaging is most appropriate.

111. The answer is d. The physical examination findings described, including the murmur and carotid pulse findings (pulsus parvus et tardus), are very suggestive of aortic stenosis. Historically, angina frequently occurs in aortic stenosis due to underperfusion of the endocardium. Syncope is typically exertional and is a late finding. While syncope associated with chest pain may be seen in aortic dissection, a PE, LVH, or mitral valve prolapse, none of these would be likely to have the classic physical examination findings described.

112. The answer is a. Based on the patient's symptoms, angina seems to be a likely diagnosis. Exercise ECG testing is the most commonly used noninvasive procedure for evaluating whether the chest pain is due to angina. Stress testing is often combined with imaging studies, but in low-risk patients without baseline ECG abnormalities, exercise ECG remains the recommended initial procedure because of its low cost and convenience. Myocardial stress imaging (scintigraphy or echocardiography) is indicated if the resting ECG makes an exercise ECG difficult to interpret, for confirmation of the results of the exercise ECG, to localize the region of ischemia, to distinguish ischemic from infarcted myocardium, or to assess the completeness of revascularization following an intervention. The electron beam CT can quantify coronary artery calcification, but is not helpful to evaluate angina.

113. The answer is c. There are several characteristics of palpitations that can help the physician determine whether or not the symptoms are from a cardiac cause. These include male sex, the description of the symptom as an "irregular heartbeat," a personal history of heart disease, and event duration greater than 5 minutes. Family history of similar symptoms would not be a risk factor for cardiac disease.

114. The answer is e. When a patient complains of palpitations that are episodic and random, the likely diagnosis is that the patient has premature beats. If unsustained and tolerated well, the risk is fairly low. If a detailed history and physical examination are unrevealing, a 12-lead ECG, TSH, hemoglobin/hematocrit, and electrolytes should be obtained. If those are normal and the patient is not high risk for arrhythmia, the most appropriate next step is to reassure the patient and continue observation. If symptoms are persistent, or the patient is extremely anxious about the diagnosis, an ambulatory ECG for 2 weeks is the next appropriate step. A 2-week test is usually adequate and more cost-effective than a traditional 4-week test.

115. The answer is a. On physical examination, when a patient's pulse is rapid and irregular, it suggests either atrial fibrillation or atrial flutter. PSVT is usually rapid and regular, as is stable ventricular tachycardia. Stimulant abuse will generally cause a sinus tachycardia. While hyperthyroidism may cause atrial fibrillation, the patient would likely have additional symptoms.

116. The answer is c. Ventricular premature beats are often random, episodic, and instantaneous beats, often described as a "flip-flopping" sensation. Atrial fibrillation is described more as a rapid and irregular heart rate or a "fluttering" in the chest. PSVT is generally rapid and regular, and lasting a longer time. Stimulant abuse would likely cause sinus tachycardia, and while hyperthyroidism can cause premature beats, the patient would likely experience other symptoms.

117. The answer is b. Hypertrophic cardiomyopathy can be associated with atrial fibrillation or ventricular tachycardia. The characteristic heart murmur associated with it is a systolic ejection murmur that worsens with Valsalva maneuver. Valsalva decreases venous return to the heart, decreasing ventricular filling. This makes the outflow tract obstruction worse, and accentuates the murmur. Mitral valve prolapse would have a characteristic click with a late systolic murmur. Dilated cardiomyopathy and CHF would likely be associated with other characteristic symptoms including dyspnea on exertion and pedal edema. Atrial fibrillation would not be associated with a regular rhythm.

118. The answer is d. Since this patient's arrhythmia only seems to occur with exercise, stress testing would be useful. Ambulatory ECG monitoring and echocardiography would not be useful. Consultation with an electrophysiologist may be appropriate, depending on the results of the stress test.

119. The answer is b. With PSVT, if mechanical maneuvers do not work, the preferred approach is to refer to electrophysiology for radiofrequency ablation. This is primarily because of the concerns regarding the safety and tolerability of antiarrhythmic medications. Cardioversion would be the treatment of choice in an unstable patient. β-Blockers are the medication of choice, but are not preferred over ablation. Second-line therapies include class Ic antiarrhythmics and class III antiarrhythmics.

120. The answer is c. The classic Wolff-Parkinson-White syndrome (pre-excitation syndrome) ECG demonstrates a short PR interval and δ-waves. Patients are treated if they have symptomatic arrhythmia. Treatment usually consists of radiofrequency ablation, but pharmacologic therapy is also an option. Medications include β-blockers and more potent antiarrhythmics (flecainide, propafenone, sotalol, or amiodarone).

121. The answer is c. Acute pericarditis, an inflammation of the pericardium, is characterized by pleuritic and postural chest pain that radiates either to the neck, shoulders, back, or epigastrium. Dyspnea, cough, and fever may also be present. The most common etiology of pericarditis is viral. Less commonly, bacterial, tuberculous-related, uremic, neoplastic, connective-tissue associated, and drug-induced pericarditis occur. Dressler syndrome, pericarditis associated with myocardial injury, can occur weeks to months after myocardial ischemia or open-heart surgery. Up to 90% of patients demonstrate generalized ST-segment elevation on ECG, whereas a myocardial infarction will demonstrate more focal abnormalities on ECG. Sinus tachycardia and nonspecific ST/T changes are associated with PE. In viral pericarditis, inflammatory markers such as sedimentation rate and C-reactive protein are often elevated, but serum troponin levels are normal. Elevations in troponin levels would suggest myocarditis or myocardial injury/ischemia. Given the patient's presentation, community-acquired pneumonia should be included in a differential diagnosis list, but wouldn't cause the ECG changes shown in the question.

122. The answer is e. Initially, treatment of acute pericarditis includes activity restriction and aspirin or NSAIDs. However, studies demonstrate a reduction in recurrence when colchicine is added to the initial regimen and continued for at least 3 months; monitoring of the CRP level can evaluate effectiveness of the treatment and indicate when it is safe to taper. Corticosteroids are not recommended for acute pericarditis unless symptoms are severe or the cause is immune-mediated.

123. The answer is d. Cardiac murmurs are present in up to 80% of children. Normal blood flow can often cause innocent murmurs and the intensity may fluctuate with positioning or conditions that increase cardiac output (febrile illness, anxiety, exertion, or anemia). Characteristics that favor a benign etiology include I-II/VI grade, changes with positioning, musical or vibratory quality, systolic, and best heard in the left lower sternal border or pulmonic area. Concerning features that should prompt cardiology referral include murmurs that are pansystolic, any diastolic murmur, the presence of a systolic click, opening snap or S_4 gallop, a murmur associated with a thrill, harsh quality, or greater than or equal to III/VI grade.

124. The answer is b. This infant is showing signs of CHF, including FTT, poor feeding, hepatomegaly, and wheezes on lung examination. Still's murmur is a benign murmur not associated with any significant pathology. Atrial septal defect is associated with a midsystolic murmur best heard at the upper left sternal border with a wide-split S_2. Aortic stenosis manifests with a systolic ejection murmur best heard at the upper right sternal border, sometimes with a systolic click if there is an associated bicuspid aortic valve. Transposition of the great vessels usually does not present with a cardiac murmur. PDA is characterized by a continuous murmur under the left clavicle that transmits to the back. The incidence of PDA increases with decreasing gestational age (it is more common with prematurity).

Recommended Reading: Cardiovascular

Bashore TM, Granger CB, Jackson MD, Patel MR. Heart disease. In: Papadakis MA, McPhee SJ, Rabow MW (eds). *Current Medical Diagnosis & Treatment 2018.* New York, NY: McGraw-Hill.

George PN, Samraj MD. Chest pain. In: Smith MA, Shimp LA, Schrager S (eds). *Family Medicine Ambulatory Care and Prevention, 6th ed.* New York, NY: McGraw-Hill.

Martchenke J, Blosser CG. Cardiovascular disorders. In: Burns CE, Dunn AM, Brady MA, Starr NB, Blosser CG (eds). *Pediatric Primary Care. 5th ed.* Philadelphia, PA: Elsevier.

Nadler PL, Gonzales R. Common symptoms. In: Papadakis MA, McPhee SJ, Rabow MW (eds). *Current Medical Diagnosis & Treatment 2018.* New York, NY: McGraw-Hill.

Rodriguez JE, Hardin MD. Palpitations. In: Smith MA, Shimp LA, Schrager S (eds). *Family Medicine Ambulatory Care and Prevention. 6th ed.* New York, NY: McGraw-Hill.

Acute Complaints—Dermatologic and Breast

125. The answer is b. The skin lesions of Rocky Mountain spotted fever are typically red macules on peripheral extremities that become purpuric and confluent. Lyme disease typically presents as a slowly spreading annular lesion—erythema chronicum migrans. Tularemia is characterized by pain and ulceration at the bite site. Brown recluse spider bites most often present as local pain and itching, then a hemorrhagic bulla with surrounding erythema and induration. The black widow bite is characterized by a mild prick followed by pain at the bite site. Left untreated, fatality rates in Rocky Mountain spotted fever are more than 70%.

126. The answer is e. The patient in the question likely has Lyme disease based on his early constitutional symptoms and rash consistent with erythema chronicum migrans. Based on his current symptoms, he likely has early disseminated disease. This is characterized by multiple system involvement, lymphadenopathy, musculoskeletal pain, arthritis, and pericarditis. Treatment of Lyme disease is dependent on the stage of the disease. Early localized disease can be treated with oral antibiotics (doxycycline for 10 to 14 days). Longer courses of therapy are indicated in more complicated disease. Amoxicillin can be used in pregnancy and cefuroxime is acceptable alternative but much more costly. Early disseminated disease is treated with oral or IV therapy for 2 to 3 weeks. Rocky Mountain Spotted Fever is treated with doxycycline that continues 2 to 3 days after the patient is afebrile, and tularemia is treated with streptomycin intramuscularly.

127. The answer is b. This case describes the typical presentation and physical examination findings of head lice, including the typical erythematous papular rash and "nits" on the hair follicles. Treatment options include permethrin and lindane. The preferred treatment is permethrin 1%. Permethrin 5% is a second option, and lindane 1% is a third option. If treatment failure occurs, a second-line medication is 0.5% malathion lotion. Extermination would be appropriate for flea infestation, not for head lice. Oral ivermectin is effective for scabies, not for head lice, but is not approved by the US Food and Drug Administration (FDA).

128. The answer is d. This case describes the classic distribution of scabies. Sarcoptes scabiei burrow into intertriginous areas, wrists, or areas where clothing is tight next to the skin. The lesions of chigger bites are similar, but bites are typically found in a linear pattern over wrists, ankles, and legs. Bedbugs typically infest unclothed areas—the neck, hands, and face. Fleas typically bite the lower extremities, and lesions from body lice would not follow the pattern described.

129. The answer is c. Zika virus is a flavivirus transmitted by the Aedes mosquito. Most infections are asymptomatic, but when they occur, symptoms can include acute fever, maculopapular rash, nonpurulent conjunctivitis, and arthralgias. Sexual transmission and vertical transmission do occur. Historically, the virus was isolated to Africa and Asia but recently has caused outbreaks in the Western Hemisphere, including a large outbreak in Brazil. Disseminated gonococcal disease causes arthralgias and tenosynovitis, but not conjunctivitis. Dengue fever and Chikungunya fever share similar features of arthralgias, rash, and fever, but Chikungunya fever is typically associated with GI and neurologic symptoms. Dengue fever is a biphasic illness with the rash and conjunctivitis appearing after resolution of the fever. Yellow fever does not cause a rash in mild cases and is characterized by jaundice and hemorrhage in more severe cases.

130. The answer is a. Insect bites are typically pruritic erythematous papules or vesicles and are sometimes difficult to differentiate. Location and distribution are helpful differentiators. Flea bites often occur in clusters, and are typically on the lower extremities, as described in this question. Bedbug bites are typically on the hands, face, and neck. Spider bites are generally not in clusters. Scabies are generally found in warm areas of the body where clothing is tight against skin (belt line, wrists) or where skin touches skin (in between fingers). The itching from lice generally begins approximately 2 to 3 weeks after infestation, and may not limit distribution to the lower extremities. Hot tub folliculitis is not clustered, and is associated with hair follicles.

131. The answer is b. Typical local reactions to stings include swelling, erythema, and pain at and around the site of the sting. In general, they resolve quickly and minimal analgesia is all that is necessary. Large local reactions include extended areas of swelling that last several days. They are not allergic in origin and carry a minimal risk of anaphylaxis upon reexposure. Toxic systemic reactions are associated with nausea, vomiting, headache, vertigo, syncope, convulsions, and fever. Pruritis, erythema, and urticaria are less common. Persons who have a toxic reaction are at risk for anaphylaxis with subsequent stings. The reaction described in the above question is not anaphylactic in nature.

132. The answer is a. Gynecomastia is a benign enlargement of the male breast. It may be asymptomatic or painful, bilateral or unilateral. It commonly occurs around the time of puberty, when sex hormone production increases and there may be a shift in the balance between estrogen and testosterone causing relative excess estrogen. If it occurs during puberty, it requires only a history, physical, examination, and reassurance if there are no abnormalities found. Most cases resolve within 1 year. Outside the pubertal period, assessment of hepatic, renal, and thyroid functions may help uncover a cause. Sex hormones are only tested if progressive enlargement is noted.

133. The answer is c. Fibrocystic changes are the most common benign condition of the breast, occurring in up to 25% of premenopausal women and 50% of postmenopausal women. Cysts may range in size from 1 mm to more than 1 cm in size. Fibroadenomas are usually rubbery, smooth, well-circumscribed, nontender, and freely mobile. Mammograms are not necessary for women younger than 30 years of age, as they are less sensitive in younger women with denser breast tissue. Mastitis generally occurs with nursing, and is characterized by inflammation, edema, and erythema in areas of the breast.

134. The answer is d. Up to 15% of breast cancers are mammographically silent. Therefore, a palpable mass deserves further workup, even if the mammogram is negative. Workup may include a US to determine if the mass is cystic or solid, and possible biopsy. Aspiration of the mass may be appropriate, but biopsy is still necessary if the mass is palpable after aspiration, if the fluid is bloody, or if the mass reappears within 1 month. The characteristics of the fluid otherwise do not dictate workup. Genetic testing is of no value in the workup of a breast mass, but can be considered based on family history, and under the direction of an experienced genetic counselor.

135. The answer is a. Spontaneous, unilateral discharge is most suspicious for breast cancer. The characteristics of the discharge cannot be used to distinguish benign versus malignant causes; however, bloody, serous, serosanguineous, or watery discharge deserves a workup.

136. The answer is d. All of the answers in this question may cause a skin infection. However, animal bites are associated with *P multocida* infection with patients typically developing signs and symptoms within 24 hours of the bite. Most other skin infections are due to *S aureus* or *S pyogenes*. *C perfringens* may produce gas, and should be considered as a cause for cellulitis that can lead to gangrene, especially if crepitus is found on clinical examination. *H influenzae* sometimes infects the skin of younger children.

137. The answer is a. Animal bites are associated with *P multocida* infection and typically develop within 24 hours of the bite. Unless the wound to the hand is superficial and does not appear infected, hospitalization is indicated. If the bite involves the tendon, joint capsule, or bone, hospitalization is also indicated. IV antibiotic therapy is with penicillin derivatives or clindamycin and a fluoroquinolone in those allergic to penicillin. Outpatient antibiotic therapy with amoxicillin/clavulanic acid is the treatment of choice if the patient is not hospitalized (5 days for prevention, 10 days for treatment). Bite wounds on the hands should never be closed primarily.

138. The answer is a. Tinea infections are common, and may be spread by close person-to-person contact (as in school wrestling). The classic tinea lesion is well-demarcated and annular with central clearing, erythema, and scaling of the periphery. This can often be confused with eczema or a bacterial skin infection, but by scraping the lesion and visualizing hyphae with microscopic examination, the diagnosis of tinea can be confirmed. Tinea cruris occurs in the groin, not on the thigh; pityriasis rosea has a different classic appearance. Most tinea infections, including tinea corporis, are treated using topical antifungals.

139. The answer is a. Acne is associated with many myths regarding its cause. The true cause is multifactorial, but familial factors are involved. The key factors are follicular keratinization, androgens, and *Propionibacterium acnes*. In acne, the keratinization pattern in the pilosebaceous unit changes, and keratin becomes more dense, blocking the secretion of sebum. The keratin plugs are called "comedones." Contributory factors to acne include certain medications, emotional stress, and occlusion and pressure on the skin, such as by leaning the face on the hands (acne mechanica). Acne is not caused by dirt, chocolate, greasy foods, or the presence or absence of any foods in the diet.

140. The answer is e. In the evaluation of acne, laboratory examinations are generally not required, unless history and physical examination indicates the need to exclude hyperandrogenism and/or polycystic ovarian syndrome. In the vast majority of acne patients, the hormone levels are normal.

141. The answer is e. For mild acne, combination therapy with topical antibiotics and benzoyl peroxide gels, with or without topical retinoids work best. While any of the individual components will work on their own, there is a synergistic effect when used in combination. It is important to let patients know that improvement occurs over a period of 2 to 5 months, and may take even longer for noninflamed comedones. Topical retinoids should be applied in the evening, and the benzoyl peroxide and topical antibiotics should be applied during the day. For moderate acne, oral antibiotics should be added to a topical regimen. Minocycline is most effective, but doxycycline is also effective. Use of oral isotretinoin has become more common to prevent scarring in moderate acne, and if listed may have also been an appropriate choice.

142. The answer is c. The indications for oral isotretinoin include nodular acne, severe acne, or moderate recalcitrant acne. The patient must have demonstrated resistance to other acne therapies, including systemic antibiotics. Isotretinoin is teratogenic, and therefore pregnancy must be prevented during its use. In addition, since both tetracycline and isotretinoin cause pseudotumor cerebri, the two medications should never be used together. Hepatotoxicity is a rare side effect in people using isotretinoin, but patients can still use Tylenol while taking isotretinoin. Transaminases should be checked before and during therapy, as some patients develop significant elevations that normalize with dosage reduction. Dry eyes are a side effect, and patients may have more difficulty with contacts, but they can still be worn. There are some reports of depression while on the medication, but there are no guidelines about screening throughout therapy, as this is a rare occurrence. Topical glucocorticoids are safe for use during therapy and are sometimes used if eczematous rashes occur during treatment.

143. The answer is e. The patient in the picture has rosacea. Although it is often considered along with acne, rosacea is a distinct entity. Comedo formation, the hallmark of acne vulgaris, is absent in rosacea. In stage I, there is persistent erythema, generally with telangiectasia formation. Stage II is characterized by the addition of papules and tiny pustules. In stage III, the erythema is deep and persistent, the *telangiectasias* are dense, and there may be edema of the central part of the face due to sebaceous hyperplasia and lymphedema (rhinophyma and metophyma). Management may include topical or oral therapies. Topical metronidazole, antibiotics, and sodium sulfacetamide can work, but oral antibiotics are more effective than topical treatments. Minocycline or doxycycline are very effective first-line therapies. Topical steroids are not generally effective.

144. The answer is d. The picture shown is classic for allergic phytodermatitis (APD) or allergic contact dermatitis caused by plants. It is caused by plants from the anacardiaceae family (poison ivy, poison oak, poison sumac) among others. When the plant brushes against exposed skin, it gives rise to linear lesions as in the picture, but most all lesions start as erythematous patches, progressing to papules or plaques, leading to vesicles and/or bullae, that may become eroded and crust. Diagnosis is by history and physical findings only. Topical therapy is effective, but for severe cases systemic therapy is more effective. Oral therapy should begin with high doses of glucocorticoid and taper over a 1- to 2-week period. Tacrolimus can be effective, but is not as effective as oral steroids.

145. The answer is c. The patient shown has a keratoacanthoma. Often, these are difficult to distinguish from basal cell cancers, nodular squamous cell cancers, or molluscum by appearance alone, but the history is quite different. Keratoacanthoma are characterized by rapid growth. Basal cell cancers and squamous cell cancers are slowly evolving. Verruca do not generally have the depressed center or the pearly borders. Molluscum do have a central dimple, but do not have such a significant keratotic plug. Keratoacanthoma were formerly considered a pseudocancer, but are now regarded as a variant of squamous cell carcinoma. Most will spontaneously regress in 6 to 12 months, but treatment by excision is often needed.

146. The answer is a. The patient described has psoriasis. While the skin lesions could be confused with eczema, fungal dermatitis, or other lesions, the history and the nail involvement should point to the correct diagnosis. For localized skin rashes, topical corticosteroids are appropriate therapeutic agent. Topical pimecrolimus is effective for inverse psoriasis (located on the perianal and genital regions) or on the face and ear canals, but is generally not used for lesions on the trunk or extremities. There is no place for antibiotics in treatment, except in the case of guttate psoriasis, a form that follows streptococcal infection and appears as multiple teardrops that erupt abruptly. Oral retinoids and methotrexate are both used to treat generalized psoriasis, and help with nail involvement, but would not be a first-line therapy for a localized rash.

147. The answer is a. The rash shown is classic for pityriasis rosea, a self-limited papulosquamous eruption. The most probable cause is a reactivation of human herpesvirus 7 or human herpesvirus 6. The classic history includes a single herald patch (an oval, slightly raised plaque with scale) followed in the next 1 to 2 weeks with a more generalized eruption. It will spontaneously resolve in 6 to 12 weeks, and recurrences are uncommon. The treatment is symptomatic, and includes antihistamines or corticosteroids to relieve itch. There is no role for the other agents listed.

148. The answer is b. The rash described is consistent with impetigo. This diagnosis should be considered in the face of well-demarcated erythematous lesions that, when disrupted, develop a secondary golden crust. The lesions have a predilection for traumatized skin, in this case where nasal discharge has disrupted the skin surface. Most cases are due to streptococci and *S aureus*. Impetigo responds well to topical antibiotics like mupirocin applied to the lesion. Treatment of the nares will help treat colonization with *S aureus*.

149. The answer is a. The patient described has "hot tub folliculitis." The infection is generally caused by exposure to water that is contaminated by *Pseudomonas aeruginosa* or *Pseudomonas cepacia*. This occurs when water is inadequately chlorinated. The condition is usually self-limited, and therefore reassurance is all that is necessary. Antibiotic therapy is only indicated in recalcitrant cases, or if patients are symptomatic. If patients are symptomatic, an oral fluoroquinolone with activity against *Pseudomonas* is an appropriate treatment.

150. The answer is c. The description and picture are consistent with a recurrence of HSV infection. Management includes topical antiviral therapy or oral antiviral therapy. Antiviral agents are more effective treating primary infections than recurrent infections. Pulse dosing (treating at the first sign of an outbreak) may shorten or reduce the severity of an eruption, but are not otherwise beneficial. Chronic suppression is best to decrease the frequency of symptomatic recurrences and asymptomatic viral shedding. Acyclovir resistance is extremely rare. Docosanol cream (Abreva) is available without a prescription. One randomized controlled trial showed a faster healing time when compared with placebo cream, but in both arms of the trial, groups healed within 10 days. If applied five times a day within 12 hours of onset, Abreva is safe and somewhat effective.

151. The answer is c. The patient described has herpes zoster, or "shingles." Antiviral therapy is the treatment of choice, and can decrease the time for lesion healing and shorten the overall duration of pain if initiated within 72 hours of onset of symptoms. The varicella (chicken pox) vaccine has not led to an increase in zoster in immunized patients or in the general population. In fact, vaccination has led to an overall decrease in zoster. Early antiviral treatment does not reduce the pain of postherpetic neuralgia at 6 months, when compared with people that did not have early antiviral treatment. While corticosteroids have not been shown to reduce the prevalence of postherpetic neuralgia, they may accelerate times to crusting and healing, return to full activity, and resumption of a good sleep pattern. Narcotic analgesics are appropriate, as the pain can be severe in the acute phase. Antiviral resistance is uncommon in this setting.

152. The answer is b. The clinical presentation and photograph are both classic for erythema infectious, otherwise known as "Fifth Disease." It is caused by parvovirus B19. The disease is common with most individuals being infected during school years. It is contagious via the respiratory route, and generally is most likely to occur in the late winter, spring, and early summer months.

153. The answer is c. Fifth disease is self-limited, and antiviral medications are not indicated. Patients with preexisting anemia or symptoms of anemia should be tested for anemia, but in otherwise healthy patients, there is no need for laboratory testing. After the viral prodrome, the patient is no longer contagious. Since the illness is biphasic with the rash in phase 2, by the time the rash appears, children are past the infectious state and can attend school and other activities. Serum testing for immunity is not necessary. The rash associated with parvovirus B19 can recur over several weeks in association with exercise, sun exposure, warm water (like in a bathtub), or stress.

154. The answer is d. The picture shows tinea capitis. Systemic therapy is necessary for a cure, but concurrent use of topical ketoconazole shampoo or selenium sulfide lotion may be used concurrently. Griseofulvin is considered the treatment of choice in the United States, and should be used for 8 to 16 weeks in children. Terbinafine can also be used, with no difference in efficacy. Fluconazole is less effective, but is the only treatment currently FDA approved for children less than 2 years old.

155. The answer is d. Tinea corporis, otherwise called "ringworm" is most commonly caused by *Trichophyton rubrum*. It appears as a well-demarcated plaque with central scaling. It is usually pruritic. Tinea infections can also be caused by *T tonsurans* (tinea capitis), *T mentagrophytes* (tinea cruris), and *M canis* (inflammatory tinea infections). Candida species are more commonly seen as a superinfection of tinea pedis. Treating tinea corporis with any of the many topical antifungal preparations will likely lead to cure. However, in the case described above, the patient had been using topical antifungals without success. In this case, an oral antifungal is necessary. Itraconazole (Sporanox), fluconazole (Diflucan), griseofulvin, ketoconazole (Nizoral), and terbinafine (Lamisil) are all reasonably effective. There is no need to use oral steroids in addition to an oral antifungal.

156. The answer is e. The patient described appears to have diaper dermatitis, likely due to candida. Satellite lesions can often differentiate candida infection from a contact dermatitis, and the concomitant thrush increases the likelihood of the diagnosis. Diaper dermatitis is the most common dermatitis of infancy. It is present in around 25% of children presenting for an outpatient visit. Treatment should include frequent diaper changes, using disposable diapers, and frequent gentle cleaning with lukewarm tap water rather than commercial wipes containing alcohol. Barrier preparations are important, with pastes better then ointments, and ointments better than creams. When candida is suspected, treatment should include a topical antifungal cream applied before the barrier preparation, as barrier preparations alone will not be enough. If there is concomitant thrush, oral nystatin should be added. If the inflammation is severe, a combination antifungal steroid agent can be used, but the steroid should not be stronger than 1% hydrocortisone cream.

157. The answer is a. Scabies is very common, with an estimated 300 million cases per year worldwide. Human scabies is caused by the mite *Sarcoptes scabiei,* with mites spending their entire life cycle (around 30 days) within the epidermis. Male mites die after copulation, with female mites burrowing under the skin to lay eggs. It is spread by direct skin-to-skin contact, and may be transmitted from animals to humans. The normal incubation period is around 3 to 4 weeks after an initial infestation. High-risk populations include young children, health care workers, homeless persons, and institutionalized individuals living in crowded conditions. Pruritis is a hallmark of the disease, and skin findings include papules, burrows, nodules, and vesiculopustules. Classic distribution includes the interdigital spaces, wrists, ankles, waist, axillae, and groin. Palms and soles may also be included. The most effective treatment is permethrin 5% cream, though scabies resistance to permethrin is increasing. Oral ivermectin is reserved for resistant cases. Other less-effective treatments include topical benzyl benzoate, lindane (no longer available in the United States), and 5% to 10% sulfur in paraffin. Tea tree oil contains oxygenic terpenoids, and has been found to have scabicidal activity. Treatment includes environmental decontamination and all household family members and contacts should be treated.

158. The answer is c. The lesion described is molluscum contagiosum. It can appear in individuals of all ages and all races. The lesion is due to an infection with a poxvirus transmitted through direct skin-to-skin contact. Lesions are common in children in a daycare or nursery school setting. However, in adults and in the pubic region, they are likely sexually transmitted. Although the lesions can be similar to those seen with basal cell cancers, the lack of telangiectasia is a diagnostic clue. The lesions can occur in immunocompetent persons, but in patients who are immunocompromised, they are generally more numerous and larger. Most lesions will resolve spontaneously within months of appearance, but they can be treated with cryotherapy, cautery, or curettage.

159. The answer is c. BCC is the most common cancer in humans. It is usually found on the head and neck, and is generally slow growing with rare metastasis. The most common type is a nodular BCC, as described in this question. Risk factors include advanced age, cumulative sun exposure, radiation exposure, family history, and genetic predisposition. The differential diagnosis is broad, and often biopsy is needed to confirm the diagnosis based on appearance, but certain historical characteristics make BCC more likely. Intradermal nevi may be nodular, dome-shaped, pearly, and have telangiectasias. However, they will present with stable size and will lack ulceration. Molluscum may have pearly edges and a central umbilication, but will be less likely to have telangiectasias and will be less likely in this age group and in this location. In an immunocompetent adult, they are more likely to be sexually transmitted, and not on the nose. Keratoacanthoma (a subtype of squamous cell carcinoma) may look very much like a nodular BCC, complete with pearly edges and telangiectasias. However, it is usually very fast growing and will change and grow more rapidly. Seborrheic keratosis is more likely to be a well-demarcated darker rough patch, rather than the type of lesion described in this question.

Recommended Reading: Dermatologic and Breast

Bacterial colonizations and infections of skin and soft tissues. In: Wolff K, Johnson RA, Saavedra AP, Roh EK (eds). *Fitzpatrick's Color Atlas and Synopsis of Clinical Dermatology.* 8th ed. New York, NY: McGraw-Hill.

Crawford-Faucher AD. Hair and nail disorders. In: Smith MA, Shimp LA, Schrager S (eds). *Family Medicine Ambulatory Care and Prevention.* 6th ed. New York, NY: McGraw-Hill.

Dailey-Garnes NJM, Shandera WX. Viral & rickettsial infections. In: Papadakis MA, McPhee SJ, Rabow MW (eds). *Current Medical Diagnosis & Treatment 2018.* New York, NY: McGraw-Hill.

Disorders of sebaceous, eccrine and apocrine glands. In: Wolff K, Johnson RA, Saavedra AP, Roh EK (eds). *Fitzpatrick's Color Atlas and Synopsis of Clinical Dermatology.* 8th ed. New York, NY: McGraw-Hill.

Eczema/dermatitis. In: Wolff K, Johnson RA, Saavedra AP, Roh EK (eds). *Fitzpatrick's Color Atlas and Synopsis of Clinical Dermatology.* 8th ed. New York, NY: McGraw-Hill.

Fungal infections of the skin, hair, and nails. In: Wolff K, Johnson RA, Saavedra AP, Roh EK (eds). *Fitzpatrick's Color Atlas and Synopsis of Clinical Dermatology.* 8th ed. New York, NY: McGraw-Hill.

Karnes J, Usatine RP. Chapter 170. Basal cell carcinoma. In: Usatine RP, Smith MA, Mayeaux EJ, Chumley HS (eds). *The Color Atlas of Family Medicine.* 2nd ed. New York, NY: McGraw-Hill; 2013.

Lewis J, Borgen P. Breast disease. In: Bope ET, Kellerman RD (eds). *Conn's Current Therapy, 2017.* Philadelphia, PA: Elsevier.

Madlon-Kay DJ. Breast lumps and other breast conditions. In: Smith MA, Shimp LA, Schrager S (eds). *Family Medicine Ambulatory Care and Prevention.* 6th ed. New York, NY: McGraw-Hill.

Malit B, Scott-Taylor J. Chapter 111. Diaper rash and perianal dermatitis. In: Usatine RP, Smith MA, Mayeaux EJ, Chumley HS (eds). *The Color Atlas of Family Medicine.* 2nd ed. New York, NY: McGraw-Hill; 2013.

Mayeaux EJ, Carter KJ. Chapter 129. Herpes simplex. In: Usatine RP, Smith MA, Mayeaux EJ, Chumley HS (eds). *The Color Atlas of Family Medicine.* 2nd ed. New York, NY: McGraw-Hill; 2013.

Mayeaux EJ. Chapter 127. Fifth disease. In: Usatine RP, Smith MA, Mayeaux EJ, Chumley HS (eds). *The Color Atlas of Family Medicine.* 2nd ed. New York, NY: McGraw-Hill; 2013.

Mayeaux EJ, Usatine RP. Chapter 124. Zoster. In: Usatine RP, Smith MA, Mayeaux EJ, Chumley HS (eds). *The Color Atlas of Family Medicine.* 2nd ed. New York, NY: McGraw-Hill; 2013.

Middeton DB. Cellulitis and other bacterial skin infections. In: Smith MA, Shimp LA, Schrager S (eds). *Family Medicine Ambulatory Care and Prevention.* 6th ed. New York, NY: McGraw-Hill.

Philip SS. Spirochetal infections. In: Papadakis MA, McPhee SJ, Rabow MW (eds). *Current Medical Diagnosis & Treatment 2018.* New York, NY: McGraw-Hill.

Powell B. Bites and stings. In: Smith MA, Shimp LA, Schrager S (eds). *Family Medicine Ambulatory Care and Prevention.* 6th ed. New York, NY: McGraw-Hill.

Precancerous lesions and cutaneous carcinomas. In: Wolff K, Johnson RA, Saavedra AP, Roh EK (eds). *Fitzpatrick's Color Atlas and Synopsis of Clinical Dermatology.* 8th ed. New York, NY: McGraw-Hill.

Psoriasis, psoriasiform, and pityriasiform dermatoses. In: Wolff K, Johnson RA, Saavedra AP, Roh EK (eds). *Fitzpatrick's Color Atlas and Synopsis of Clinical Dermatology.* 8th ed. New York, NY: McGraw-Hill.

Usatine RP, Chamoine P, Smith MA. Chapter 143. Scabies. In: Usatine RP, Smith MA, Mayeaux EJ, Chumley HS (eds). *The Color Atlas of Family Medicine.* 2nd ed. New York, NY: McGraw-Hill; 2013.

Usatine RP. Chapter 135. Fungal overview. In: Usatine RP, Smith MA, Mayeaux EJ, Chumley HS (eds). *The Color Atlas of Family Medicine.* 2nd ed. New York, NY: McGraw-Hill; 2013.

Usatine RP, Hunter-Anderson K. Chapter 117. Folliculitis. In: Usatine RP, Smith MA, Mayeaux EJ, Chumley HS (eds). *The Color Atlas of Family Medicine.* 2nd ed. New York, NY: McGraw-Hill; 2013.

Usatine RP, Jimenez A. Chapter 138. Tinea corporis. In: Usatine RP, Smith MA, Mayeaux EJ, Chumley HS (eds). *The Color Atlas of Family Medicine.* 2nd ed. New York, NY: McGraw-Hill;2013.

Viral diseases of skin and mucosa. In: Wolff K, Johnson RA, Saavedra AP, Roh EK (eds). *Fitzpatrick's Color Atlas and Synopsis of Clinical Dermatology.* 8th ed. New York, NY: McGraw-Hill.

Acute Complaints—Gastrointestinal

160. The answer is b. The first priority when evaluating abdominal pain is to determine whether the pain is acute or chronic. Sudden and/or severe onset of pain should lead the clinician toward an emergent evaluation. Right lower quadrant pain is suspicious for an acute appendicitis, but by itself is not specific enough to warrant an emergent workup. A "gnawing" sensation is often described with ulcer disease, while pain that worsens after eating is associated with many conditions—pancreatitis, gallbladder disease, or even reflux. In the absence of hemodynamic instability, those causes are less likely to warrant emergent workup. Emesis with pain is not enough, by itself, to warrant emergent workup.

161. The answer is d. The location and radiation of pain is often helpful in determining the cause of abdominal pain. Pancreatitis generally settles in the midepigastric region with radiation to the back and is associated with nausea and vomiting. The most common causes of acute pancreatitis in the United States are biliary tract disease (gallstones) or alcohol intake. Only 15% to 25% cases of acute pancreatitis are idiopathic. A congenital anomaly in which the dorsal and ventral pancreatic ducts fail to fuse, pancreatic divisum, can predispose patients to acute pancreatitis, but it is much less common. Overeating and NSAID use are contributors to GERD and NSAID use is a common cause of gastric ulcers, but is not associated with acute pancreatitis.

162. The answer is d. Plain abdominal x-rays are often used in the workup of the acute abdomen due to availability and cost advantages, however, they have poor specificity (< 15%) and are not recommended for the initial evaluation of suspected acute pancreatitis. X-ray findings that may suggest pancreatitis included a segment of air-filled small bowel (sentinel loop) or an abrupt end at the pancreas of the gas-filled colon (colon cutoff sign). While abdominal US can identify biliary tract abnormalities such as gallstones, bowel gas can obscure the abnormal pancreas. Abdominal MRI may evaluate the pancreas adequately, but is expensive and often difficult to obtain in the acute setting. An MRCP is helpful to rule out stones of the common bile duct. In the acute setting, an abdominal contrast-enhanced CT is the most suitable test to detect acute pancreatitis and rule out other causes of acute abdominal pain.

163. The answer is b. Advanced age can change the presentation and perception of abdominal pain. In fact, studies estimate that there is a 10% to 20% reduction in the perceived intensity of the pain per decade after the age of 60. Only 22% of elderly patients with appendicitis present with classic symptoms, making the diagnosis more difficult. Therefore, a high index of suspicion is necessary. Small-bowel obstruction and constipation may cause bilateral lower quadrant pain and decreased appetite, but fever indicates something different. IBS is chronic and generally not associated with fever. Pancreatitis is associated with food intolerance but the associated pain is usually in the epigastric region.

164. The answer is b. The patient describes the classic presentation for peptic ulcer disease (PUD). The two major causes of peptic ulcers are *H. pylori* infection and the use of NSAIDs. Alcoholism and gallstones can cause pancreatitis, but are not associated with PUD. Gastroparesis may cause dyspepsia, but is a less likely cause for ulcer disease. A significant weight loss can predispose a patient to gallstones, but not PUD. This patient's most likely cause is NSAID use to manage her osteoarthritis symptoms. While *H. pylori* infection is responsible for 70% to 90% of duodenal ulcers, its association with gastric ulcers is less. Duodenal ulcers typically occur in patients 30 to 55 years of age, while gastric ulcers are more common in patients 55 to 70. *H. pylori* eradication is responsible for a significant decline in the prevalence of duodenal ulcers.

165. The answer is a. Reflux can be appropriately diagnosed by medical history and by evaluating the response to treatment after 4 to 8 weeks. Those who respond are likely to have the diagnosis. Upper endoscopy fails to reveal GERD in 36% to 50% of the patients who have been found to have GERD by a pH probe. EGD should be performed if bleeding, weight loss, or dysphagia is present, especially in an elderly patient. The other tests have not been shown to be sensitive or specific enough to replace response to treatment as a diagnostic tool.

166. The answer is b. In many cases of GERD, the diagnosis can be made using the medical history and trying treatment to assess for response. Symptomatic improvement after treatment is indicative of GERD and further workup is usually unnecessary. However, endoscopy should always be performed if alarm symptoms are present. These symptoms include bleeding, abdominal mass, weight loss, dysphagia, or vomiting, especially if these symptoms are present in an elderly patient.

167. The answer is d. ERCP is the gold standard for diagnosis and treatment of choledocholithiasis, and is usually performed in the setting of an acute cholecystitis with increased liver enzymes, amylase, or lipase. US shows stones, but is less sensitive for choledocholithiasis or for complications (abscess, perforation, and pancreatitis). CT or MRI is better for those. Cholescintigraphy can be used, and a negative test rules out cholecystitis, but in the setting of increased liver enzymes, an ERCP is a better choice.

168. The answer is d. This patient has a classic presentation of acute diverticulitis, which can present along a spectrum from mild to severe disease. Patients with mild symptoms and absence of peritoneal signs may be managed as outpatients with a clear liquid diet. Antibiotics have not been shown to be beneficial in patients with uncomplicated diverticulitis. Moderate symptoms can be treated with oral or IV antibiotics with coverage for anaerobic and Gram-negative bacteria. Abdominal CT examination is useful in patients with moderate and severe disease or those who fail to improve after conservative management. Colonoscopy is not indicated in the acute phase of illness due to the risk of perforation. Surgical consultation is indicated in patients with severe symptoms, peritoneal signs, or evidence of perforation or abscess on CT examination.

169. The answer is b. Ranson criteria assess the severity and prognosis of pancreatitis. On admission, five criteria are considered. It is a poor prognostic sign if the patient has the following: age more than 55 years, WBC is greater than $16,000/mm^3$, glucose is greater than 200 mg/dL, LDH is greater than 350 IU/L, or AST is greater than 250 U/L. Three or more of these criteria predict severe disease. Six other criteria reflect the development of complications and include a decrease in hematocrit greater than 10 mg/dL, a BUN increase greater than 5 mg/dL, calcium less than 8 mg/dL, PaO_2 less than 60 mm Hg, base deficit greater than 4 mEq/L, and a fluid sequestration greater than 6 L. These are assessed during the first 48 hours of admission. 0-2 criteria correlate with a 1% mortality risk, while 5-6 criteria indicate a 40% risk of mortality.

170. The answer is c. Henoch-Schönlein purpura is the most common vasculitis in children and usually presents with abdominal pain, palpable purpura, joint pain, and sometimes hematuria. The underlying pathophysiology is a leukocytoclastic vasculitis with IgA deposition. Joint pain most commonly involves the ankles or knees. Poststreptococcal glomerulonephritis also can cause hematuria but is typically preceded by a febrile illness with pharyngitis, lymphadenopathy, and generalized body aches. Reiter syndrome, also known as reactive arthritis, typically follows a gastrointestinal or genitourinary infection and presents with asymmetrical arthritis of the large joints, sacroiliitis or ankylosing spondylitis, balanitis, and conjunctivitis. Fingernail and skin involvement can mimic psoriatic disease. This is less likely in our patient, as he has not had any diarrhea or urethral discharge and describes a rash inconsistent with a psoriatic appearance. Renal lithiasis is unlikely in this young patient without the intermittent pain typical of renal colic and lithiasis does not cause a rash. Disseminated gonococcal disease typically presents as a purulent arthritis or a triad of rash, tenosynovitis, and arthralgias. However, this patient does not have a history of urethral discharge or tenosynovitis and gonococcal disease does not usually cause abdominal pain in men.

171. The answer e. Dyspepsia refers to a set of symptoms that can encompass a variety of diseases and the etiologies associated with them. Most clinicians describe dyspepsia as chronic or recurrent discomfort centered around the upper abdomen. Dyspepsia can be associated with heartburn, belching, bloating, nausea, or vomiting, and while common causes include PUD and GERD, no specific etiology is found for 50% to 60% of patients who present with dyspepsia. Only 15% to 25% of patients with dyspepsia have ulcer disease, and only 5% to 15% have GERD. Rare causes include gastric or pancreatic cancers.

172. The answer is a. Constipation may mean different things to different patients, but is generally defined as infrequent bowel movements or straining to achieve a bowel movement. A thorough history is generally all that is needed to rule out secondary causes and define the underlying process. Laboratory testing is only indicated if alarm symptoms are present, if a specific medical disorder is likely given history and physical, or if the person does not respond to initial treatment. Alarm symptoms include hematochezia, family history of colon cancer, family history of inflammatory bowel disease, positive fecal occult blood test or fecal immunochemical test, weight loss, or new onset of constipation in people older than 50 years. In some instances, TSH, serum electrolytes, calcium, or CBC may be indicated, but in this case, they would not be necessary and an initial trial of therapy would be indicated.

173. The answer is b. With secondary constipation not responsive to increased fluid intake and fiber, laxatives are a good first choice. They may be given intermittently or on a chronic basis, and there is no evidence that long-term use of these agents is harmful. Osmotic laxatives like magnesium hydroxide, a nondigestible carbohydrate (sorbitol, lactulose), or polyethylene glycol are all effective and safe, and are a good first-line therapy. Stimulant laxatives can be used as a "rescue" therapy for patients with limited or no response to osmotic laxatives. Chloride secretory agents like lubiprostone (Amitiza) and linaclotide (Linzess) stimulate chloride secretion, resulting in increased intestinal fluid and accelerated colonic transit. Because these agents are expensive, they should be reserved for patients that have not responded to less-expensive alternatives. Opioid receptor antagonists should be used for opioid-induced constipation. Because the patient described does not have alarm symptoms, referral to gastroenterology is not yet indicated.

174. The answer is a. Chronic constipation is a common problem, and pharmacologic treatments may be employed when nonpharmacologic measures fail. Bulk-forming agents (like psyllium) are a well-tolerated alternative and are not a problem if taken regularly. Magnesium hydroxide works well, but chronic use may cause hypermagnesemia. Stimulant laxatives like bisacodyl work well in acute settings, but research is not available to support their routine use for the treatment of chronic constipation. Enemas are usually the treatment of choice for impaction, but not chronic constipation. Lubiprostone is beneficial in the treatment of adults with chronic constipation, but not as a first line. It should be reserved for those refractory to other treatments.

175. The answer is e. Patients with constipation should be referred to gastroenterology for a colonoscopy if they are over 50 or have alarm symptoms. Alarm symptoms include hematochezia, weight loss, anemia, or a positive fecal occult blood test or fecal immunochemical test. Since the patient described reports weight loss, he should be referred.

176. The answer is a. IBS is a functional bowel disorder in which abdominal pain is associated with a change in bowel habits. There is not an identified organic cause. The Rome Consensus Committee for IBS identify the criteria as two of the following three features:

- Abdominal pain relieved with defecation
- Onset of pain associated with a change in stool frequency
- Onset of pain associated with change in form or appearance of the stool

IBS is a clinical diagnosis, and signs or symptoms of an anatomic disease should be absent. These features include fever, gastrointestinal (GI) bleeding, unintentional weight loss, anemia, or abdominal mass.

177. The answer is c. Crohn disease is a chronic illness with characteristic exacerbations and periods of remission. Treatment is directed toward symptomatic improvement and control of the disease process. During acute illness, specific drug therapy should be used to help quiet the symptoms. Mesalamine has long been used as an initial therapy for active disease, but meta-analyses of published and unpublished trial data suggest that it is of limited value in either treatment or maintenance of remission. Current treatment guidelines do not recommend its use. Antibiotics like metronidazole or ciprofloxacin are commonly used because they are thought to reduce inflammation through alteration of the gut flora. Meta-analyses of controlled trials suggest they have little or no efficacy, despite their widespread use. Corticosteroids dramatically reduce inflammation and suppress the acute clinical symptoms. Ileal release budesonide induces remission in 50% to 70% of patients. Prednisone can be used in those that fail budesonide, or in very severe cases. Azathioprine is an immune modulator, and is best used after therapy with corticosteroids to allow their withdrawal (especially in patients who are steroid dependent for symptom relief). Methotrexate is generally a less-preferred immunomodulatory agent. It is used in those intolerant to azathioprine or mercaptopurine, and does not seem to be effective in inducing remission.

178. The answer is c. Anti-TNF agents are recommended as first-line agents to induce remission in patients with moderate to severe disease. The best data support the use of anti-TNF agents early in the course of disease, but in combination with an immunomodulatory agent. A large trial in 2010 compared treatment with combination therapy (infliximab and azathioprine) with single-agent treatment (both infliximab alone and azathioprine alone) and found that combination therapy outperformed either single agent. "Step-up" therapy is considered obsolete, as adding an anti-TNF agent is thought to positively alter the course of the disease. Postsurgical patients can use an anti-TNF agent to maintain remission, but this is not the only use for these agents. Side effects from anti-TNF agents include serious infections, but the increased risk for this seems to be attributable to severe disease and concomitant use of corticosteroids. There is also an increased risk for opportunistic infections, though these risks are relatively small when appropriate screening is done prior to the use of the agents.

179. The answer is a. The agents used to treat ulcerative colitis are the same as those used to treat Crohn disease, even though the diseases are distinct entities. For mild to moderate colitis, 5-ASA agents like mesalamine are excellent first-line treatment options, resulting in symptomatic improvement in 50% to 75% of patients. Corticosteroids are used in patients with mild to moderate disease who do not improve within 4 to 8 weeks of 5-ASA therapy. Immunomodulating agents are used for patients who do not respond to corticosteroids or are unable to tolerate corticosteroid tapering. Anti-TNF agents are used in patients with inadequate response to conventional therapies.

180. The answer is a. Acute diarrhea is defined as an increased number or decreased consistency of stool lasting 14 days or less. Most acute diarrhea is due to infection and usually occurs after the ingestion of contaminated food or water, or direct person-to-person contact. Viral infections account for 70% to 80% of acute infectious diarrhea, with rotavirus being the most frequent cause. Enteric adenoviruses are the second most common type. Rotavirus occurs in the winter months, and most cases occur between the ages of 3 months and 2 years. Contaminated water, salads, or shellfish may transmit Norwalk virus. Giardiasis is less common in the general population, but may be more prevalent in children in daycare centers. *Salmonella* is generally due to raw or undercooked meat, and enterotoxigenic *E coli* is the most common cause of traveler's diarrhea.

181. The answer is c. Approximately one-third of travelers to underdeveloped countries will develop travelers' diarrhea. Of those, 40% will alter their plans because of the symptoms, 20% will be bed-bound for at least 1 day, and 1% will require hospitalization. Most cases of travelers' diarrhea are benign and self-limited. The illness usually subsides within 1 to 5 days, although 10% will remain symptomatic for more than 1 week. Symptomatic therapy with loperamide is all that is generally necessary.

182. The answer is b. Traveler's diarrhea unresponsive to supportive care and loperamide after 7 days should be treated with antimicrobials. The treatment of choice is loperamide and a single dose of ciprofloxacin (750 mg). Levofloxacin (500 mg) or ofloxacin (200 mg) can also be used. Azithromycin (1000 mg) should be used if diarrhea is associated with bloody stools, or is persistent after a single dose of a fluoroquinolone. Rifaximin is a nonabsorbable agent that should be reserved for diarrhea found in travelers where invasive bacteria more commonly cause diarrhea or where fluoroquinolone-resistant campylobacter is prevalent (Indian subcontinent and Asia).

183. The answer is a. The growth chart raises concern for failure to thrive (FTT). While there are several definitions, concern should be raised when a child drops more than two percentile brackets on a growth curve and does not maintain at that area. In the United States, the vast majority of FTT is secondary to inadequate nutrition and a thorough dietary history is most likely to reveal the cause. Albumin has a long half-life and is a poor indicator of recent undernutrition. Prealbumin is decreased in acute inflammation and undernutrition and is therefore insensitive. Organic disease, including hypothyroidism, is found in less than 10% of cases of FTT. IgA levels are sensitive to undernutrition and would be decreased in FTT.

184. The answer is d. The most accurate assessment for FTT is median weight for age. It can be determined by using the most accurate growth chart for where the child lives, and should not be adjusted for race or ethnicity. Mild undernutrition is defined by 76% to 90% of the expected median weight for age, and means that the child is in no immediate danger. The child can be safely observed in this case over time. If the child's median weight for age is 61% to 75% of what is expected, the child has moderate undernutrition. This warrants immediate evaluation and intervention with close outpatient follow-up. A value of less than 61% of expected median weight indicates severe undernutrition. That patient should be hospitalized for evaluation and nutritional support.

185. The answer is d. In a child with FTT, diarrhea and recurrent respiratory infections, cystic fibrosis must be considered, and a sweat chloride test should be ordered. The other tests may be indicated in the workup of FTT, but only with a reasonable degree of clinical suspicion. With the history given, the most useful test would be the sweat chloride test.

186. The answer is b. The infant in this question is most likely to have esophageal reflux contributing to his FTT. The history in this case often will be positive for "wet burps," and the child will frequently have emesis or cough with eating and occasional wheezing. The best laboratory test to diagnose this in children is an esophageal pH probe. If the history were positive for diarrhea or melena, inflammatory bowel disease may be considered, and a hemoccult test would be necessary. If the history were positive for diarrhea, abdominal pain, and foul-smelling stools, lactose intolerance may be considered, and a lactose tolerance test would be a good choice. If pyloric stenosis were being considered, the patient would likely have projectile vomiting, abdominal distension, and perhaps a palpable mass. In that case, an ultrasound would be helpful. It is important to note that an organic cause is only identified in 10% of cases of FTT. The family physician that diagnoses GERD as the cause for FTT risks making one of two mistakes. First, GERD is found is around 70% of those infants tested and therefore may be a normal finding in a child who has FTT for a different reason. Second, poor nutrition causes decreased lower esophageal segment tone, leading to reflux being an effect of FTT rather than a cause.

187. The answer is a. Children with familial short stature have a growth curve that shows simultaneous changes in height and weight. Characteristics of familial short stature include a proportional decrease in weight and length, bone age consistent with chronological age, a family history of short stature, and a normal annual growth rate without deceleration. A child's growth potential can be estimated for girls by adding the father's and mother's height, subtracting 5 inches and dividing by 2. For a boy, it can be estimated by adding the father's and mother's height, adding 5 inches and dividing by 2. In FTT and constitutional growth delay, weight decreases first, then height. In hypothyroidism, height velocity slows first and may plateau before weight changes. In breast-fed infants, weight decreases relative to peers after 4 to 6 months, but catches up after 12 months.

188. The answer is e. When children with FTT present with hypotension and bradycardia, hospital admission is indicated. These are signs of severe malnutrition. Other interventions may be appropriate, but with vital sign abnormalities, it is important to admit the patient. Patients like this are generally not neglected, especially since he has been seen all along for well-child checks.

189. The answer is d. The child in the question has signs and symptoms suggestive of intussusception. It is the second most common cause of significant lower GI bleeding in children and is caused by the involution of one bowel segment into another bowel segment. The diagnosis can be confirmed by US or other abdominal imaging, but an air or barium enema can be both diagnostic and therapeutic. In children, a barium enema can fix the intussusception in

90% of the cases. If the barium enema is not successful, surgical referral would be indicated. It can reoccur around 10% of the time and treatment may need to be repeated.

190. The answer is c. Upper endoscopy is the best diagnostic testing option in the setting of an acute upper GI bleed. It can localize the source of bleeding, potentially allow therapeutic intervention, and allow for tissue diagnosis when necessary. Gastric lavage is less useful, and a barium study might interfere with subsequent intervention. Red cell scans can only localize bleeding to a general area and intervention requires additional procedures. Angiography may miss slower bleeds.

191. The answer is c. The most common cause of upper GI bleeding is PUD; however, it typically occurs in patients with chronic NSAID use, alcohol use, or *Helicobacter pylori* infection. This patient most likely has a Mallory-Weiss tear of the esophagus, caused by repeated or forceful vomiting. Acute gastritis can cause bleeding, but it would not be expected so soon after alcohol ingestion. Esophageal varices account for about 6% of all upper GI bleeds and tend to occur in people with a chronic history of alcohol ingestion. Aortoenteric fistulas are uncommon, seen in less than 1% of patients who undergo aortoiliac bypass surgery.

192. The answer is c. Up to 15% of patients with colonic diverticulosis develop an episode of diverticular bleeding. However, the bleeding resolves spontaneously in 80% of cases. While many believe it may be triggered by the ingestion of certain foods, this has never been proven by studies. It is unusual to find the source of bleeding during colonoscopy. If colonoscopy does not localize the bleeding, a tagged RBC scan should be the next step, and will help guide segmental resection if necessary. In patients without signs of diverticulitis, colonoscopy is the preferred initial modality. A subtotal colectomy is only necessary for recurrent severe bleeding with no source identified.

193. The answer is e. The condition described is a thrombosed external hemorrhoid. External hemorrhoids are defined as hemorrhoids arising distal to the dentate line. When they thrombose, they are associated with acute pain and are hard and nodular on physical examination. The excision can be safely done in the office with local anesthesia in patients who present within 72 hours of symptoms. It eliminates pain immediately and eliminates the risk of reoccurrence. In patients who present after 72 hours, conservative treatment with sitz baths and stool softener is recommended. Hydrocortisone would not be helpful. Rubber-band ligation and sclerotherapy should be reserved for internal hemorrhoids. Incision and drainage of the hemorrhoid increases the risk of reoccurrence and can lead to infection of the retained clot.

194. The answer is a. An anal fissure is a split in the anoderm of the anal canal. It generally occurs after the passage of a hard bowel movement. Patients present with excruciating pain on defecation with blood found on the toilet paper. After the bowel movement, the patient may complain of an ache or spasm that resolves after a couple of hours. Thrombosed external hemorrhoids would generally be visible on examination. Internal hemorrhoids are generally not painful, unless they are thrombosed because of an unreducible prolapse. If that were the case, the pain would not resolve. A perianal abscess may not present with bleeding, but would likely be associated with systemic signs of infection.

195. The answer is c. Hepatitis A is the most commonly reported hepatitis virus. It is spread via the fecal-oral route, most commonly through the ingestion of contaminated food or water. Hepatitis A causes acute hepatitis only and never results in chronic hepatitis. Lifelong immunity is expected for all patients that recover, therefore relapses are uncommon. Fecal shedding of the virus occurs early, and declines once jaundice develops. When patients are jaundiced, they are less infectious than during the prodrome. Symptoms of infection change with age. Ninety percent of those infected before the age of 10 years are asymptomatic, but up to 70% of infected adults have symptoms.

196. The answer is a. Transmission of hepatitis B may occur through the transfer of blood or body fluids, but can also occur perinatally (vertical transmission). If the virus is acquired early in life, the infection is silent, but up to 90% of those infected develop chronic disease. Those with a compromised immune system may also develop chronic disease easier than healthy patients. Healthy adults infected have spontaneous resolution more than 95% of the time. As with infection with hepatitis A, less than of 1% those infected will develop fulminant liver disease.

197. The answer is c. The hepatitis B surface antigen, or HBsAg, is the first marker to appear after acute infection and, if the body is able to clear the virus, it disappears as the hepatitis B surface antibody (HepBsAb) appears. The presence of HBsAg after 6 months is indicative of chronic infection. HBeAg is a form of HBsAg and its presence indicates viral replication and infectivity. IgM antibodies are immediate-response antibodies indicating acute infection while the presence of IgG antibodies indicates a more chronic infection or immunity. This patient has + HBsAg and only IgG antibodies, indicating chronic infection. The presence of HBeAg is consistent with replication.

Serologic Marker	Interpretation
HBsAg	First marker to appear after acute infection; resolves as HBsAb appears
HBsAg	Appearance of this antibody indicates either recovery or immunity
HBeAg	It's presence indicates replication and infectivity
Anti-HBc	IgM = "immediately" or acute infection antibodies IgG = long-term antibodies (chronic infection or recovery)

198. The answer is e. The positivity of the anti-HBs indicates either exposure with immunity, recovery phase, or vaccination. If the patient had exposure and subsequent acute hepatitis, the IgM antibodies could be positive, but the longer term IgG antibodies would not be present. Because the IgG anti-HBc is negative, there is no evidence of past exposure or infection.

199. The answer is a. The HBsAg positivity in this case indicates either chronic infection or early infection. The presence of HBeAg is consistent with replication. The positivity of the IgM anti-HBc indicates early infection, and is negative in chronic infection. Additionally, if the patient were in the recovery phase, his HBsAg would be negative.

200. The answer is e. In evaluating childhood jaundice, it's important to differentiate between conjugated and unconjugated hyperbilirubinemia. If jaundice occurs in childhood and is associated with unconjugated hyperbilirubinemia, hemolytic diseases (G6PD deficiency and spherocytosis), Gilbert disease, and Crigler-Najjar syndrome should be considered. If associated with conjugated hyperbilirubinemia, viral hepatitis is the most common cause. Less common causes of conjugated hyperbilirubinemia include Wilson disease and milder forms of galactosemia.

201. The answer is c. Adult-onset jaundice is always concerning, and understanding the likelihood of disease states will help guide the workup. Hemolytic anemia causes an unconjugated hyperbilirubinemia, and is therefore not a consideration in this patient. Viral hepatitis accounts for up to 75% of jaundice in patients younger than 30, but only accounts for 5% of jaundice in patients older than 60 years. Extrahepatic obstruction (gall stones, strictures, and most importantly pancreatic cancer) accounts for more than 60% of jaundice in patients older than 60 years. CHF accounts for around 10% of jaundice in patients older than 60, and metastatic disease accounts for around 13%.

202. The answer is d. In the setting of suspected obstruction with normal initial testing, it is sometimes difficult to determine the next steps. When obstruction is suspected, US or CT scan is the appropriate initial test. If dilated bile ducts are seen, then ERCP or PTC should be done, followed by appropriate intervention. If bile ducts are not dilated but the likelihood of obstruction is low, the patient should be evaluated for hepatocellular or cholestatic liver disease. If obstruction is still considered likely after a negative US or CT scan, MRCP is a reasonable next option. It has excellent sensitivity and specificity, will evaluate anatomy appropriately, and unlike ERCP, does not induce postprocedure pancreatitis. A HIDA scan is used to evaluate the filling and function of the gall bladder and is used if a US study is inconclusive.

203. The answer is c. While all of the medications listed have antiemetic properties, the patient described most likely has gastroparesis as a result of her longstanding diabetes. The prokinetic agent metoclopramide can improve gastric motility and help her symptoms more than the other antiemetics listed. Antiemetics can cause a variety of side effects. The phenothiazines, antihistamines, and scopolamine can cause drowsiness, dry mouth, and dizziness. Tigan causes similar side effects. Zofran is a serotonin receptor antagonist, and may cause dizziness and headache. Reglan is a prokinetic agent and can cause diarrhea and extrapyramidal reactions. Extrapyramidal reactions can be serious.

204. The answer is c. A careful history and physical examination can often distinguish between potential causes for nausea and vomiting. In this case, mild pain, followed by the acute onset of distension, nausea, and vomiting is consistent with ileus or obstruction. High pitched or hyperactive bowel sounds lead one to think of obstruction; with an ileus, bowel sounds are absent. Gastroenteritis begins acutely, but is usually not preceded by mild abdominal pain. Diverticulosis and diverticulitis would cause pain, but would be less likely to present with nausea, vomiting, and distension.

205. The answer is b. Psychogenic vomiting should be suspected in patients who are able to maintain adequate nutrition despite chronic symptoms. It is usually seen during times of social stress or in patients with a past history of physical or sexual abuse, post-traumatic stress disorder, and eating disorders. Chronic gastroenteritis is an unlikely condition. While young girls in this age group are at risk of anorexia and bulimia, sufferers usually do not seek medical attention or treatment until concerned others bring the condition to medical attention. A central nervous system malignancy is possible, if the lesion involves the vomiting center, but one would expect to see a nutritional deficit in that case.

206. The answer is e. The situation described is consistent with viral gastroenteritis, a common clinical condition. The Norwalk virus, reoviruses, and adenoviruses are common causes. Symptoms typically begin acutely and are consistent with typical viral syndrome symptoms. Generally, these illnesses are self-limited, and will resolve within 5 days. Unless symptoms are severe, no testing is necessary.

207. The answer is b. In cases of gastroenteritis, oral rehydration is indicated as long as there are no signs of severe dehydration. IV rehydration and antiemetics may have a role, but only in more severe cases. There is no role for antibiotic therapy.

208. The answer is d. Based on her age and history, the patient described has pancreatitis, likely due to gallstones. Biliary tract stones account for 70% to 80% of the cases of acute pancreatitis. If the gall bladder is not eventually removed, pancreatitis will reoccur in 30% to 60% of patients. While the laboratory findings in acute pancreatitis are often nonspecific, elevated serum amylase in the right clinical setting is often suggestive. Radiographic evidence can help confirm the diagnosis. In establishing a cause for pancreatitis, history is key, but some laboratory findings are helpful. Elevated ALT is more suggestive of gallstone pancreatitis and is less likely when alcohol or hypertriglyceridemia is the cause. ACE-inhibitors are an uncommon cause of pancreatitis. Hypercalcemia is also a rare cause, and is unlikely in this case.

209. The answer is c. Hypertrophic pyloric stenosis is the most common surgical condition seen in the first 2 to 8 weeks of life. Risk factors include a positive family history and male gender. Children with pyloric stenosis usually present with weight loss, dehydration, and occasionally a palpable "olive" mass in the epigastric area. It is usually identified before 7 weeks of age. Breast milk allergies are uncommon. Reflux may be possible, but is less likely to be associated with weight loss and dehydration. Intussusception is associated with significant abdominal pain, and hemoccult positive stools. Small-bowel obstruction is less likely, and would be associated with high-pitched bowel sounds.

210. The answer is d. The patient described likely has cholelithiasis. Nausea, vomiting, and pain occur after eating fatty meals. The diagnostic test of choice would be a right upper quadrant US to identify stones in the gallbladder. Amylase and lipase may be positive if the patient develops secondary pancreatitis, but are unlikely to be elevated until that point. Hemoccult testing, abdominal x-rays, and upper endoscopy are all likely to be normal.

Recommended Reading: Gastrointestinal

Barter CM, Dunne L, Jardim C. Abdominal pain. In: South-Paul JE, Matheny SC, Lewis EL (eds). *Current Diagnosis & Treatment Family Medicine.* 4th ed. New York, NY: McGraw-Hill.

Chin-Hong PV, Guglielmo BJ. Common problems in infectious diseases & antimicrobial therapy. In: Papadakis MA, McPhee SJ, Rabow MW (eds). *Current Medical Diagnosis & Treatment 2018.* New York, NY: McGraw-Hill.

Contratto EC, Jennings MS. Gastrointestinal bleeding. In: Smith MA, Shimp LA, Schrager S (eds). *Family Medicine Ambulatory Care and Prevention.* 6th ed. New York, NY: McGraw-Hill.

Dewar JC, Dewar SB. Failure to thrive. In: South-Paul JE, Matheny SC, Lewis EL (eds). *Current Diagnosis & Treatment Family Medicine.* 4th ed. New York, NY: McGraw-Hill.

Dirkx TC, Woodell T, Watnick S. Kidney disease. In: Papadakis MA, McPhee SJ, Rabow MW (eds). *Current Medical Diagnosis & Treatment 2018.* New York, NY: McGraw-Hill.

Friedman LS. Liver, biliary tract & pancreas disorders. In: Papadakis MA, McPhee SJ, Rabow MW (eds). *Current Medical Diagnosis & Treatment 2018*. New York, NY: McGraw-Hill.

Garber J, Pratt, DS. Acute and chronic viral hepatitis. In: Bope ET, Kellerman RD (eds). *Conn's Current Therapy, 2017*. Philadelphia, PA: Elsevier.

Gerhart JL, Kamens C. Failure to thrive. In: Smith MA, Shimp LA, Schrager S (eds). *Family Medicine Ambulatory Care and Prevention*. 6th ed. New York, NY: McGraw-Hill.

Hellmann DB, Imboden J. Rheumatologic, immunologic & allergic disorders. In: Papadakis MA, McPhee SJ, Rabow MW (eds). *Current Medical Diagnosis & Treatment 2018*. New York, NY: McGraw-Hill.

Krishnan K, Pandolfino JE. Dysphagia and esophageal obstruction. In: Bope ET, Kellerman RD (eds). *Conn's Current Therapy, 2017*. Philadelphia, PA: Elsevier.

McQuaid KR. Gastrointestinal disorders. In: Papadakis MA, McPhee SJ, Rabow MW (eds). *Current Medical Diagnosis & Treatment 2018*. New York, NY: McGraw-Hill.

Melton-Meaux GB, Kwaan MR. Hemorrhoids, anal fissure, and anorectal abscess and fistula. In: Bope ET, Kellerman RD (eds). *Conn's Current Therapy, 2017*. Philadelphia, PA: Elsevier.

Philip SS. Spirochetal infections. In: Papadakis MA, McPhee SJ, Rabow MW (eds). *Current Medical Diagnosis & Treatment 2018*. New York, NY: McGraw-Hill.

Ramakrishnan K. Abdominal pain. In: Smith MA, Shimp LA, Schrager S (eds). *Family Medicine Ambulatory Care and Prevention*. 6th ed. New York, NY: McGraw-Hill.

Ramakrishnan K, Schweibert LP. Jaundice. In: Smith MA, Shimp LA, Schrager S. (eds). *Family Medicine Ambulatory Care and Prevention*. 6th ed. New York, NY: McGraw-Hill.

Roberts JR, Castell DO. Gastroesophageal reflux disease (GERD). In: Bope ET, Kellerman RD (eds). *Conn's Current Therapy, 2017*. Philadelphia, PA: Elsevier.

Shah NR, Wilson GR. Nausea and vomiting. In: Smith MA, Shimp LA, Schrager S (eds). *Family Medicine Ambulatory Care and Prevention*. 6th ed. New York, NY: McGraw-Hill.

Van Buren G, Fisher WE. Acute and chronic pancreatitis. In: Bope ET, Kellerman RD (eds). *Conn's Current Therapy, 2017*. Philadelphia, PA: Elsevier.

Acute Complaints—Urogenital

211. The answer is d. Many types of cervical and vaginal abnormalities can be detected using the Pap smear. Certain oncogenic sub-types of HPV, a sexually transmitted DNA virus, are highly associated with the development of cervical cancer. However, young women with HPV infections often "clear" them over time and, therefore, management of women less than 25 years of age is different from that of older women. Due to the high clearance rate of young women, The American Society for Colposcopy and Cervical Pathology (ASCCP) recommends against HPV "co-testing" with HPV screening in women less than 30 years of age. For a women less than 25 years of age, a Pap result of "atypical squamous cells of undetermined significance," is preferably followed by another pap smear in 1 year.

212. The answer is e. In women over 30 years of age, the preferred routine screening regimen is co-testing (cytology + HPV testing) every 5 years. For cytology to be considered "sufficient," there must be adequate numbers of cells and the presence of transformational zone cells. In women with unknown or positive HPV status, normal but insufficient cytology should be followed by repeat testing. However, in a woman with negative HPV, the risk of significant cytologic abnormality is low and should be followed by routine screening (co-testing in 5 years).

213. The answer is a. According to the ASCCP, women aged 21 to 24 years of age with ASC-US or LSIL should have repeat cytology in 1 year. If that repeat cytology is negative, ASC-US or LSIL, the clinician should repeat cytology in another 12 months. If the repeat cytology shows high-grade atypical squamous cells (ASC-H), atypical glandular cells (AGC), or high-grade squamous intraepithelial lesions (HSIL), the clinician should proceed to colposcopy at that time. Once there are two consecutive negative cytologies, normal screening can be resumed. If the repeat cytology (on the third Pap) is ASC-US or greater, it is recommended to proceed to colposcopy.

214. The answer is d. According to the current ASCCP guidelines, any result of ASC-H should be followed by colposcopy. This should happen regardless of HPV result in a woman more than 25 years of age due to the possibility of significant cytologic abnormality. Treatment with estrogen is not recommended as it could delay a diagnosis.

215. The answer is c. HPV virus has many sub-types with infection of at least 50% of sexually active women and men by 50 years of age. However, most infections with low-risk sub-types will clear over time. Continued infection with high-risk subtypes is associated with the development of cervical cancer. Types 16 and 18 are particularly correlated with cervical cancer and should prompt more frequent monitoring. Women more than 30 years of age with normal cytology and the presence of high-risk sub-types of HPV should have repeat co-testing (cytology and HPV testing) at 1 year. If the high-risk sub-type is still present at that time or the cytology is ASC-US or greater, clinicians should proceed with colposcopy.

216. The answer is c. AGC can be associated with a wide variety of conditions, from polyps to neoplasia. However, the risk of endometrial, cervical, or ovarian neoplasia is greater in patients with AGC reported and should prompt further assessment. All subcategories of AGC should proceed with colposcopy with endo*cervical* sampling and endo*metrial* sampling in women who are 35 years of age or older, OR at risk for endometrial neoplasia. Age more than or equal to 35 years, obesity, chronic anovulation, and unexplained vaginal bleeding are all risk factors for endometrial neoplasia. Although HPV status is useful in the management of abnormal cervical pathology, it is not predictive of endometrial cancer and AGC should prompt endometrial biopsy even in the absence of HPV infection.

217. The answer is c. The preferred action in this step is to proceed to colposcopy without endocervical sampling during this pregnancy. Deferring until 6 weeks postpartum is an option, but not the preferred recommendation, due to the risk of significant cytologic abnormality. The current guidelines do not recommend repeat co-testing in this situation due to the higher likelihood of significant abnormality. HPV high-risk sub-types other than 16 or 18 are often reported as "other high-risk" HPV. However, the presence or absence of HPV does not influence the recommendation in this case.

218. The answer is a. If a woman with a prior history of uncomplicated UTI presents with classic symptoms of a UTI, clinicians can consider empirically treating the patient. This has been shown to be effective and decrease health care costs. A useful flow chart for evaluating women with symptoms is below:

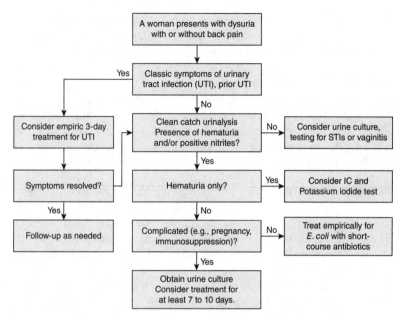

```
A woman presents with dysuria
with or without back pain
            │
            ▼
Yes   Classic symptoms of urinary
      tract infection (UTI), prior UTI
            │ No
            ▼
Consider empiric 3-day    Clean catch urinalysis     No    Consider urine culture,
treatment for UTI         Presence of hematuria     ───▶   testing for STIs or vaginitis
                          and/or positive nitrites?
            │                   │ Yes
            ▼                   ▼
Symptoms resolved?        Hematuria only?      Yes    Consider IC and
                                              ───▶    Potassium iodide test
   │ Yes                        │ No
   ▼                            ▼
Follow-up as needed       Complicated (e.g., pregnancy,   No    Treat empirically for
                          immunosuppression)?            ───▶   E. coli with short-
                                                                course antibiotics
                                │ Yes
                                ▼
                          Obtain urine culture
                          Consider treatment for
                          at least 7 to 10 days.
```

(Reproduced with permission from Smith MA, Shimp LA, and Schrager S. Family Medicine: Ambulatory Care and Prevention. 6th ed. New York, NY: McGraw-Hill Education; 2014: Figure 21-1, p. 168.)

219. The answer is d. In many women with postcoital UTIs, symptoms develop within 24 hours of sexual intercourse. If measures like voiding after intercourse, acidification of the urine, and discontinuing diaphragm do not work, prophylaxis is indicated for women with frequent infections. Single-dose postcoital antibiotic use is often helpful. If that does not decrease infections, daily single-dose antibiotic prophylaxis may be appropriate for 3 to 6 months. If symptoms reoccur after discontinuation of daily prophylaxis, it may need to continue for up to 2 years.

220. The answer is c. Dysuria without pyuria is common. In the postmenopausal years, atrophy is a usual cause. In younger women, a careful history can reveal a bladder irritant (caffeine and acidic foods are common irritants). When hematuria without pyuria is present in patients with recurrent symptoms, interstitial cystitis should be suspected. The potassium iodide sensitivity test involves a catheter infusion of sterile water into the bladder, with the patient rating pain and urgency. After draining, the test is repeated with 40 mg of potassium solution and 100 mL of water. The test is positive if pain with infusion of the potassium solution is rated higher. Lack of evidence regarding the benefit of cystoscopy has led to consensus that it is not needed to confirm the diagnosis of interstitial cystitis.

221. The answer is b. The American College of Obstetrics and Gynecology recommends treating asymptomatic bacteriuria in pregnancy, as 20% to 35% of the cases eventually develop into overt UTIs. In the other cases above, treatment of asymptomatic bacteriuria is not indicated, as it has not been shown to decrease morbidity and may increase the likelihood of developing resistant microorganisms.

222. The answer is a. The patient described is eligible for over-the-phone treatment with first-line antibiotics. If she is not symptom-free in 3 days, she would need to be seen. If the patient had never had a UTI in the past, or if she had fever, vaginal discharge, back pain, or hematuria, she would also need to be seen. Ciprofloxacin is a second-line treatment and therefore not appropriate in this case. Obtaining a urinalysis or culture after antibiotics is not useful and increases the costs of care. If no treatment is initiated, infection can worsen. Home collection of urine specimen is likely to be contaminated, and not useful.

223. The answer is e. In men with urinary symptoms and a normal urinary tract, cystitis and pyelonephritis are uncommon. Urethritis would be unlikely to cause this systemic illness. The patient described above has acute bacterial prostatitis. Acute prostatitis is most commonly seen in 30- to 50-year-old men, and symptoms include frequency, urgency, and back pain. The patient generally appears acutely ill, and has pyuria. The prostate examination would reveal a boggy, tender, and warm prostate.

224. The answer is b. While the cause of nocturnal enuresis is unknown, it is felt to be due to decreased production of nocturnal antidiuretic hormone. Risk factors include family history (there is a 5-7X risk if one parent was eneuretic), preterm birth, male gender (3X more common in males), and smaller bladder capacity. Most children presenting will have a normal physical examination, and in that case, the only testing necessary is a urinalysis and an estimation of bladder capacity. This estimate is most easily done by measuring a post-void residual. The normal capacity is age (in ounces) plus 2, and a post-void residual should be less than 10% of maximum bladder capacity.

225. The answer is a. In the child with monosymptomatic nocturnal enuresis, no further evaluation is needed, other than a thorough voiding history, physical examination, urinalysis, and potentially a post-void residual. X-rays of the lumbar and sacral spine are indicated if there is suspicion of spina bifida occulta, and renal US/VCUG are indicated if there are suspected anatomic abnormalities that would lead to enuresis. Observation is appropriate because treatment should not be considered until the age of 7, or when the child can be relied upon to be an active participant in his/her therapy.

226. The answer is b. Enuresis alarms have been shown to be an effective treatment for nocturnal enuresis. The alarms need to be used appropriately, with parental involvement in order to be effective. Frequent night-time wakening may be effective, but compliance is a barrier to effectiveness. DDAVP can also be effective, but relapse rate is high once the medication is discontinued. Tricyclics have a lower initial cure rate and a high relapse rate. They can also be lethal, if overdosed and are therefore not used for this purpose. Oxybutynin has a high relapse rate and has not been proven to be efficacious when compared with placebo.

227. The answer is e. Lifestyle modifications should be tried for 3 to 6 months prior to initiating pharmacologic therapy. Effective interventions include:

- Goal-setting for the child to get up and urinate at night, using an alarm
- Stopping use of diapers or pull-ups so the child can notice the sensation of wetness
- Improving access to the toilet, including the use of a bedside potty
- Emptying bladder before bedtime
- Including the child in cleanup activities, as long as it's done non-punitively
- Positive reinforcement with the use of stickers or other methods

Fluid restriction after dinner is often advocated, but not effective. However, avoiding excessive fluids at night is appropriate.

228. The answer is a. Moisture-sensitive alarms can be a very successful behavioral treatment for nocturnal enuresis. The first drops of urine complete a circuit, activating an alarm that will wake the child (and the parents). The parents then help the child complete voiding in the toilet. Over time, a conditioned response develops, and the child awakens voluntarily with the sensation of a full bladder. There is no gender difference in success rates, and with appropriate use and parent involvement, success rates are around 66%. It may take weeks or months to be successful, and requires a sizeable commitment from the parents and child involved. The child should not take responsibility for this treatment, because without parental involvement, success rates drop.

229. The answer is e. Painless hematuria without other symptoms is the most common presentation of bladder carcinoma. Risk factors include being male, smoking, and working with aromatic amines that are often used in the dye, paint, aluminum, textile, and rubber industries. Acute prostatitis and UTIs are usually associated with dysuria, fever, and urinary frequency and urgency. Chronic prostatitis is associated with urinary symptoms as well. Stones are associated with pain.

230. The answer is d. In a patient with hematuria and signs and symptoms consistent with infection, an empiric course of antibiotics for cystitis is the best next step. Urine culture should be considered if the urinalysis does not support the patient's symptoms, if symptoms of upper UTI are present (flank pain, fever), or the patient has recurrent infections. Renal US can be helpful in the evaluation of hematuria or recurrent UTIs, but is not indicated for an isolated episode of cystitis. Urine cytology is used to evaluate the urine for the presence of malignant cells and would be unnecessary in this young patient with low risk for bladder cancer. In a patient with suspected genital infection or possible pregnancy, a speculum and bimanual examination should be carried out. However, this patient denies being sexually active and is not having any symptoms consistent with pregnancy or vaginal infection.

231. The answer is a. In patients younger than 40 years with hematuria, but a normal IV pyelogram, urine culture and cytology, periodic monitoring, and reassurance are appropriate. In a patient older than 40 years, cystoscopy would be appropriate. A diagnosis of poststreptococcal glomerulonephritis would be unlikely in this age group and no recent infection is reported in his history, so an ASO titer would not be helpful. A renal biopsy would not be needed if the creatinine is normal and is typically only utilized if there is evidence of progressive disease.

232. The answer is d. Imaging studies to evaluate hematuria should be ordered based on the differential diagnosis. In the absence of infectious symptoms, the urinary tract should be evaluated to rule out neoplasms, urolithiasis, cystic disease of the kidneys, and/or obstructive lesions. This patient doesn't have any symptoms, so urolithiasis and obstructive lesions are less likely. IVP was traditionally used for this purpose, but its use of nephrotoxic contrast dye has limited its use recently. An unenhanced or spiral CT of the abdomen is the test of choice to detect renal calculi and small masses and is the best test in this situation. The use of contrast is not needed for this evaluation. A renal US is helpful to identify large masses (> 3 cm) but is unlikely to find small neoplasms. A KUB is not typically used in the workup of hematuria due to its low sensitivity for masses and small stones.

233. The answer is d. Asymptomatic bacteriuria is common in otherwise well elderly, and does not cause incontinence—whereas, a symptomatic infection may. Hyperglycemia can cause secondary incontinence because of polyuria, and continence can be restored by more tightly controlling the patient's sugar. Diuretics also may cause secondary incontinence, and may need to be avoided unless necessary. Stool impaction is thought to be a causative factor in up to 10% of patients with incontinence, and disimpaction may restore continence. Atrophic vaginitis may also be causative, and treatment may improve the situation.

234. The answer is d. Stress incontinence is much more commonly seen in women than in men, and is most often caused by urethral hypermobility resulting from weakness of the pelvic floor musculature. Patients complain of involuntary loss of urine associated with increase in intra-abdominal pressure (when sneezing, coughing, laughing, or exercising). Functional incontinence refers to a limitation that does not allow the patient to void in the bathroom (bed rest, paralysis, severe dementia) and does not generally relate to the urinary tract. Urge incontinence is the loss of urine following a strong urge to void, and overflow incontinence is due to overdistention of the bladder. Senile incontinence is a fictional term.

235. The answer is e. After ruling out secondary causes of incontinence, a post-void residual measurement should be taken. This can be done through catheterization or via US. A post-void residual less than 50 mL is normal. A post-void residual greater than 200 mL indicates inadequate bladder emptying and is consistent with overflow incontinence. Between 50 and 200 mL is indeterminate.

236. The answer is b. Kegel exercises are designed to strengthen the pelvic floor musculature. Patients are asked to squeeze the muscles in the genital area as if they were trying to stop the flow of urine from the urethra. They hold this contraction for 10 seconds, and repeat this many times in the day. Patients are then taught to contract these muscles and hold them during situations where incontinence may occur. They are most useful to treat stress incontinence, but may help with mixed incontinence as well. It is not helpful for functional, urge, or overflow incontinence.

237. The answer is a. Pharmacologic therapy is indicated for incontinence if a behavioral approach is ineffective. For urge incontinence, anticholinergic medications are the drugs of choice with oxybutynin (Ditropan) and tolterodine (Detrol) both indicated for symptoms. Pseudoephedrine has been shown to help stress incontinence, trimethoprim-sulfamethoxazole has been shown to help in the case of prostatitis, and finasteride and terazosin will help frequent voiding caused by prostatic hyperplasia.

238. The answer is c. Pharmaceuticals are a common cause of incontinence. There are many neural receptors involved in urination and, therefore, many medications that are used to treat other medical issues can often cause problems. Antihypertensives are especially problematic. α-Blockers cause urethral sphincter relaxation and can cause urinary leakage, but not urgency. Calcium channel blockers can cause urinary retention. Diuretics can cause increased frequency and urgency, but usually not leakage. β-Blockers inhibit bladder relaxation and therefore can cause both urinary leakage and urgency.

239. The answer is e. Many nonprescription agents may contribute to urinary symptoms. Alcohol has a diuretic effect and may cause polyuria or incontinence. Decongestants and diet pills may cause urinary retention if they include α-agonists. Antihistamines can cause urinary retention or functional incontinence. Caffeine has a diuretic effect and can cause polyuria. Marijuana abuse is not known to contribute to urinary symptoms.

240. The answer is a. Primary amenorrhea is defined as the absence of menses at age 15 in the presence of normal secondary sex characteristics, or absence of menses at age 13 in the absence of secondary sex characteristics. It is usually the result of a genetic or anatomic abnormality. Gonadal dysgenesis is the most common cause of primary amenorrhea, responsible for about 50% of the cases. The most well-known type is Turner syndrome (45 XO). Hypothalamic failure is often a result of anorexia nervosa, excessive exercise, chronic or systemic illness, and severe stress, and results from a suppression of hypothalamic gonadotropin-releasing hormone (GnRH) secretion. Pituitary failure may result from inadequate GnRH stimulation and is often associated with a history of head trauma, shock, infiltrative processes, pituitary adenoma, or craniopharyngioma. These patients will often display deficiency of other pituitary hormones as well. Polycystic ovarian syndrome may cause primary amenorrhea, but is generally associated with normal breast development. Constitutional delay of puberty, although common in boys, is an uncommon cause of amenorrhea in girls, but clinically is very hard to distinguish from other more common causes.

241. The answer is c. Pregnancy is the most common cause of secondary amenorrhea, and can even occur in a patient who claims that she has not been sexually active or says that she only has intercourse during "safe" times. Polycystic ovarian syndrome is common and is responsible for about 30% of the cases of secondary amenorrhea. It is characterized by androgen excess, and symptoms include irregular or absent menses, hirsutism, acne, and virilization. Functional hypothalamic amenorrhea is usually a result of anorexia, rapid weight loss, rigorous exercise, or significant emotional stress. Hypothyroidism and hyperprolactinemia can both be associated with secondary amenorrhea, but are less common causes.

242. The answer is c. Anovulatory bleeding is caused by continuous unopposed endometrial estrogen stimulation. Since these patients do not ovulate, progesterone from the corpus luteum is not secreted, the withdrawal from which would normally cause endometrial sloughing. When women are within 2 years of menarche, this is especially common, and can be followed expectantly. Alternatively, oral contraceptives can be used to regulate periods. Pregnancy should be ruled out, even in women who deny sexual activity. Ovulatory bleeding due to fluctuations in estrogen and progesterone levels is also a cause of abnormal bleeding, but accounts for only about 10% of cases. Leiomyomas and polyps may cause bleeding, but usually not in this age group.

243. The answer is d. If a postmenopausal woman has vaginal bleeding, she needs an endometrial biopsy to rule out endometrial cancer. In fact, this is usually the first step in the evaluation of this problem, after performing the examination and ruling out sexually transmitted infections or anatomic abnormalities. US evaluation may be needed, but this would not be the next step in the evaluation of this condition. Contraindications to this procedure include pregnancy, acute infection, PID, or known bleeding disorder (including Coumadin use).

244. The answer is a. Primary dysmenorrhea is caused by the release of prostaglandin from the endometrium at the time of menstruation. Treatment focuses on the reduction of endometrial prostaglandin production. This can occur either by using medications that inhibit prostaglandin synthesis, or by suppressing ovulation. NSAIDs are generally the first-line therapy, given their favorable risk to benefit ratio and effectiveness. They should be started a day before menstruation, if possible. Daily use of NSAIDs does not increase effectiveness and is associated with an increase of side effects. While opiate use may help with pain control, it does not inhibit prostaglandin synthesis and may lead to addiction. SSRI therapy is sometimes used for premenstrual dysphoric disorder, but is not a first-line therapy for dysmenorrhea. Oral contraceptive pills can be used and are effective, but are thought of as second-line therapy.

245. The answer is b. Many medications can cause hyperprolactinemia leading to amenorrhea. When hyperprolactinemia is related to medication, the measured prolactin level is usually less than 100 ng/mL. Many psychotropic medications can cause this, including benzodiazepines, SSRIs, tricyclic antidepressants, phenothiazines, and buspirone. Neurologic drugs that can increase prolactin levels include sumatriptan, valproate, and ergot derivatives. Estrogens and contraceptives can also elevate prolactin, as can some cardiovascular drugs (atenolol, verapamil, reserpine, and methyldopa). This is a less likely side effect in proton pump inhibitors, diuretics, ACE-inhibitors, and thyroid replacement.

246. The answer is a. When evaluating primary amenorrhea in patients with normal secondary sexual characteristics and a normal initial laboratory evaluation (pregnancy test, TSH assessment, and prolactin level), it is appropriate to perform a progestin challenge test. When there is no withdrawal bleeding, it either indicates inadequate estrogen production or an outflow tract obstruction. An estrogen-progestin challenge can differentiate between the two. No withdrawal bleeding after an estrogen-progestin challenge indicates an outflow tract obstruction or an anatomic defect.

247. The answer is c. Classically, ovarian cysts present with a unilateral dull pain that can become diffuse and severe if the cyst ruptures. On physical examination, the examiner feels a smooth mobile adnexal mass with peritoneal signs if the cyst ruptures. PID is associated with fever and vaginal discharge. Ectopic pregnancy may present with similar symptoms, but menses would not be normal. Uterine leiomyoma are generally asymptomatic if present in this age group, and if symptomatic would classically be associated with low midline pressure and menorrhagia or metrorrhagia. Appendicitis would be associated with fever, nausea, and anorexia.

248. The answer is d. PID is classically described as lower abdominal pain that is gradual in onset and bilateral. Fever, vaginal discharge, dysuria, and occasionally abnormal vaginal bleeding may be associated symptoms. Treatment should provide coverage for likely etiologic agents (*N gonorrhoeae, C trachomatis*, anaerobes, and enteric Gram-negative rods). The Center for Disease Control and Prevention (CDC) recommended outpatient regimen is ceftriaxone 250 mg IM plus doxycycline 100 mg BID for 14 days with or without metronidazole 500 mg BID for 14 days. Inpatient treatment with parenteral antibiotics is recommended for pregnant women, patients with severe illness with fever and vomiting, and cases where surgical emergencies can't be ruled out. Inpatient therapy may be necessary for those who fail an appropriate outpatient regimen as well.

249. The answer is b. The pain associated with ectopic pregnancy is often described as colicky, and may radiate to the shoulder if there is a significant hemoperitoneum. Nausea and breast tenderness, symptoms of pregnancy, are diagnostic clues.

250. The answer is d. The patient described has symptoms and signs suggestive of endometriosis. Endometriosis is found in 45% to 50% of women with chronic pelvic pain. Risk factors include family history, cigarette smoking lack of exercise, vaginal stenosis, and uterine abnormalities among others. Endometriosis can be treated medically or surgically (through laparoscopic ablation). Medications include oral contraceptives as first-line therapy, but this patient is trying to conceive. A levonorgestrel intrauterine system can also be effective, though not FDA approved for this use. An antispasmodic would be used if you thought the pelvic pain were caused by IBS. Adhesiolysis would be considered if pelvic adhesions were the cause of her symptoms.

251. The answer is c. Eighty percent of ovarian masses in girls younger than 15 years are malignant. Because of the high potential for malignancy, any adnexal mass should be evaluated by transvaginal US and referral for surgical removal. In many women of childbearing years, adnexal masses are commonly cysts. If the pain is not acute or recurrent, palpable cysts less than 6 cm in size may be monitored with repeat pelvic examination. US is reserved for those masses that do not resolve, or those that increase in size. CT and MRI may be useful in some cases, but the US is the best first test.

252. The answer is a. Epididymitis commonly occurs in sexually active males. It is generally caused by retrograde spread of prostatitis or urethral secretions through the vas deferens. In sexually active men younger than 35 years, it is usually associated with urethritis and caused by *N gonorrhoeae* or *C trachomatis*. It is less commonly caused by *Ureaplasma* or *Mycoplasma* in this age group. In men older than 35 who are sexually monogamous, it is more commonly caused by *E coli* and other enteric coliform bacteria.

253. The answer is b. Testicular torsion occurs most frequently in neonates or adolescent boys. In torsion, the cremasteric reflex (elicited by pinching or brushing the inner thigh which causes the ipsilateral testicle to retract toward the inguinal canal) is absent. If pain is relieved upon elevation of the testicle when the patient is supine, it is called a positive Prehn sign. This does not occur with testicular torsion, and in fact, elevation of the testicle often increases the pain. The cremasteric reflex and Prehn sign are positive in cases of epididymitis, hernias, orchitis, or cancer. When testicular torsion is confirmed, or when there is high clinical suspicion, immediate urologic referral is indicated, as the sooner surgery happens, the more likely you are to salvage the affected testis. If surgery is performed within 6 hours of the onset of pain, 90% of testicles will remain viable. If it occurs at 24 to 48 hours, only 10% remain viable.

254. The answer is d. Undescended testicle(s) or cryptorchidism occurs in 3% to 5% of term newborns, but occurs in up to 30% of premature infants. In most cases, the testis will descend on its own with time. Cryptorchidism does increase the risk of testicular cancer and can decrease fertility, so urologic consultation is indicated between the age of 6 to 12 months. The prevalence decreases to 1% by 1 year of age, so waiting that long is advisable.

255. The answer is a. The patient in this question has vulvovaginal candidiasis (VVC). For an uncomplicated infection, azole creams, ointments, suppositories, and oral antifungals all share similar efficacy and cure rates. Single-dose fluconazole is less expensive, better tolerated, and at least as effective as a 3 to 7 day intravaginal regimen, but relief of itching is slower than with topical azole antifungals. Metronidazole, clindamycin, or doxycycline would not be used to treat VVC.

256. The answer is c. The history and physical described are classic for trichomonas vaginalis. The classic "strawberry cervix" is a strong diagnostic clue. Trichomonads are seen on high power in the saline preparation, and appear as triangular cells with long tails, slightly larger than WBC. "Studded" epithelial cells (clue cells) are more consistent with bacterial vaginosis; "moth-eaten" cells (pseudo-clue cells) are seen in an acid-base disturbance of the vagina. Bacterial vaginosis will have few WBCs visible, whereas trichomonas vaginalis will present with many WBCs, and hyphae are consistent with vaginal candidiasis.

257. The answer is a. The condition described is bacterial vaginosis. Clue cells, epithelial cells studded with bacteria, are diagnostically helpful. The treatment of choice is topical or oral metronidazole, with oral or topical clindamycin being an acceptable alternative. Doxycycline is used to treat *Chlamydia*. Clotrimazole is used to treat fungal infections. Imiquimod is an immunomodulating agent approved to treat HPV infection, and acyclovir treats herpetic infections.

Recommended Reading: Urogenital

American Society for Colposcopy and Cervical Pathology Guidelines, ACSCCP.org, published 04/06/2016, last modified on 12/22/2017. Available at http://www.asccp.org/asccp-guidelines.

Carr RJ. Urinary incontinence. In: South-Paul JE, Matheny SC, Lewis EL (eds). *Current Diagnosis & Treatment Family Medicine.* 4th ed. New York, NY: McGraw-Hill.

Evans P. Vaginal bleeding. In: South-Paul JE, Matheny SC, Lewis EL (eds). *Current Diagnosis & Treatment Family Medicine.* 4th ed. New York, NY: McGraw-Hill.

Grasso-Knight G, Goodwin MA, Khanna N. Pelvic pain. In: Smith MA, Shimp LA, Schrager S (eds). *Family Medicine Ambulatory Care and Prevention.* 6th ed. New York, NY: McGraw-Hill.

Kaufman A. Amenorrhea. In: Smith MA, Shimp LA, Schrager S (eds). *Family Medicine Ambulatory Care and Prevention.* 6th ed. New York, NY: McGraw-Hill.

Krueger MV. Menstrual disorders. In: South-Paul JE, Matheny SC, Lewis EL (eds). *Current Diagnosis & Treatment Family Medicine*. 4th ed. New York, NY: McGraw-Hill.

Nduati MN, Heydt JA. Scrotal complaints. In: Smith MA, Shimp LA, Schrager S (eds). *Family Medicine Ambulatory Care and Prevention*. 6th ed. New York, NY: McGraw-Hill.

Paladine HL, Shah, PA. Abnormal vaginal bleeding. In: Smith MA, Shimp LA, Schrager S (eds). *Family Medicine Ambulatory Care and Prevention*. 6th ed. New York, NY: McGraw-Hill.

Ramakrishnan K. Enuresis. In: Smith MA, Shimp LA, Schrager S (eds). *Family Medicine Ambulatory Care and Prevention*. 6th ed. New York, NY: McGraw-Hill.

Reilly K, Fox A. The abnormal Pap smear. In: Smith MA, Shimp LA, Schrager S (eds). *Family Medicine Ambulatory Care and Prevention*. 6th ed. New York, NY: McGraw-Hill.

Rew KT, Walker, LL. Urinary symptoms in men. In: Smith MA, Shimp LA, Schrager S (eds). *Family Medicine Ambulatory Care and Prevention*. 6th ed. New York, NY: McGraw-Hill.

Schwiebert LP. Dysuria in women. In: Smith MA, Shimp LA, Schrager S (eds). *Family Medicine Ambulatory Care and Prevention*. 6th ed. New York, NY: McGraw-Hill.

Schwiebert LP. Vaginal discharge. In: Smith MA, Shimp LA, Schrager S (eds). *Family Medicine Ambulatory Care and Prevention*. 6th ed. New York, NY: McGraw-Hill.

Waickus CM. Hematuria. In: Smith MA, Shimp LA, Schrager S (eds). *Family Medicine Ambulatory Care and Prevention*. 6th ed. New York, NY: McGraw-Hill.

Acute Complaints—Hematologic and Other Causes of Fatigue

258. The answer is c. Anemias can often be classified by cell size. Causes of microcytic anemias include iron deficiency, anemia of chronic disease, thalassemia, and sideroblastic anemias. In iron deficiency, the RDW would be elevated due to variation in cell size. Vitamin B_{12} deficiency causes a macrocytic anemia not a microcytic anemia. In thalassemia, the RDW would be normal because the red cells are uniformly small. Aplastic anemia and anemia due to chronic renal insufficiency are generally normocytic. In a patient with mild to moderate microcytic anemia due to iron deficiency, a trial of iron therapy is indicated. Iron comes in various preparations including ferrous sulfate, gluconate, or fumarate. Up to 180 mg of elemental iron can be given daily; 300 mg of ferrous sulfate is equivalent to 60 mg of elemental iron while 300 mg of ferrous gluconate contains 34 mg of elemental iron daily. Erythropoietin is useful to treat anemia of chronic disease and B_{12} supplementation is indicated in B_{12} deficiency, but not iron deficiency. A bone marrow biopsy is not indicated in a stable patient with mild iron-deficiency anemia.

259. The answer is a. The laboratory evaluation in this patient clearly indicates iron-deficiency anemia. The most common cause is blood loss. Poor nutrition and/or inadequate absorption are less common causes. In females, menstrual blood loss is an important cause of iron-deficiency anemia. Chronic disease would lead to a high or normal ferritin and a low TIBC. Folic acid deficiency would lead to an elevated MCV.

260. The answer is d. The patient described has a laboratory profile suspicious for thalassemia minor. These patients have low hemoglobin and MCV, but in contrast to iron deficiency, the patients have an elevated RBC and normal RDW. Additionally, the MCV is low out of proportion to the anemia. Given that the patient is asymptomatic, he should be treated only if necessary. Iron supplementation should be avoided as it can lead to iron overload. Treatment includes transfusion if blood loss leads to significant anemia. The patient should have genetic counseling if planning a family.

261. The answer is c. Some clinical features are common to all megaloblastic anemias—anemia, pallor, weight loss, fatigue, and glossitis to name a few. Neurologic symptoms are specific to vitamin B_{12} deficiency. Typically, treatment has been with parenteral vitamin B_{12} replacement weekly for 1 month, often with concurrent administration of folic acid. However, recent studies have shown that oral replacement of vitamin B_{12} at levels of 1000 to 2000 mgc daily is equivalent to IM treatment.

262. The answer is e. Most often, vitamin B_{12} deficiency is a result of inadequate absorption. Since vitamin B_{12} is present in all animal products, only strict vegans or people not ingesting animal products would be deficient from a dietary standpoint. Vitamin B_{12} deficiency is not a side effect of hydrochlorothiazide. Alcohol can impact intracellular processing of folic acid, but not vitamin B_{12}.

263. The answer is b. The slide shows sickle-cell anemia, an autosomal recessive trait seen in those of African, Mediterranean, or Asian heritage. It is found before the age of 6 in 90% of patients, with acute pain crises as the most common presentation. Prophylaxis for pain crises involves ensuring adequate oxygenation and hydration. Immunization against streptococcal infection is appropriate, as most patients are functionally asplenic. The patients often have daily prophylaxis with penicillin until the age of 5. Immunization and antibiotic prophylaxis do not, however, prevent pain crises. Chronic analgesics and scheduled transfusions have not been shown to reduce pain crises. Hydroxyurea, a myelosuppressive agent, has been proven to reduce the frequency of painful episodes.

264. The answer is d. Mononucleosis is often mistaken for streptococcal pharyngitis. Both have symptoms of sore throat, fatigue, fever, and adenopathy. Lymphadenopathy is more widespread in mononucleosis and usually confined to the anterior nodes in streptococcal pharyngitis. If patients with mononucleosis are given ampicillin (and other penicillin derivatives), up to 100% may develop the rash described above, sometimes confused as an allergic reaction to penicillin. The rash of scarlet fever is more confluent, and has a sandpaper-like texture. The rash of rubella is similar in appearance to that of mononucleosis, but exudative pharyngitis is absent.

265. The answer is a. Fatigue is a subjective complaint, and is the seventh most common symptom in primary care, accounting for more than 10 million office visits annually. Fatigue lasting 1 month or less is likely the result of a physical cause (infections, endocrine imbalances, cardiovascular disease, anemia, or medications), while fatigue lasting 3 months or more is more likely to be related to psychologic factors (depression, anxiety, stress, or adjustment reactions). Physiologic fatigue is because of overwork, lack of sleep, or a defined physical stressor like pregnancy. Depression is one of the most common diagnoses in patients presenting with fatigue, especially when denying weakness or hypersomnolence, lasting more than 3 months, and not becoming progressively worse. Once the complaint is defined, the practitioner should screen for depression. Screening for sleep apnea, anemia, hypothyroidism, and pregnancy should occur if the depression screen is negative.

266. The answer is d. The initial laboratory workup for an uncertain diagnosis of fatigue included a CBC, sedimentation rate, urinalysis, chemistry panel, thyroid testing, pregnancy testing (for women of childbearing age), and age/gender appropriate cancer screening. In a 55-year-old African-American man, a prostate screen would be appropriate. Chest x-ray, ECG, HIV test, and a drug screen would be appropriate if the initial screen is negative.

Recommended Reading: Hematologic and Other Causes of Fatigue

Dailey-Garnes NJM, Shandera WX. Viral & rickettsial infections. In: Papadakis MA, McPhee SJ, Rabow MW (eds). *Current Medical Diagnosis & Treatment 2018*. New York, NY: McGraw-Hill.

Jones AD, Clarke CL. Anemia. In: Smith MA, Shimp LA, Schrager S (eds). *Family Medicine Ambulatory Care and Prevention*. 6th ed. New York, NY: McGraw-Hill.

Primack BA, Mahaniah KJ. Anemia. In: South-Paul JE, Matheny SC, Lewis EL (eds). *Current Diagnosis & Treatment Family Medicine*. 4th ed. New York, NY: McGraw-Hill.

Valdini AF. Fatigue. In: Smith MA, Shimp LA, Schrager S (eds). *Family Medicine Ambulatory Care and Prevention*. 6th ed. New York, NY: McGraw-Hill.

Acute Complaints—Musculoskeletal

267. The answer is d. Achilles tendon rupture usually causes acute onset pain in the posterior heel. Examination will usually reveal a palpable tear of the Achilles tendon, but you will also see swelling and ecchymosis over the posterior heel. The Thompson test (no plantar flexion when the calf is squeezed) is positive. Treatment is surgical, and the patient should be immediately referred to orthopedics. A Lisfranc injury is a severe mid foot sprain to the tarsometatarsal articulation. Pain and swelling over the area and inability to bear weight on the tiptoes are clues to the injury. A tarsal navicular bone fracture should be considered when the patient has tenderness over the navicular bone and increased pain with hopping on the affected foot. Plantar fasciitis should be suspected when the patient has dull achy pain in the inferior heel, especially after a period of rest. Rupture is unusual. A calcanea fracture will present with pain over the fracture site.

268. The answer is b. The patient described has symptoms consistent with classic plantar fasciitis. Most times, the condition is caused by overuse and/or excessive weight. Signs and symptoms include dully achy pain in the inferior heel, worse with weight bearing after a period of rest. The symptoms actually improve with use, as the plantar fascia stretches. Physical examination findings include tenderness over the calcaneal tubercle and arch, and no imaging is generally necessary until conservative treatment fails. Conservative treatment includes stretching and strengthening of the plantar fascia and Achilles tendon, arch support or a heel cup, and a night splint. NSAIDs are also helpful for symptomatic relief. Physical therapy can help if there is no improvement after a few weeks of conservative treatment, and a planar fascia injection may be necessary if there is no response to NSAIDs. Referral to a foot specialist should occur if there is no improvement after 6 months of conservative therapy.

269. The answer is a. Neck pain is commonly seen in family medicine. In fact, the lifetime prevalence of at least one episode of neck pain in the adult population is estimated to be between 40% and 70%. Pain aggravated by movement, worse after activities, associated with a dull ache and with limited range of motion is consistent with spondylosis or osteoarthritis. If the pain were due to chronic mechanical problems, there would be tenderness to palpation on examination. If cervical nerve root irritation were the diagnosis, there would be radiation of symptoms, weakness, numbness, or paresthesias. With a whiplash injury, one would expect a history of an acceleration injury. And, with cervical dystonia (torticollis), the neck would be laterally flexed and rotated.

270. The answer is b. The patient likely has spinal stenosis. He is an older individual, and describes axial stiffness and paresthesias over several dermatomes (C7-T1). In this case, a CT scan is the best choice. C-spine radiographs are indicated after injury, or if there are red-flags identified (see next question). MRI provides the best anatomic assessment of disk herniation and soft tissue or spinal cord abnormalities. EMG would help localize radiculopathy, but that is not necessary in this case.

271. The answer is b. The Canadian cervical spine rules help determine who should receive radiography. There are three questions to ask:

- Is there one high-risk factor? High-risk factors include age more than 65 years, dangerous mechanism (including high-speed motor vehicle accident), or numbness/tingling in the extremities. A "yes" answer to any of the above requires radiography.

- Is there one low-risk factor? Low-risk factors include a simple rear-end collision, if the patient was ambulatory at any time at the scene, if there was absence of neck pain at the scene, and if there was absence of C-spine tenderness on examination. A "no" answer to any of the above would require radiography.
- Is the patient able to voluntarily actively rotate the neck 45 degrees to the left and right regardless of pain? A "no" answer to that question would require radiography.

Since the answer to the first question is "yes" in this case, the patient would require C-spine radiography.

272. The answer is d. The Spurling test is also called the neck compression test. It requires the patient to bend his/her head to the side and rotate the head toward the side of pain while the tester exerts downward pressure. The maneuver reproduces symptoms in the affected upper extremity in the case of nerve root injury. It has a high specificity, but a low sensitivity for cervical radiculopathy. Nonspecific mechanical pain should be considered to be the diagnosis if the maneuver results in neck discomfort only.

273. The answer is a. There are several findings that are clues to serious underlying conditions or diseases that warrant further workup for neck pain. They include:

- The presence of radiculopathy: if the patient has sensory or motor changes, spasticity or bladder/bowel changes, further workup is indicated.
- The concern for infection: patients with fever or chills, an immunocompromising condition, or alcohol/drug abuse, further workup is indicated.
- The concern for a fracture: patients with significant trauma or a history of osteoporosis should be further evaluated.
- The concern for a tumor: patients with a history of unexplained weight loss, a history of cancer, or age less than 20 or more than 49 should be further evaluated.

274. The answer is d. Treatment for a shoulder dislocation consists of pain management and relocation. After relocation, the shoulder should be immobilized for up to 3 weeks to allow for capsular healing. Then, range of motion exercises and strengthening should be started. Younger patients may have a higher recurrence rate, and surgical referral should be entertained, but it is not necessary immediately. Immediate return to play would likely result in recurrence. An MRI is not necessary in this setting.

275. The answer is c. Rotator cuff tendonitis is most common in men between the ages of 40 and 50. Hawkins test, which is positive when the patient has pain and/or diminished motion when the shoulder is passively moved into internal rotation and forward flexed to 90 degrees, has almost 90% sensitivity but only ~40% specificity for diagnosing rotator cuff tendonitis. The cross-arm maneuver is specific for acromioclavicular (AC) joint pathology and is performed by passively moving the extended arm across the body toward the other shoulder. Spurling maneuver, axial compression of the cervical spine, is used to diagnose cervical spine pathology and/or radicular symptoms cause by cervical spine dysfunction. The sulcus test, a noticeable gap between the acromion and humeral head with a caudal load, is a sign of glenohumeral joint instability. The O'Brien test is useful to diagnose labral pathology and AC joint pathology. The evaluator asks the patient to forward flex their extended arm to 90 degrees and then internally rotates the arm and slightly adducts. A positive test occurs if downward pressure applied to the arm results in pain. This test has been shown to have close to 100% positive and negative predictive value.

276. The answer is b. Adhesive capsulitis is characterized by painful loss of shoulder motion in all planes. The etiology is not well understood, but the condition is more commonly seen in patients with diabetes. It often resolves spontaneously, but is exquisitely painful for many patients. Treatment should be directed at reducing symptoms and improving range of motion. Physical therapy with gentle range of motion exercises, stretching, and graded resistance training is effective in directing recovery. Corticosteroids, which can improve pain, do not seem to hasten recovery. If steroid injection is desired to reduce pain, it would be placed in the glenohumeral joint, not the subacromial space. While MRI of the shoulder is useful to rule out other conditions, it is not the most useful next step to improve the patient's condition. Finally, manipulation under anesthesia should be reserved for patients whose symptoms are refractory to other treatment modalities.

277. The answer is a. Iliotibial band syndrome is the most common cause of lateral knee pain in an athlete. It is most commonly seen in athletes who participate in repetitive knee flexion activities like distance runners, dancers, tennis players, and cyclists. The patient will present with pain or ache over the lateral aspect of the knee that worsens with activity, and on examination has pain and tightness over the IT band. Patellofemoral pain syndrome would present with diffuse knee pain and a positive patellar grind test. MCL sprains, ACL sprains, and meniscal tears would not present with lateral pain.

278. The answer is b. The twisting injury, feeling of a "pop," and immediate effusion while still being able to bear weight are consistent with an ACL tear. The sense of instability also helps lead toward that diagnosis. Patellofemoral pain would generally not occur acutely or after an injury. The mechanism of a PCL injury is through direct force to the knee. Meniscal injuries also cause knee pain, and are frequently associated with ACL tears, but are more likely to cause locking, catching, or giving way. Medial collateral ligament sprains are generally caused by a valgus stress to a partially flexed knee. The sprain would present with pain over the medial aspect of the knee, but does not have swelling of the joint.

279. The answer is c. Once the diagnosis of ACL tear is confirmed in an athlete who wants to return to a high level of activity, ACL reconstruction is likely needed. This is because the blood supply to the ACL is poor, and ACL tears are not likely to repair on their own. Timing of reconstruction is important, and experts recommend surgery 3 to 4 weeks after injury to allow for decreased swelling, increased range of motion, and improved strength before surgery. During the presurgical time, physical therapy to focus on knee strengthening may shorten recovery time.

280. The answer is c. The symptoms described are consistent with patellofemoral pain syndrome, one of the most common diagnosis for patients with anterior knee pain presenting to their primary care physician. The pain is typically worse with walking, running, ascending or descending stairs, or squatting or sitting for prolonged periods of time (the theatre sign). The goal of treatment is pain reduction and return to previous levels of activity. Strengthening the quadriceps muscles has been found to reduce pain. Strengthening the hip abductors, internal rotators, and knee flexors is generally treatment for iliotibial band syndrome, but would not generally help patellofemoral syndrome. Bracing and taping have not been shown to have better outcomes than physical therapy alone.

281. The answer is a. The Ottawa ankle rules are a useful guide to use when determining if radiographs are necessary after an ankle injury. Films should be obtained if there is an inability to bear weight both immediately after an injury and in the office, OR for the following findings:

- Pain is present near the malleoli PLUS there is bone tenderness in the posterior half of the lower 6 cm of the tibia or fibula.
- Pain is present in the midfoot PLUS there is bone tenderness at the navicular or the base of the 5th metatarsal.

Rest, ice compression, and elevation are mainstays of therapy, but the x-ray is imperative in this case. Early mobilization is recommended unless there is a fracture present. NSAIDs or acetaminophen can be used for pain control, but the x-ray is the most important next step. Physical therapy may expedite the return to activity, but only after a fracture has been ruled out.

282. The answer is d. The treatment for mallet finger is continuous extension splinting of the DIP joint for at least 6 weeks. At the end of the 6-week period, it is recommended to continue with nighttime splinting and activity splinting for another 6 weeks to ensure healing and to avoid surgery. If the finger is allowed to flex at any time during the initial 6 weeks of splinting, the 6-week clock starts over. If it is not completely healed after the initial 6 weeks, splinting for another 6 weeks should be tried prior to surgical referral.

283. The answer is d. Acute low back pain is commonly encountered by the family physician. Most patients do not have evidence of serious pathology and 70% of patients improve within 2 weeks. In patients without red flags for serious pathology (such as history of trauma, age > 50 years, history of cancer, unexplained weight loss, severe or progressive neurologic deficit, fever, or immunosuppression), imaging is not helpful in the first 2 to 4 weeks of treatment. Treatment options should be aimed at reducing pain and restoring function. Graded, or reduced activity has not been shown to improve pain or function and bed rest beyond 24 hours should be avoided. NSAIDs are effective in the short- term at reducing acute low back pain symptoms. The addition of muscle relaxants to NSAIDs has not been shown to provide any additional relief and the drowsiness associated with these agents may limit the patient's activity and ambulation.

284. The answer is c. Spondylolysis is the most commonly identifiable cause of low back pain in adolescent athletes, occurring in up to 45% of these patients. It is caused by a unilateral defect in the pars interarticularis, most frequently in the lumbar spine and usually a result of overuse and repetitive extension of the lumbar spine. Onset is usually insidious, but the condition can also occur as the result of trauma. Spondylolisthesis occurs when a bilateral defect allows the vertebral body to slide forward on the vertebral body below it. Pain with extension of the lumbar spine is the cardinal finding of spondylolysis. Single-photon emission computed tomography (SPECT) scan is the best diagnostic test for spondylolysis. MRI can alternatively be considered if avoiding radiation exposure is paramount; however, it's not as sensitive for the detection of pars defect compared to SPECT imaging. Plain radiographs can be useful in the evaluation of spondylolysis, but the large radiation load of the oblique views and limited sensitivity has caused this to fall out of favor. Plain CT of the lumbar spine is quite accurate at diagnosing spondylolysis but is not recommended in children and adolescents due to the high radiation exposure.

Recommended Reading: Musculoskeletal

Barrett JR. Foot conditions. In: Smith MA, Shimp LA, Schrager S (eds). *Family Medicine Ambulatory Care and Prevention*. 6th ed. New York, NY: McGraw-Hill.

Bowen JE, Malanga GA, Tutankhamen P, et al. Physical examination of the shoulder. In: Malanga GA, Nadler SF. *Musculoskeletal Physical Examination: An Evidence-Based Approach*. Philadelphia, PA: Elsevier.

Coleman BR. Arm and shoulder complaints. In: Smith MA, Shimp LA, Schrager S (eds). *Family Medicine Ambulatory Care and Prevention*. 6th ed. New York, NY: McGraw-Hill.

Criswell D. Low back pain. In: Smith MA, Shimp LA, Schrager S (eds). *Family Medicine Ambulatory Care and Prevention*. 6th ed. New York, NY: McGraw-Hill.

Palmer PR. Ankle injuries. In: Smith MA, Shimp LA, Schrager S (eds). *Family Medicine Ambulatory Care and Prevention*. 6th ed. New York, NY: McGraw-Hill.

Porter AST. Common sports injuries. In: Bope ET, Kellerman RD (eds). *Conn's Current Therapy, 2017*. Philadelphia, PA: Elsevier.

Rodriguez V, Kaminski MA. Knee complaints. In: Smith MA, Shimp LA, Schrager S (eds). *Family Medicine Ambulatory Care and Prevention*. 6th ed. New York, NY: McGraw-Hill.

Rowane MP. Neck pain. In: Smith MA, Shimp LA, Schrager S (eds). *Family Medicine Ambulatory Care and Prevention*. 6th ed. New York, NY: McGraw-Hill.

Standaert CJ, Herring SA. Expert opinion and controversies in spots and musculoskeletal medicine: the diagnosis and treatment of spondylolysis in adolescent athletes. *Archives of Physical Medicine and Rehabilitation*. 2007;88(4):537-540.

Acute Complaints—Neurological

285. The answer is a. "Dizziness" is a subjective symptom, often meaning different things to different people. It is imperative that this complaint be better characterized to develop an appropriate differential diagnosis and treatment plan. Vertigo is a rotational sensation, in which the room spins around the patient. Patients will often say that the room is "spinning" or that they feel a sense of falling forward or backward. Orthostasis refers to light-headedness upon arising, common with orthostatic hypotension. Presyncope is a feeling of impending faint. Disequilibrium is a sensation of unsteadiness, or a loss of balance. Light-headedness is often vaguely described as a "floating" sensation.

286. The answer is e. The patient described has benign positional vertigo (BPV). While symptom relief can occur with medications, treatment involves physical therapy protocols (including the Epley maneuver or Brandt-Daroff exercises). Oral meclizine and diazepam may be helpful to treat other causes of vertigo, including Meniere Syndrome, acute labyrinthitis, vestibular neuritis, or traumatic vertigo. Migraine prophylactic therapies including β-blockers or valproate may be used to treat migrainous vertigo, but would be less helpful here. Intratympanic corticosteroids are used for refectory cases of Meniere Syndrome.

287. The answer is c. Acoustic neuromas typically present with unilateral tinnitus and hearing loss. The symptoms are constant and slowly progressive. They are among the most common intracranial tumors. Most are unilateral, with benign lesions arising within the internal auditory canal, and gradually growing to involve the cerebellopontine angle. Nonclassic presentations are fairly common, and any individual with a unilateral or asymmetric sensorineural hearing loss should be evaluated. Vestibular neuronitis presents with an acute onset of severe vertigo lasting several days, with symptoms improving over several weeks. Benign positional vertigo typically involves symptoms with position changes only. Meniere disease presents with discrete attacks of vertigo lasting for several hours, associated with nausea and vomiting, hearing loss, and tinnitus. A cerebellar tumor would typically present with disequilibrium as opposed to tinnitus.

288. The answer is a. The Dix-Hallpike maneuver, described in the question, is often useful to distinguish central from peripheral causes of vertigo. With a peripheral cause of vertigo, the latency time for the onset of symptoms of vertigo or nystagmus is 3 to 10 seconds, the symptoms are severe, and the direction of the nystagmus is fixed. In addition, repeating the maneuver lessens the symptoms. With a central cause of vertigo, there is no latency to onset of symptoms, no lessening of symptoms with repeat maneuvers, the direction of the nystagmus changes, and the symptoms are of mild intensity. Of the above answers, all are peripheral causes of vertigo, except the correct answer, stroke.

289. The answer is b. Once diagnosed with a peripheral vestibular disorder, antihistamines are the first-line therapy for symptomatic relief. They suppress the vestibular end-organ receptors and inhibit activation of the vagal response. Meclizine (Antivert), 25 mg orally every 4 to 6 hours and diphenhydramine (Benadryl), 50 mg orally every 4 to 6 hours are commonly recommended choices. Antiemetics may be used if nausea and vomiting are prominent symptoms. Benzodiazepines may be helpful in symptom reduction, but are usually second-line agents. NSAIDs and antibiotics are not helpful.

290. The answer is a. While many agents, including some anticonvulsants, have been used as prophylactic agents to prevent migraines, β-blockers are the most studied, and are effective. Propranolol, metoprolol, valproic acid, and topiramate all have data to support their efficacy. Amitriptyline has some data to say it is "probably" effective, while there is insufficient evidence for or against the use of gabapentin. Clonazepam has not been shown to be effective in migraine prophylaxis.

291. The answer is a. The goal of prophylactic migraine therapy is to reduce the frequency of headache by 50%. Of the antidepressants, the strongest evidence for efficacy involves amitriptyline. Therapy begins with a low dose (10 mg at night) and can be titrated up to the most effective dose that does not cause prohibitive side effects (up to 150 mg). SSRIs, MAOIs, and other antidepressants have been variably studied, but the best evidence supports the use of amitriptyline, a tricyclic antidepressant.

292. The answer is a. Warning signs include a headache that has its onset after the age of 50 years, a very sudden onset, increase in severity or frequency, with signs of systemic disease, new-onset headache in a patient with an immunocompromising condition, focal neurologic symptoms (except those consistent with a visual aura typical for a known migraine sufferer), papilledema, or a headache after trauma. Migraines often occur in a consistent location, are severe and frequent, include a visual aura, and may be associated with severe nausea.

293. The answer is c. Abortive or acute therapy for migraines is appropriate monotherapy if attacks occur less than two to four times per month. The most effective approach will be tailored to the individual and his/her needs; however, an abortive medication with receptor-specific action (a triptan) should be the first choice if possible. Ergot alkaloids are a good alternative. If triptans or ergot alkaloids fail or are contraindicated, rescue medications (simple analgesics) may be tried. Although frequently used in emergency settings, narcotics are rarely needed in the treatment plan for migraine sufferers.

294. The answer is b. Tension-type headaches (TTHs) are typically unilateral, described as a tightening or pressure sensation, and not associated with nausea/vomiting or photo/phonophobia. Initially, acetaminophen or NSAID treatment is recommended for episodic headaches. However, prophylactic therapy should be considered in patients who take medication more than 9 days per month in order to avoid medication rebound headaches. Amitriptyline and SSRIs have been shown to improve headaches and decrease analgesic use. Butalbital and opioid drugs should be avoided since they come with a significant risk of dependence and medication overuse headaches. Topiramate has not been well studied in TTH and sumatriptan is an abortive agent used in the treatment of migraine headaches.

295. The answer is d. Cluster headaches characteristically develop rapidly, and tend to recur frequently in a period of time or "cluster." Usually, the headaches are intensely painful and last for about 45 to 90 minutes without treatment. The mainstay of treatment is acute abortive therapy is oxygen. In general, oral medications are not helpful, including the oral serotonin antagonists. Subcutaneous or intranasal triptans and ergotamine have been shown to be more efficacious. For prophylactic management, nifedipine has been shown to be effective, as has prednisone, indomethacin, and lithium. However, the medication should not be given daily, just during the symptomatic period. Fluoxetine has not been shown to be beneficial.

296. The answer is b. TTH have a formal definition, with positive and negative criteria for diagnosis, but many physicians diagnose this type of headache by exclusion (after ruling out more interesting or rare etiologies for headache). They are in fact, the most frequent of all headaches encountered in clinical practice. The episodes last from 30 minutes to several days, and headaches should occur less than 15 times per month. It requires at least two of the following characteristics:

- Pressure/tightness
- Bilateral
- Mild to moderate
- Not aggravated by activity

There is generally no nausea. Either photophobia or phonophobia may be present, but not both. If criteria for this classification of headache are met, a trial of NSAIDs may be appropriate, with follow-up if there is no improvement. Narcotics should be avoided, since the condition is generally chronic, and overuse is likely. Imaging would not be helpful or indicated at this stage.

297. The answer is e. Drug- and alcohol-related sleep disturbances are common, and can take many forms. Some medications cause excessive somnolence, some cause nightmares or other problems that inhibit sleep, and others cause excessive wakefulness making it difficult to fall or stay asleep. Obesity is a risk factor for sleep apnea, but that generally does not cause inability to return to sleep after waking. Propranolol is known to cause nightmares, but not the problems described by this patient. Hydrochlorothiazide can cause nocturia that inhibits sleep, and naproxen is not known to interfere with sleep. Alcohol is known to cause excessive wakefulness, and often allows people to fall asleep, but interferes with the ability to stay asleep.

298. The answer is c. Good sleep hygiene is essential for treating insomnia. Important aspects of sleep hygiene include awakening at a regular hour, exercising daily (but not too close to bedtime), control the sleep environment, eat a light snack before bedtime (not a meal), limit or eliminate alcohol, caffeine and nicotine, go to bed when sleepy, use your bed for sleep and intimacy only (not for reading or watching television), and get out of bed if you aren't asleep within 15 to 30 minutes.

Pharmacologic agents may be used in select cases of transient sleep disorders unassociated with more serious problems. Before using any agents, it is important to make sure the patient maintains excellent sleep hygiene. Zolpidem (Ambien), eszopiclone (Lunesta), or zaleplon (Sonata) may be used to decrease sleep latency. Only zaleplon can be redosed, due to its shorter half-life and they can be taken in the middle of the night to help with sleep maintenance. Melatonin has been shown to help with adjustments to the sleep-wake cycle (as with jet lag or shift work). Benadryl can cause excessive somnolence, and may help with sleep onset, but not maintenance.

299. The answer is c. Dementia is an acquired, persistent, and progressive impairment in intellectual function with compromise of memory and at least one other cognitive domain. This may be aphasia, apraxia, agnosia, or impaired executive function. In dementia, the level of consciousness is not clouded, but disorientation may occur later in the illness. Hypertension and diabetes may be seen with both delirium and dementia. The inability to complete serial sevens (count backward from 100 by 7s) may be related to dementia, but may also have to do with the patient's baseline educational level. Although his symptoms have appeared recently, it is often difficult to pinpoint the exact onset of dementia. Delirium is seen as being more abrupt in onset.

300. The answer is a. Delirium and dementia are often clinically difficult to distinguish, especially if you are unfamiliar with the patient. Disorientation is characteristic of both processes, as is a disturbed sleep-wake cycle. His history of hypertension would lead one to think of multi-infarct dementia, rather than delirium. Responsiveness to questions may be a feature of either process, though patients with delirium often have a shortened attention span. Delirium and dementia both can cause disorientation in the early morning hours, and therefore timing does not point to one or the other diagnosis. The abrupt onset of a mental status change is consistent with delirium as opposed to dementia, which occurs insidiously.

301. The answer is e. Management of delirium is largely supportive and includes reassurance and reorientation, treatment of underlying causes, eliminating unnecessary medications, and avoidance of restraints. Pharmacologic therapies should be reserved for severely agitate patients, psychotic patients, or those who are likely to harm themselves or others. Medical management is best accomplished by antipsychotic agents like haloperidol, 0.5 to 1 mg orally, or quetiapine, 25 mg orally. The other medications listed are known to increase the risk of delirium, as are other sedative/hypnotics, anticholinergics, benzodiazepines, and antihistamines.

302. The answer is c. The patient described has a hypertensive encephalopathy. With his severe hypertension, a stroke may be considered, but unlikely without focal neurologic deficits. Sixth nerve palsy may be seen in a stroke. Pinpoint pupils would be more consistent with narcotic excess, unlikely given his vital signs and history. Dilated pupils suggests sympathetic outflow, and may be consistent with delirium tremens, but the history and physical is not consistent with this. Papilledema is seen with hypertensive encephalopathy. Anisocoria of 1 mm is a nonspecific finding that can be seen in normal individuals.

303. The answer is d. When patients exhibit signs of delirium, defining the subtype can help to determine the cause. Hypoactive delirium requires four of the following symptoms: unawareness, decreased alertness reduced or delayed speech, lethargy, slowed movements, apathy, diminished appetite, or new incontinence. Hyperactive delirium requires three of the following symptoms: hypervigilance, restlessness, fast/loud speech, irritability, combativeness, impatience, swearing, singing, laughing, uncooperativeness, euphoria, anger, wandering, distractibility, and others. Mixed delirium is a combination of both behaviors. The patient described has hyperactive confusion, and this is common with alcohol withdrawal. Withdrawal from levothyroxine would cause hypothyroidism, and would present with psychomotor slowing. Fluoxetine usually does not cause a withdrawal syndrome, but may be associated with depressive symptoms. Opiate withdrawal does not present with a confusional state. Amphetamine withdrawal would be associated with psychomotor slowing.

304. The answer is e. Conjunctivitis is the most common cause of red eye seen in the primary care office. Symptoms of conjunctivitis include increased redness, irritation, tearing, discharge, and/or itching. The character of the eye discharge is sometimes useful in distinguishing bacterial from viral conjunctivitis, with bacterial causes associated with purulent discharge and viral causes associated with more watery discharge. However, one meta-analysis recently failed to find evidence that discharge character is diagnostically useful. Eye pain is suggestive of a more serious problem, possibly acute angle closure glaucoma, uveitis, scleritis, keratitis, a foreign body, or a corneal abrasion.

305. The answer is e. Of the symptoms of conjunctivitis, itching is more specific for allergic conditions. Irritation, tearing, and discharge are more general symptoms, and not useful in differentiating allergic conjunctivitis from other causes. Allergic conjunctivitis is more characteristically bilateral; therefore, single-eye involvement in this case would not point to allergic conjunctivitis.

306. The answer is c. Viral conjunctivitis is most commonly caused by members of the Adenovirus family. It can be transmitted through ocular and respiratory secretions and less commonly from fomites on towels or equipment. Typically it starts in one eye, and spreads to the other after a few days. The natural course is self-limiting, lasting around 10 to 14 days. It is highly contagious, and people diagnosed should avoid close contact with others for up to 2 weeks. Supportive treatment is indicated. Although topical antibiotics have been prescribed to try to prevent bacterial superinfection, there is no good evidence that it makes any significant impact.

307. The answer is d. Bacterial conjunctivitis is most commonly caused by *Streptococcus* and *Staphylococcus*. However, there are increasing reports of conjunctivitis caused by methicillin-resistant *S aureus* (MRSA). MRSA conjunctivitis manifests as bacterial conjunctivitis resistant to conventional therapy, and is treated with the same drugs used to treat MRSA in other parts of the body. Cultures should be obtained when MRSA is suspected. It is likely that the other oral or topical antibiotics listed would not cure MRSA, and an ophthalmology referral is not necessary unless treatment is unsuccessful.

308. The answer is a. The patient described in the question has conjunctivitis-otitis media syndrome. It is a common condition in which children with otitis media also have a purulent ocular discharge and bilateral conjunctivitis. It responds to treatment for the otitis media, and therefore no additional treatment for the conjunctivitis is necessary.

309. The answer is d. The patient in this question has a subconjunctival hemorrhage. In this condition, the redness of the eye is localized and sharply circumscribed, with the underlying sclera not being visible. There is generally no discharge, no pain, and no vision disturbance. These hemorrhages can be spontaneous, but can also arise from trauma, hypertension, bleeding disorders, or from straining (as with severe coughing, retching, or straining during defecation). In this case, the intrathoracic pressure increase from patient's vomiting is the likely cause. Referral to an ophthalmologist is only indicated if the hemorrhage is from trauma, or if it does not spontaneously resolve in 2 to 3 weeks. If there are recurrent episodes, consideration of other causes should be included in the differential.

310. The answer is c. In the evaluation of patients with syncope, a systematic history and physical examination alone can elucidate the cause in up to 45% of cases. Since cardiac syncope has a 2-year mortality rate of 30% compared to 6% of all other causes, testing should be directed at differentiating cardiac from noncardiac causes. As such, initial testing should include an ECG always. Although the diagnostic yield is low (around 5%), the ECG can reveal structural heart diseases and can be helpful in uncovering arrhythmogenic causes of syncope.

311. The answer is a. In syncopal patients who present with a heart murmur, echocardiography should be obtained. It will help rule out valvular heart disease, but will also identify hypertrophic cardiomyopathy (the likely cause in this question). Holter monitoring and long-term ambulatory loop ECG testing will help identify arrhythmias, stress testing will help identify ischemia and/or exercise-induced arrhythmias, and tilt table tests are indicated in patients with unexplained recurrent syncope in whom cardiac causes are ruled out.

312. The answer is d. The patient in this scenario had exertional dyspnea and diaphoresis. As a diabetic, she is at high risk for silent ischemia, often signaled by anginal equivalents such as dyspnea and diaphoresis. A hypoglycemic event could have also caused diaphoresis and syncope, but serum glucose testing 1 day later would not help identify that as a cause. In addition, glycosylated hemoglobin would not be helpful in determining the cause of the event. An echocardiogram would not be helpful without physical examination findings consistent with cardiomyopathy or valvular disease, and a Holter monitor would be less helpful without evidence of palpitations or ECG abnormalities.

313. The answer is e. Tilt table testing is recommended in patients with unexplained recurrent syncope in whom cardiac causes including arrhythmias have been ruled out. An abnormal result suggests vasovagal syncope. Psychiatric evaluation should be considered if the tilt table is normal, especially if associated with other psychiatric symptoms (anxiety, depression, fear, or dread). Carotid Dopplers and MRI of the brain should be reserved for people with bruits or focal neurologic signs. Stress testing is indicated if there is high risk for, or symptoms of, ischemic disease.

314. The answer is a. The ability to characterize movement disorders appropriately will help with diagnosis and management. Ataxia refers to a wide-based unsteady gait associated with cerebellar dysfunction.

It can occur secondary to stroke, trauma, alcoholic degeneration, multiple sclerosis, or may be inherited. Chorea is an unpredictable irregular, non-rhythmic, brief, jerky, flowing, or writhing movement. Chorea has several causes (including stroke), but it may also be drug related. It is the classic movement disorder associated with Huntington disease. Dystonia is a syndrome that includes a sustained contraction of opposing muscles that cause twisting, repetitive movements, and abnormal postures. It can be inherited or may be caused by drugs or many other causes. Myoclonus is a brief, sudden movement caused by involuntary muscle contractions. It's generalized if it occurs in many body parts, or focal if it impacts a single body part.

315. The answer is a. The patient described in the question has an essential tremor, the most common movement disorder. It is characteristically bilateral, starts in the hands, and will change with age. It is more noticeable in times of stress or fatigue. Alcohol ingestion has a positive effect, and sometimes eliminates the tremor completely. Laboratory testing in this case is not for diagnosis, but primarily to rule out other causes, or when a patient presents with atypical symptoms. Routine laboratory tests that should be ordered include thyroid function testing, liver function tests, electrolytes, calcium, magnesium, phosphorous, and blood glucose levels. Other lab tests or imaging studies should be ordered based on the clinical scenario. If the tremor starts before 40 years of age, blood and urine should be checked to rule out Wilson disease. A CT or MRI should be used if there are suspicions for MS or Parkinson disease, and an EMG might be ordered to assist with diagnosis in an atypical presentation or to measure severity over time.

316. The answer is e. Seizures are alarming for all those involved. The patient described in this question had a classic febrile seizure (the most common seizure disorder), and no further workup would be indicated. In fact, the majority of evidence fails to support routine testing for first-time tonic-clonic seizures, regardless of suspected cause. Laboratory tests would be necessary if the child is less than 6 months old, fails to arouse, has continued focal seizures, or physical findings suggestive of meningitis. Primary treatment would consist of parental reassurance that the seizures will not cause permanent damage, and letting them know that there is a relatively high recurrence rate (around 30%). Despite this, only 3% of patients will go on to develop epilepsy. If the seizure is prolonged, IV lorazepam is the drug of choice, and hospitalization is indicated if the seizure lasts beyond

30 minutes or becomes recurrent. A seizure uninterrupted by consciousness for more than 5 minutes is termed *status epilepticus* (SE). Around 5% of children with febrile convulsions will have SE at least once. First-line treatment for SE is a parenteral benzodiazepine, but poorly controlled SE may respond to IV phenytoin. In adults with SE, immediate treatment should include thiamine, glucose, and naloxone.

Recommended Reading: Neurological

Clinch CR. Evaluation & management of headache. In: South-Paul JE, Matheny SC, Lewis EL (eds). *Current Diagnosis & Treatment Family Medicine*. 4th ed. New York, NY: McGraw-Hill.

Close KR. Delirium. In: Bope ET, Kellerman RD (eds). *Conn's Current Therapy, 2017*. Philadelphia, PA: Elsevier.

Criswell DF. Headaches. In: Smith MA, Shimp LA, Schrager S (eds). *Family Medicine Ambulatory Care and Prevention*. 6th ed. New York, NY: McGraw-Hill.

Dorsch JN. Red eye. In: Bope ET, Kellerman RD (eds). *Conn's Current Therapy, 2017*. Philadelphia, PA: Elsevier.

Falleroni J. Insomnia. In: Smith MA, Shimp LA, Schrager S (eds). *Family Medicine Ambulatory Care and Prevention*. 6th ed. New York, NY: McGraw-Hill.

Gallagher RM. Headache. In: Bope ET, Kellerman RD (eds). *Conn's Current Therapy, 2017*. Philadelphia, PA: Elsevier.

Halstater BH, Ragsdale J, White LC, Horng F. Syncope. In: Smith MA, Shimp LA, Schrager S (eds). *Family Medicine Ambulatory Care and Prevention*. 6th ed. New York, NY: McGraw-Hill.

Harper GM, Johnston CB, Landefeld CS. Geriatric disorders. In: Papadakis MA, McPhee SJ, Rabow MW (eds). *Current Medical Diagnosis & Treatment 2018*. New York, NY: McGraw-Hill.

Lustig LR, Schindler JS. Ear, nose & throat disorders. In: Papadakis MA, McPhee SJ, Rabow MW (eds). *Current Medical Diagnosis & Treatment 2018*. New York, NY: McGraw-Hill.

Madlon-Kay DJ. Dizziness In: Smith MA, Shimp LA, Schrager S (eds). *Family Medicine Ambulatory Care and Prevention*. 6th ed. New York, NY: McGraw-Hill.

Middleton DB. Seizures. In: South-Paul JE, Matheny SC, Lewis EL (eds). *Current Diagnosis & Treatment Family Medicine*. 4th ed. New York, NY: McGraw-Hill.

Sutters M. Systemic hypertension. In: Papadakis MA, McPhee SJ, Rabow MW (eds). *Current Medical Diagnosis & Treatment 2018*. New York, NY: McGraw-Hill.

Walling A. Migraine headache. In: Bope ET, Kellerman RD (eds). *Conn's Current Therapy, 2017*. Philadelphia, PA: Elsevier.

Xia Y. Movement disorders. In: South-Paul JE, Matheny SC, Lewis EL (eds). *Current Diagnosis & Treatment Family Medicine*. 4th ed. New York, NY: McGraw-Hill.

Yaman A, Yaman H, Rao, G. Tremors and other movement disorders. In: Smith MA, Shimp LA, Schrager S (eds). *Family Medicine Ambulatory Care and Prevention*. 6th ed. New York, NY: McGraw-Hill.

Acute Complaints—Respiratory Tract

317. The answer is a. The most common causes of a chronic cough are asthma, postnasal drainage, smoking, and GERD. Given that he did not respond to a bronchodilator, asthma is an unlikely diagnosis. Sore throat, combined with symptoms that are worse when lying down or with ingestion of caffeine or alcohol make GERD a likely diagnosis. Therefore, treatment with a proton-pump inhibitor would be most likely to help his symptoms. Antihistamines could treat asthma or post-nasal drip due to allergies. A steroid inhaler would help with asthma, and an antibiotic might be helpful if an infection were the underlying cause. ACE-inhibitors have cough as a side effect, and would not be used in this case. If the cough were acute, the differential diagnosis would include asthma exacerbation, acute bronchitis, aspiration, exposure to irritants (cigarette smoke, pollutants), allergic rhinitis, uncomplicated pneumonia, sinusitis with postnasal drip, and viral upper respiratory infection. Of these usual causes, viral upper respiratory infection is by far the most common cause. Viral upper respiratory infection is the most frequent illness in humans with a prevalence of up to 35%.

318. The answer is b. Because the patient reports a productive cough for at least 3 months of the year for at least 2 consecutive years, she meets the criteria for chronic bronchitis. This is a common cause of chronic cough in smokers. Chronic bronchitis is a useful clinical designation, but falls under the broad category of chronic obstructive pulmonary disease (COPD). While it is true that her smoking may cause irritation of her airways, it wouldn't explain why the cough isn't present year-round (since she continues to smoke throughout the year). The most common cause of chronic cough in nonsmokers is postnasal drainage, but since this patient has a significant smoking history, chronic bronchitis is more likely. Lung cancers rarely present solely with cough. Associated signs and symptoms include weight loss and hemoptysis. Asthma is less likely to present with a productive cough.

319. The answer is e. The Centers for Disease Control and Prevention published guidelines for treating acute bronchitis. The guidelines state that antibiotics are not indicated for uncomplicated acute bronchitis, regardless of the duration of the cough. Antibiotics should be reserved for patients with significant COPD and CHF, those who are very ill-appearing, or the elderly. This patient likely has hyper-responsive airways, sometimes called a postinfectious cough. In this case, the best treatment would be an inhaled steroid and a bronchodilator or antihistamine. If the cough persists, an oral steroid taper can be used. Anti-inflammatory medications and nasal steroids are not effective.

320. The answer is e. The causes of cough can range from a self-limited viral upper respiratory infection to severe infections. Patient signs and symptoms will define the approach to take. The first factor to consider is whether or not the patient has symptoms, signs, or risk factors that would warrant a chest radiograph. Symptoms that a chest radiograph is necessary include dyspnea, high fever, rigors, pleuritic chest pain, and altered mental status. Signs include a temperature greater than 38°C, heart rate greater than 100 beats/min, a respiratory rate greater than 24 breaths/min, and an abnormal lung examination. Risk factors include elderly patients, those with known COPD, heat failure, renal failure, or diabetes. Since the patient in this question has dyspnea, a high fever, and an abnormal lung examination, the next thing to do would be to obtain a PA and lateral chest x-ray to confirm the diagnosis of pneumonia.

321. The answer is b. Pneumonia is the most common cause of infectious death in the United States. *Streptococcus pneumonia* is the most commonly identified community-acquired pathogen in hospitalized patients, with *M pneumoniae* also commonly identified. Other less common pathogens include *Chlamydia, H influenzae, Legionella,* and respiratory viruses like influenza, parainfluenza, respiratory syncytial virus, and adenovirus. While the overall prognosis is good, there is an 8% hospitalization rate and a 1.2% mortality rate.

322. The answer is e. Those at risk for obstructive lung disease include pediatric patients (asthma, bronchitis, bronchiolitis), adults with asthma, and adults with chronic cigarette smoking. Dyspnea due to restrictive lung disease is more likely with occupational exposures (for farmers, cotton dust, grain dust, and hay mold), and in those with severe scoliosis, the morbidly obese, and the pregnant patients.

323. The answer is a. In evaluating patients with dyspnea, the first thing to do is establish whether it is severe enough to warrant hospitalization. With signs and symptoms suggesting severity, it's appropriate to obtain a PEFR using a peak flow meter. If the PEFR is less than 150 L/min, the dyspnea is considered severe, and the patient should be evaluated for life-threatening causes of dyspnea. Pulmonary causes include severe pneumonia, status asthmatics, and tension pneumothorax. The patient's PEFR indicates his condition is too severe to treat as an outpatient or in the office. Obtaining additional tests in the ambulatory setting would waste valuable time.

324. The answer is e. A PEFR between 400 and 600 L/min is considered normal, and indicates that the dyspnea is not severe enough to warrant oxygen and immediate transportation to the hospital. The next step would be to conduct a history and physical examination. If the results of that indicate a pulmonary cause is likely, an appropriate diagnostic and treatment plan should be followed based on the cause. In the case described in this question, the patient has risk factors for a cardiac cause of his dyspnea, and an ECG is an appropriate next step. A D-dimer would potentially be appropriate if a PE were suspected, but given that the patient has a normal extremity examination and risk factors for cardiac disease, it would not be the appropriate next step.

325. The answer is a. B-type natriuretic peptide evaluates for the presence of CHF. Studies indicate that a value less than 80 pg/mL has a high (99%) negative predicative value and helps rule out CHF. Values less than 100 pg/mL make CHF unlikely. Values in between 100 and 500 pg/mL require clinical judgment and further diagnostic testing. Values greater than 500 pg/mL make CHF a likely diagnosis.

326. The answer is e. A D-dimer test is useful in determining the risk for a DVT or PE. The test is highly sensitive, but not very specific; therefore, if the test is negative, no further workup is necessary. If the result were high, a confirmatory test would be appropriate. A spiral CT scan has become a standard validated test. A V/Q scan, often used in the past, can be used when a spiral CT is unavailable, but is often indeterminate. A pulmonary angiogram is the gold standard. Doppler flow studies are used to verify a DVT. If positive, a PE can be assumed in the correct clinical setting.

327. The answer is b. The patient has temporomandibular joint dysfunction, a common cause of referred otalgia. First-line therapies include treatment with NSAIDs, heat, a mechanical soft diet, and referral to the dentist if there is no improvement in 3 to 4 weeks. Antibiotic therapy is not indicated. Obtaining an MRI would not add value to the diagnosis or treatment plan at this stage. An ESR may be elevated in temporal arteritis, another cause of referred ear pain, but would not be likely to be useful in this setting.

328. The answer is d. A reddened tympanic membrane, by itself, is not a sufficient finding to diagnose acute otitis media. It may be due to increased intravascular pressure associated with crying. More reliable findings include an opaque tympanic membrane (indicating a purulent effusion), a bulging tympanic membrane, and impaired tympanic membrane mobility. When all three of those characteristics are present, the positive predictive value is very high. Purulent discharge in the ear canal may indicate a tympanic membrane perforation, and in the face of an otherwise normal canal is more indicative of acute otitis media than otitis externa.

329. The answer is a. Effusions may take up to 3 months to resolve. Antibiotics are not indicated for persistent effusions in the absence of acute otitis media. Effusions persisting beyond 3 months require evaluation by an otolaryngologist. Decongestants or antihistamines have never been documented to help effusions, and a Cochrane review found no clinical benefit for their use. In fact, subjects treated with decongestants or antihistamines had 11% more side effects than nontreated subjects.

330. The answer is c. The picture represents acute otitis media. The child should be treated with a first-line antibiotic. In most cases, amoxicillin is used as first-line therapy. However, in patients with severe illness (moderate to severe otalgia and/or fever > 102°F), therapy should be initiated with high-dose amoxicillin-clavulanate (90 mg/kg/d of amoxicillin in two divided doses). Azithromycin is often used as a first-line choice in 1-day, 3-day, or 5-day doses, but it should be reserved as a second-line therapy.

331. The answer is c. Fundamental to the treatment of external otitis is protection from additional moisture and avoidance of further mechanical injury from scratching. Otic drops containing antibiotics and corticosteroids are very effective. Oral antibiotics or steroids would be reserved for recalcitrant cases, as the process is generally localized, not systemic, and demonstrates a good response to topical therapy. Any case of persistent otitis externa in an immunocompromised or diabetic individual should be referred for specialty evaluation.

332. The answer is a. Pharyngitis is common and accounts for more than 7 million outpatient visits for children annually. The estimated total cost for pharyngitis in children is $540M per year. Around 30% of pharyngitis in children is caused by group A β-hemolytic *Streptococcus*, while another 30% to 40% are caused by viruses. Rhinovirus is the most common of the viral causes. The type of pharyngitis cannot be identified by history alone, and if treatment is to be initiated with antibiotics, microbiologic confirmations are necessary. However, if clinical symptoms suggest viral pharyngitis and the pretest probability of GABHS infection is low, a diagnostic test need not be performed. In this question, the patient's hoarseness and cough are more likely associated with a viral cause, therefore symptomatic care is appropriate. There is no need to treat with antibiotics or antivirals, and testing is unnecessary. A modified Centor score can be used to help evaluate probability. Patients are given one point each for

- Absence of cough
- Swollen and tender anterior cervical lymph nodes
- Temperature more than 100.4°F
- Tonsillar exudate or swelling

If the patient has an age of 3 to 14 years, a point is added. For people between 15 and 44 years old, no points are added, and for patients 45 years old and older, a point is taken away. Patients with a score of zero or 1 are at very low risk for streptococcal infection. Patients with a score of 2 or 3 should be tested. Patients with a score of 4 or higher are at high risk. In those high-risk patients, empiric treatment may be considered.

333. The answer is d. It is necessary to obtain microbiologic confirmation of infection before treating GABHS pharyngitis. If the clinical symptoms suggest GAHBHS, an RADT is the appropriate next step. A culture would not be necessary unless the rapid test were negative. The RADT has high specificity but low sensitivity. The use of the RADT has allowed clinicians to begin antibiotic therapy early in those with a positive test, decreasing the risk of spread and allowing an earlier return to school or work. Students can return to school 24 hours after starting antibiotics.

334. The answer is c. Infectious mononucleosis should be suspected when a teen or young adult (ages 15-25) present with the classic triad of severe sore throat, lymphadenopathy, and fever (which can be up to 104°F). In general, mononucleosis begins with a prodrome of chills, sweats, and malaise. Clinical signs include enlarged tonsils, cervical adenopathy (posterior and anterior), and sometimes hepatosplenomegaly. A CBC would show absolute lymphocytosis with more than 10% atypical lymphocytes. It would not show erythrocytosis, and although neutropenia can be seen with viral infections, atypical lymphocytes are more likely. A throat culture would be negative, unless the person was a carrier, and the heterophile antibody test would not be positive for 2 to 3 weeks after symptoms began.

335. The answer is a. Approximately 20% of school age children are carriers of group A β-hemolytic *Streptococcus*. In the past, it was felt that these children needed to be treated to eradicate the bacteria. The antibiotics used to eliminate group A streptococcal carriage from oropharyngeal secretions were oral respiratory quinolones or oral clindamycin. Recent studies have shown that these carriers do not need to be identified or treated, as they do not develop complications from infection and have not been found to be important in the spread of group A β-hemolytic *Streptococcus* to others.

336. The answer is c. The goal of antibiotic treatment for GABHS is to decrease infectivity and prevent complications, especially rheumatic fever. Even without treatment, symptoms generally improve in 3 to 5 days. Delay of treatment does not appear to increase the risk of rheumatic fever, but early treatment does reduce infectivity, lessen morbidity, and promote early return to normal activities. The choice of antibiotic is determined by the bacteriology of the GABHS, clinical efficacy, patient adherence, adverse effects, and cost. Penicillin remains the antibiotic of choice for GABHS pharyngitis. There has been no reported resistance to penicillin. First-generation cephalosporins and macrolides can be used in patients allergic to penicillin. There is no need to observe once a test is positive, and a throat culture is not necessary to confirm a positive rapid antigen test.

337. The answer is e. Despite the fact that acute bacterial rhinosinusitis affects more than 20 million Americans per year, there are no agreed-upon criteria for the diagnosis of acute bacterial rhinosinusitis in adults. This is because so many of the symptoms mimic other diseases ranging from a common cold to allergic rhinitis. Some feel that the presence of two major criteria or one major and two minor criteria allow a clinician to diagnosis sinusitis in adults. Major criteria are:

- Purulent anterior nasal discharge or postnasal discharge
- Nasal congestion or obstruction
- Facial congestion or fullness
- Facial pain or pressure
- Hyposmia/anosmia and fever

Minor criteria include:

- Headache
- Ear pain/pressure
- Halitosis
- Dental pain
- Cough
- Fatigue

Bacterial rhinosinusitis can sometimes be distinguished from viral rhinitis by persistence of symptoms for more than 10 days after onset, or worsening symptoms within 10 days after an initial improvement. This bimodal presentation can be helpful in diagnosis.

338. The answer is d. *S pneumoniae* is the most common bacterial pathogen in bacterial sinusitis. Other causes include *H influenzae, M catarrhalis,* and group A β-hemolytic streptococci. Pathogens vary regionally in both prevalence and drug resistance. Complicating the situation further is that if the sinus aspirates of healthy adults are cultured, bacteria colonization will be found in around one quarter of them.

339. The answer is e. Between 40% and 70% of patients with acute bacterial rhinosinusitis improve symptomatically within 2 weeks without antibiotic therapy. Antibiotic treatment is controversial in uncomplicated cases of clinically diagnosed sinusitis because only around 5% of patients will note a shorter duration of symptoms with treatment, and antibiotics have nearly twice the number of adverse events as compared with placebo. Antibiotics should be considered when symptoms are severe, or when cases are complicated. In these cases, antibiotics reduce the incidence of clinical failure by 50%.

340. The answer is b. In general, most patients with acute sinusitis do not benefit from imaging studies. However, imaging may be helpful in uncertain or recurrent cases, as in this question. Sinus films, though not helpful for initial evaluation, may be abnormal in acute rhinosinusitis, but are actually most helpful when negative. A normal series has a negative predictive value of 90% to 100%. The positive predictive value is around 80%, but its sensitivity is only around 60%. CT scans have superior sensitivity (95% to 98%) when compared with sinus films, so can be valuable in acute settings. That said, they are particularly valuable in establishing the diagnosis of chronic sinusitis or in equivocal cases before starting long-term antibiotic therapy. MRI is used when fungal sinusitis or tumors are suspected, but are not used for routine evaluation. US is not helpful.

341. The answer is a. Acute viral respiratory tract infections cause up to 50% of wheezing episodes in children less than 2 years of age. Risk factors include fall or winter season, history of atopy, daycare attendance, and passive smoke exposure. Pneumonia causes 33% to 50% of wheezing episodes in children, and most are also caused by viruses as well. Bronchiolitis accounts for less than 5% of all episodes of wheezing, but is important, especially in preterm infants. Aspiration is uncommon, and is less likely in the setting of viral infection symptoms. Asthma is common in children, but is not diagnosed after one episode of wheezing.

342. The answer is b. Patients with a first episode of wheezing require a chest x-ray. Peak flow testing may be helpful in monitoring control of asthma, but are not useful in evaluating a first episode. Pulmonary function testing and a CBC may be needed, but a chest x-ray is an absolute necessity.

343. The answer is e. Physiologic gastroesophageal reflux is a passive return of gastric contents into the esophagus. It peaks at 1 to 4 months and usually resolves by 12 months. Children affected often wheeze and will have more spitting up after eating. The gold standard test for GERD is a 24-hour pH probe in children. Given the symptoms in this question, this is the most likely test to reveal the diagnosis. A chest x-ray would be better if pulmonary or cardiac causes were suspected. A child of this age cannot participate in PFTs. An upper GI barium swallow can reveal structural defects, and upper endoscopy is usually reserved for older patients unresponsive to medical management of GERD.

Recommended Reading: Respiratory Tract

Berkson D, Naini G, DiSalvo C. Earache. In: Smith MA, Shimp LA, Schrager S (eds). *Family Medicine Ambulatory Care and Prevention.* 6th ed. New York, NY: McGraw-Hill.

Carlson JM, Stiles M, Quattlebaum Rg, Diaz VA, Mains AG. Rhinitis and sinus pain. In: Smith MA, Shimp LA, Schrager S (eds). *Family Medicine Ambulatory Care and Prevention.* 6th ed. New York, NY: McGraw-Hill.

Chesnutt JC, Stephan MR, Fields SA, Toffler WL. Dyspnea. In: Smith MA, Shimp LA, Schrager S (eds). *Family Medicine Ambulatory Care and Prevention.* 6th ed. New York, NY: McGraw-Hill.

Chronic obstructive pulmonary disease. In: Smith MA, Shimp LA, Schrager S (eds). *Family Medicine Ambulatory Care and Prevention.* 6th ed. New York, NY: McGraw-Hill.

Cough, fever, and respiratory infections. In: Stern SC, Cifu AS, Althorn D (eds). *Symptom to Diagnosis: An Evidence-Based Guide.* 3rd ed. New York, NY; McGraw-Hill; 2014.

Hudson SA, Tingen JM. Venous thromboembolism. In: Smith MA, Shimp LA, Schrager S (eds). *Family Medicine Ambulatory Care and Prevention.* 6th ed. New York, NY: McGraw-Hill.

Lochner JE, Holmes D. Cough. In: Smith MA, Shimp LA, Schrager S (eds). *Family Medicine Ambulatory Care and Prevention.* 6th ed. New York, NY: McGraw-Hill.

Lustig LR, Schindler JS. Ear, nose & throat disorders. In: Papadakis MA, McPhee SJ, Rabow MW (eds). *Current Medical Diagnosis & Treatment 2018.* New York, NY: McGraw-Hill.

Schwiebert LP. Sore throat. In: Smith MA, Shimp LA, Schrager S (eds). *Family Medicine Ambulatory Care and Prevention.* 6th ed. New York, NY: McGraw-Hill.

Taggart C, Kerber-Frazier J. Wheezing. In: Smith MA, Shimp LA, Schrager S (eds). *Family Medicine Ambulatory Care and Prevention.* 6th ed. New York, NY: McGraw-Hill.Vogt HB.

Weber R. Pharyngitis. In: Bope ET, Kellerman RD (eds). *Conn's Current Therapy, 2017.* Philadelphia, PA: Elsevier.

Chronic Conditions

Questions

Adult Sexual Issues

344. A 48-year-old man is seeing you to discuss sexual concerns. He complains of being unable to achieve an erection, despite having strong interest in sexual activity. Which of the following is true?

a. This is most often because of an unrecognized mood disorder.
b. This is most often because of a lack of attraction for his partner.
c. This is most often because of stressors in the home and interpersonal conflict.
d. This is most often because of a vascular problem.
e. This is most often because of alcohol abuse.

345. A 36-year-old man sees you to discuss a lack of sexual interest. He is not having sexual fantasies and is unmotivated to begin sexual activity. He does not report depressive symptoms and has no other physical complaints. His physical examination is normal. Which of the following laboratory tests is most appropriate?

a. Total testosterone
b. Free testosterone
c. Thyroid-stimulating hormone (TSH)
d. Prolactin
e. Prostate-specific antigen (PSA)

346. You have diagnosed a 30-year-old woman with depression. She is concerned that medical treatment may cause sexual dysfunction. In order to avoid sexual side effects, which antidepressant would be the best choice?

a. Amitriptyline
b. Paroxetine
c. Citalopram
d. Sertraline
e. Bupropion

347. A 23-year-old man comes to your office to discuss premature ejaculation. He has had this condition since beginning sexual activity at 17 years of age. He has tried behavioral methods, but these have not been successful. Which of the following medications is most likely to help this condition?

a. Alprostadil
b. Fluoxetine
c. Bupropion
d. Sildenafil
e. Atenolol

348. You are evaluating a 47-year-old man with erectile dysfunction. After a thorough history and physical examination, you order a morning free testosterone level. His level was low. What is the most appropriate next step?

a. Begin testosterone injections
b. Begin topical testosterone replacement
c. Obtain follicle-stimulating hormone (FSH), luteinizing hormone (LH), and prolactin levels
d. Confirm the low level with repeat testosterone testing
e. Perform a nocturnal penile tumescence evaluation

349. You are caring for a woman who describes primary orgasmic dysfunction and comes to you for advice. Which of the following therapies has shown to be the most effective in treating this condition?

a. Directed self-stimulation
b. The "stop-start" technique
c. Group therapy
d. Hypnotherapy
e. Sensate focus

Addiction

For questions 350 to 354, use the following scenario: You are evaluating a 28-year-old man who is concerned about depression. He reports increased irritability, depressed mood, decreased enjoyment from usual activities, and sleep and appetite disturbances for 6 weeks. His wife reports an increasing history of alcohol use; he currently drinks 6 beers a day on the weekdays, with up to 12 per day on the weekends. The patient feels his wife is exaggerating.

350. Which of the following laboratory tests would be the most sensitive to detect excess alcohol use?

a. Mean corpuscular volume (MCV)
b. Alanine aminotransferase (ALT)
c. Aspartate aminotransferase (AST)
d. γ-Glutamyl transferase (GGT)
e. Ethyl glucuronide (EtG)

351. Which of the following is the most appropriate next step in treating his depression?

a. Treat with a selective serotonin reuptake inhibitor (SSRI)
b. Treat with bupropion
c. Recommend detoxification and abstinence
d. Recommend detoxification and abstinence and start an SSRI
e. Recommend detoxification and abstinence and start bupropion

352. After you facilitate a brief intervention for this patient and his family, he agrees to an inpatient detoxification program. You are concerned about alcohol withdrawal seizures. Which of the following is the cornerstone of therapy for alcohol withdrawal seizures?

a. Naltrexone
b. Buprenorphine
c. Clonidine
d. β-blockers
e. Benzodiazepines

353. Your patient returns to the office after completing his inpatient detoxification program. His counselor recommended trying naltrexone to help with sobriety, and he asks you how that medication works in alcoholism. Which of the following is the best answer for your patient?

a. If the person taking naltrexone ingests alcohol, it causes an adverse reaction.
b. Naltrexone reduces the reinforcing effects of alcohol.
c. Naltrexone blocks the effects of alcohol by binding to alcohol-receptor sites on cells.
d. Naltrexone saturates the alcohol-receptor sites on cells by acting as an alcohol agonist.
e. Naltrexone changes the binding sites on alcohol, making it unable to bind to cells.

354. His wife has been reading about these medications and wants him to try disulfiram, and he asks you how that medication works in alcoholism. Which of the following is the best answer for your patient?

a. If the person taking disulfiram ingests alcohol, it causes an adverse reaction.
b. Disulfiram reduces the reinforcing effects of alcohol.
c. Disulfiram blocks the effects of alcohol by binding to alcohol receptor sites on cells.
d. Disulfiram saturates the alcohol receptor sites on cells by acting as an alcohol agonist.
e. Disulfiram changes the binding sites on alcohol, making it unable to bind to cells.

355. You are caring for a patient who would like to quit smoking. She failed nicotine patches. Which of the following is an appropriate next step?

a. Add nicotine gum to the patch
b. Use clonidine
c. Use a tricyclic antidepressant
d. Use an SSRI
e. Use a selective serotonin and norepinephrine reuptake inhibitor

356. You are currently evaluating a patient for unstable angina. He takes phenytoin for a seizure disorder, has high cholesterol, and is a current smoker. Which of the following would be the best therapeutic option to help with his smoking cessation plan?

a. Behavioral intervention
b. Nicotine replacement
c. Bupropion
d. Varenicline
e. Clonidine

For questions 357 to 359, consider the following scenario: You are seeing an otherwise healthy 42-year-old female patient in the office for a routine physical examination. She confides in you that she has become dependent on oxycodone. In fact, she recently lost her job due to poor performance and has been using her savings to buy oxycodone off the street.

357. The patient is considering outpatient treatment and using Narcotics Anonymous (NA) as the cornerstone of her therapy. Which of the following is true regarding 12-step programs such as NA?

a. She cannot attend NA unless she practices a Christian religion.
b. NA is only available to her if her physician refers her.
c. If she chooses to go to NA, she will be included in research protocols to assess its effectiveness.
d. NA has resources to her find a new job.
e. NA is funded through member contributions alone.

358. Your patient is interested in pursuing pharmacologic treatment for her opiate use disorder, and would like to consider the combination of buprenorphine and naloxone (Suboxone). Which of the following is true regarding its mechanism of action?

a. Buprenorphine/naloxone therapy displaces opioids at receptor sites and binds to μ-opiate receptors.
b. Buprenorphine/naloxone therapy inhibits opiate metabolism, so it can't be absorbed.
c. Buprenorphine/naloxone therapy increases serotonin levels in the brain to inhibit opiate craving.
d. Buprenorphine/naloxone therapy affects GABA transmission in the brain to block the effect of opiates in the brain.
e. Its mechanism of action is unknown.

359. Your patient is admitted for induction therapy and medication-assisted treatment for her opiate use disorder. Which of the following symptoms would you expect to see as the patient begins to withdraw from opioids?

a. Fatigue, depressed mood, and increased appetite
b. Abdominal cramping, diaphoresis, vomiting, and chills
c. Anxiety, restlessness, tremor, nystagmus, and tachycardia
d. Seizures, psychosis, and delirium
e. Lethargy, slowed movements, and increased sleep

Arthritis and Joint Issues

For questions 360 to 362, use the following scenario: A 64-year-old woman comes to see you as a new patient. She is interested in finding the cause of her hand deformities. Upon inspection, you see that the joints in her hands are nodular and enlarged as in the picture below. She does not complain of significant disability.

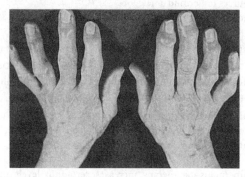

(Reproduced, with permission, from South-Paul J. Current Diagnosis & Treatment in Family Medicine. 1st ed. New York, NY: McGraw-Hill; 2004: 266).

360. Which of the following laboratory findings is likely in her case?

a. Her laboratory evaluation will likely be normal.
b. Her serum uric acid level will likely be elevated.
c. Her sedimentation rate will likely be elevated.
d. Her C-reactive protein level will likely be elevated.
e. Her rheumatoid factor will likely be elevated.

361. For this patient, what changes would you expect to see on radiographs of the hand?

a. Small erosions on the lateral aspects of the phalanges.
b. No abnormalities would be seen on plain radiographs.
c. Loss of joint space, subchondral sclerosis, and osteophyte formation of the proximal and distal interphalangeal joints.
d. Effusion and sclerosis of the metacarpal joints symmetrically.
e. Loss of joint space, subchondral sclerosis, and calcium deposition within the surrounding cartilage of the proximal and distal interphalangeal joints.

362. Your patient is seeking relief from the chronic, daily pain she is experiencing in her hands. Which of the following would be the best first step to treat her pain?

a. Acetaminophen 3 to 4 times daily
b. Naproxen twice daily
c. Short-acting opiates 2 to 3 times daily
d. Methotrexate once weekly until symptom relief is achieved
e. Corticosteroid injections up to 2 to 3 times yearly

For questions 363 to 364 use the following scenario: A 43-year-old obese patient comes to your office with a painful, inflamed, swollen elbow. He reports that the pain began suddenly last evening, without a known precipitant or trauma. The pain is exquisite, and does not allow him to move his elbow at all—in fact, last evening even the pressure of his bed sheet on his elbow was painful. On examination, he has an elbow effusion with warmth, erythema, and intense pain with movement.

363. Which of the following is most likely the cause?

a. Rheumatoid arthritis (RA)
b. Osteoarthritis (OA)
c. Gout
d. Stress fracture
e. Cellulitis

364. What is the most appropriate initial treatment for this condition?

a. IV antibiotics
b. Nonsteroidal anti-inflammatory drugs (NSAIDs)
c. Methotrexate once weekly
d. Colchicine 0.6 mg twice daily
e. Allopurinol 100 mg daily, increasing to 300 mg daily

365. A 66-year-old diabetic man comes to your office with acute monoarticular arthritis. You suspect gout. Which of the following tests is the most helpful in establishing the diagnosis?

a. Sedimentation rate
b. C-reactive protein
c. Serum uric acid levels
d. Evaluation of joint aspirate
e. Twenty-four-hour urine collection to measure uric acid excretion

366. For the patient described in the above question, you perform an arthrocentesis. The fluid analysis reveals rhomboid-shaped positively bire-fringent crystals. Which of the following is the most likely diagnosis?

a. Gout
b. Pseudogout
c. Infectious arthritis
d. OA
e. RA

367. You are evaluating a patient with a painful, swollen knee. You per-form arthrocentesis and find cloudy fluid. Analysis reveals a white blood cell (WBC) count of 50,000/mm^3 with more than 90% identified as poly-morphonuclear (PMN) leukocytes. The glucose level in the joint fluid is decreased. Which of the following is the most likely diagnosis?

a. Gout
b. Pseudogout
c. Infectious arthritis
d. OA
e. RA

368. You are evaluating a 56-year-old patient with a painful, swollen knee. Joint aspirate reveals clear fluid with a WBC count of 5000/mm^3, 20% of which are PMN leukocytes. Which of the following is the most likely diagnosis?

a. Gout
b. Pseudogout
c. Infectious arthritis
d. OA
e. RA

369. You are caring for a 42-year-old woman who was diagnosed with RA 8 years ago. You are concerned about potential extra-articular manifesta-tions of her disease. Which of the following signs or symptoms, if present, would signal extra-articular manifestations of RA?

a. Cough
b. Congestive heart failure (CHF)
c. Gastrointestinal (GI) distress
d. Peripheral neuropathy
e. Renal failure

Asthma

For questions 370 to 373, use the following scenario: You are seeing a 13-year-old patient in the office for the first time. She has had recent episodic shortness of breath and her mother is concerned that she has developed asthma. As you explore this patient's history, you learn that she has been having 2 to 3 months of daytime symptoms, including coughing, wheezing, and shortness of breath more than 2 days per week but not daily. She wakes up once weekly at night with coughing spells and the teacher at school just told her mother that the patient is often not participating in her normal recess activities because of her symptoms. She has never been to the emergency department (ED) or hospitalized for these symptoms and has not had any workup at this point.

370. Which of the following features, if present, is the strongest predisposing factor in the development of asthma in children?

a. Family history of asthma
b. History of atopy
c. Caucasian race
d. Exposure to cigarette smoke
e. Exposure to environmental pollution

371. Based on this patient's history, how would you categorize her symptoms?

a. Intermittent asthma
b. Mild persistent asthma
c. Moderate persistent asthma
d. Severe persistent asthma
e. Cough variant asthma

372. In order to more fully understand this patient's symptoms, you order pulmonary function testing (PFT). What finding is consistent with moderate persistent asthma?

a. Peak flow 80% of personal best
b. Forced expiratory volume in 1 second/forced vital capacity (FEV1/FVC) 88% predicted
c. FEV1 less than 75% predicted
d. FVC less than 80% predicted
e. Volume-time curve of less than 4 seconds

373. The history and PFTs for this patient are consistent with moderate persistent asthma. What is the best first course of action for this patient?

a. Initiate a low-dose inhaled corticosteroid alone
b. Initiate a short-acting bronchodilator alone
c. Initiate a medium-dose inhaled corticosteroid and a long-acting bronchodilator
d. Initiate a low-dose inhaled corticosteroid, a long-acting bronchodilator, and a short-acting bronchodilator rescue inhaler
e. Initiate a low-dose inhaled corticosteroid and a leukotriene receptor antagonist

For questions 374 to 376, use the following scenario: You are caring for a 30-year-old woman who has had asthma since childhood. Currently, she reports symptoms 2 to 3 times a week, but never more than once a day. Sometimes, her symptoms cause her to skip her usual exercise regimen. She wakes in the night approximately 3 or 4 times a month to use her inhaler and return to bed.

374. Which of the following classifications best characterizes her asthma?

a. Mild intermittent
b. Moderate intermittent
c. Mild persistent
d. Moderate persistent
e. Severe persistent

375. The patient has updated PFTs consistent with her above asthma categorization and she is only using a short-acting β_2-agonist rescue inhaler to treat her asthma. Given her severity of asthma, what would be the next best course of action for controlling her symptoms?

a. Addition of a low-dose inhaled corticosteroid
b. Addition of a leukotriene receptor antagonist
c. Addition of a medium-dose inhaled corticosteroid
d. Addition of a medium-dose inhaled corticosteroid plus a leukotriene receptor antagonist
e. Addition of a low-dose inhaled corticosteroid plus a long-acting bronchodilator

376. You have developed an asthma action plan for this patient, including the use of home peak flows. When is it recommended to reassess this patient's condition?

a. 1 week
b. 2 weeks
c. 2 months
d. 3 months
e. When her peak flow readings fall in the green zone

377. You are caring for a 19-year-old man who has been treated for mild intermittent asthma since childhood. He has been controlled using a short-acting bronchodilator as needed. Over the past month, he has been using his inhaler more than 4 times a week, and has had to wake up in the middle of the night to use his inhaler on three occasions. In the past, he was intolerant of the side effects associated with an inhaled corticosteroid. Which of the following is the most appropriate treatment option?

a. Long-acting β-agonist
b. Leukotriene receptor antagonist
c. Cromolyn (Intal)
d. Theophylline
e. Oral corticosteroids

378. You are caring for a 22-year-old with moderate persistent asthma who has been well-controlled for several months. He developed an upper respiratory infection and his control worsened. He has not had a fever, but is coughing up sputum. In addition to stepping up his therapy, which of the following is true?

a. You should begin a course of amoxicillin.
b. You should begin a course of amoxicillin/clavulanate.
c. You should begin a course of azithromycin.
d. You should begin a course of ciprofloxacin.
e. No antibiotics are necessary.

Back Pain

For questions 379 to 381, use the following scenario: A 22-year-old man is seeing you to discuss his low back pain. He is athletic and exercises regularly. He denies any inciting event, does not have pain with movement, and denies radiation of the pain. You suspect spondylolisthesis.

379. Your patient reports low back pain for 4 weeks. Which of the following characteristics, if present, would suggest the need for early imaging in a patient with acute low back pain?

a. Radicular pain down the right leg
b. A 20-pound weight gain over the last 6 months
c. Recurrent fevers
d. Pain that worsens with physical activity and improves with rest
e. Numbness in his left great toe

380. This patient has tried acetaminophen for 2 days without relief. On examination, his range of motion is limited, and he has tenderness to palpation of the lumbar paraspinal muscles. Which of the following treatment options is best?

a. NSAIDs and return to normal activity
b. Opiate analgesia and limited activities
c. Oral corticosteroids
d. Bed rest for 3 to 5 days
e. Facet joint injection

381. You prescribed an appropriate conservative regimen for your patient. Today, he is following up after 6 weeks of this therapy. His neurologic examination is normal, but his history and physical examination do not demonstrate any improvement as a result of the treatment plan. Plain x-rays are normal. Which of the following is the most appropriate next step?

a. Flexion and extension radiographs
b. Magnetic resonance imaging (MRI)
c. Electromyography
d. Bone scan
e. A complete blood count (CBC) and erythrocyte sedimentation rate (ESR)

382. You are caring for a 48-year-old construction manager with a history of chronic back pain due to OA of the lumbar spine. His symptoms have been controlled on NSAIDs for several years, but they are no longer as effective as they once were. Imaging studies have not changed and his laboratory work is normal. You are considering adjusting his pain control regimen. Of the following, which would be the best option?

a. Add a muscle relaxant to his NSAID
b. Add an opioid to his NSAID
c. Add a tricyclic antidepressant to his NSAID
d. Add an SSRI to his NSAID
e. Schedule him for facet joint corticosteroid injections

Chronic Obstructive Pulmonary Disease

For questions 383 to 385, use the following scenario: You are assessing a 59-year-old patient with an 80-pack-year history of smoking cigarettes. He stopped smoking 1 year ago. He reports a cough productive of white frothy sputum for the past 4 months. Reviewing his chart, you discover that he had a similar presentation last winter, with a cough that lasted more than 3 months.

383. Given this information, which of the following tests is necessary for him?
a. CBC
b. Arterial blood gas measurements
c. Office spirometry
d. Computerized tomographic scans of the chest
e. An electrocardiogram

384. Treatment modalities for chronic obstructive pulmonary disease (COPD) are based on a patient's category of disease. What combination of factors is used in the Global Initiative for Chronic Obstructive Lung Disease (GOLD)?
a. Duration of symptoms and pack years smoking
b. FEV_1 and nocturnal oxygen levels
c. Spirometry and symptom severity
d. Number of exacerbations and breathlessness scale
e. Pack years smoking and changes on chest x-ray (CXR)

385. Which of the following measurements is most sensitive to diagnose COPD in this patient?
a. Total lung capacity (TLC)
b. FVC
c. FEV_1
d. Forced expiratory flow rate over the interval from 25% to 75% of the total FVC ($FEF_{25\%-75\%}$)
e. FEV_1:FVC

386. You have diagnosed a 66-year-old female patient of yours with COPD. Which of the following therapies has been shown to improve the natural history of COPD?

a. Bronchodilators
b. Inhaled steroids
c. A combination of bronchodilators and inhaled steroids
d. Antibiotics
e. Supplemental oxygen

387. You are seeing a 59-year-old patient in the office for a chief complaint of "COPD exacerbation." GOLD recommends the use of antibiotics in patients with acute exacerbations of COPD who have which of the following three symptoms?

a. Hypoxia, fever, and lethargy
b. Increase in dyspnea, cough, and fever
c. Increase in dyspnea, pleuritic pain, and sputum volume
d. Decrease in SpO_2, energy level, and FEV_1
e. Increase in dyspnea, sputum volume, and sputum purulence

388. The patient described in the question above required admission to the hospital for his exacerbation. Which of the following treatment plans will be likely to result in the shortest hospitalization and lowest rate of reexacerbation?

a. Treatment with antibiotics only
b. Treatment with antibiotics and β-agonists only
c. Treatment with antibiotics, β-agonists, and an antimuscarinic agent (like ipratropium bromide) only
d. Treatment with antibiotics, β-agonists, an antimuscarinic agent, and a short course of steroids (5 days)
e. Treatment with antibiotics, β-agonists, an antimuscarinic agent, and a long course of steroids (14 days)

Renal Disease

For questions 389 to 390, use the following scenario: You are seeing a 65-year-old woman with a history of diabetes and hypertension. She is overweight and does not exercise regularly. Her medications include metformin, amlodipine, and omeprazole. You are concerned that she may have renal failure, given her risk factors.

389. Which of the following is the best test to detect the presence of renal insufficiency in this patient?
a. Her blood urea nitrogen (BUN) level
b. Her serum creatinine level
c. Her BUN to creatinine ratio
d. Her calculated or estimated glomerular filtration rate (GFR)
e. Her urine microalbumin level

390. Her laboratory values are as follows:

BUN	11 mg/dL	Microalbumin/creat ratio	30 mg/g Creatinine
Cr	1.08 mg/dL	GFR	49 mL/min/1.73 m^2

Assuming her values are steady and present for at least 3 months, which of the following interventions is most likely to slow the progression of chronic kidney disease (CKD)?
a. Avoiding NSAIDs such as ibuprofen
b. Tightly controlling blood pressure
c. Adding a statin to her current regimen
d. Adding a thiazide diuretic to her current regimen
e. Adding lisinopril to her current regimen

391. You are following a 54-year-old patient with hypertension and diabetes in your office. Despite good blood pressure and glycemic control, his GFR has started to decrease. His GFR measurement was 74 mL/min/1.73 m^2 3 months ago. At this visit, his GFR is 55 mL/min/1.73 m^2. His creatinine is within normal limits, and his serum potassium is 5.2 mmol/L (normal is up to 5.1 mmol/L). The patient denies any changes in urination or other problems. Which of the following is most appropriate at this stage?
a. See the patient more frequently, at least monthly
b. Increase his angiotensin-converting enzyme (ACE)-inhibitor
c. Add diuretic therapy
d. Refer to a nephrologist
e. Refer to a vascular surgeon for fistula placement

For questions 392 to 394, use the following clinical scenario: You are treating a 67-year-old patient with chronic and progressing renal disease. His GFR is decreasing and you fear he will need dialysis soon. He states he feels well, besides some fatigue and decreased appetite, and he does not want to discuss dialysis. He has lost 5 pounds since his last visit 3 months ago, and his current body mass index (BMI) is 19.8 kg/m^2. His laboratory values are as follows:

BUN	62 mg/dL	K	6.3 mmol/L
Cr	6.17 mg/dL	Na	137 mmol/L
GFR	13 mL/min/1.73 m^2	Phosphorus	6.3 mg/dL
Hemoglobin A1C	8.5%	Parathyroid Hormone (intact)	126.5 pg/mL
Hemoglobin	9.3 g/dL	Calcium	9.0 mg/dL

392. Which of the following will be the most likely cause of death in this patient?

a. Renal failure
b. Liver failure
c. Neurovascular disease
d. Cardiovascular disease (CVD)
e. Coagulopathy

393. Based on the patient's symptoms and laboratory values, which action should you consider next?

a. Call his nephrologist to discuss emergent dialysis
b. Increase his insulin to ensure better glycemic control
c. Start an erythropoietin-stimulating agent
d. Order an electrocardiogram (EKG), stop his ACE-inhibitor, and add a loop diuretic
e. Order a parathyroid scan

394. You are concerned that this patient has metabolic bone disease. What is the best first course of action to treat this in your patient?

a. Continue his low-phosphorus diet and add calcium carbonate
b. Continue his low-phosphorus diet and cinacalcet
c. Add calcitriol
d. Add vitamin D
e. Refer to endocrinology to evaluate for secondary hyperparathyroidism

Chronic Pain

For questions 395 to 399, consider the patient scenarios described and choose the best option for chronic pain management using the following key:

a. Tramadol
b. Anticonvulsants
c. Antidepressants
d. Muscle relaxants
e. Steroids

395. You are treating a 48-year-old breast cancer survivor who reports peripheral neuropathy ever since she completed her chemotherapy. She denies allergies, and has not found relief with nonsteroidal anti-inflammatories or other over-the-counter analgesics.

396. You are treating a 46-year-old man with chronic back pain without neurologic symptoms. He is participating in a multimodal treatment plan including physical therapy and rehabilitation. He is using nonsteroidal anti-inflammatory agents, but they are not enough to manage his pain at certain times. He is looking for occasional pain relief.

397. You are caring for a 59-year-old patient with low back pain due to spinal stenosis. He has no neuropathic symptoms. He has failed conservative treatment with physical therapy, nonsteroidal anti-inflammatory agents, and wants to postpone surgery as long as possible.

398. You are seeing a 70-year-old patient who had shingles 4 months ago, and is struggling with pain from postherpetic neuralgia.

399. You are caring for a 32-year-old woman with chronic headaches and fibromyalgia. She reports that her symptoms are interfering with her desire to engage in her usual leisure activities, and she is feeling desperate for some relief.

400. You are treating a 48-year-old woman with arthritis in her knees. The pain keeps her from exercising, and she is becoming concerned about the limitations in her activity. Of the following, which would be the most appropriate first-line agent for her pain control?

a. Ibuprofen, 600 mg tid
b. Celecoxib, 200 mg daily
c. Tramadol, 50 mg q4-6h
d. Amitriptyline, 50 mg at night
e. Gabapentin, 300 mg tid

401. You are treating a 55-year-old obese diabetic for his neuropathy. It's extremely painful and not responsive to NSAID therapy. Of the following, which is the best option for pain control?

a. Celecoxib, 200 mg daily
b. Tramadol, 50 mg q4-6h
c. Amitriptyline, 50 mg at night
d. Oxycodone 15-30 mg q4-6h
e. Fentanyl patch, 25 µg/q72h

402. You are treating a patient for chronic pain. She is taking NSAIDs, anticonvulsants, and a fairly high dose of long-acting opioid, but her pain is becoming increasingly hard to control. Although you don't have any concern for aberrant behavior, you are reluctant to increase her dose of narcotic, and she is already on maximal doses of her other therapies. Which of the following options is most appropriate?

a. Discontinue the opioids
b. Increase the opioids
c. Change to a lower dose of a different opioid
d. Add a second anticonvulsant
e. Add an antidepressant

Chronic Liver Disease

403. You are evaluating a 48-year-old man with liver disease. His laboratory evaluation is as follows:

AST:	268 U/L (high)
ALT:	114 U/L (high)
Alkaline phosphatase:	140 U/L (high)
Bilirubin:	2.3 mg/dL (high)
GGT:	220 U/L (high)

Which of the following is the most likely cause of his liver disease?

a. Autoimmune hepatitis
b. Hepatitis B
c. Hepatitis C
d. Hemochromatosis
e. Alcoholic hepatitis

404. You are evaluating a 45-year-old man with liver disease. His laboratory evaluation reveals the following:

AST:	52 U/L (high)
ALT:	56 U/L (high)
Alkaline phosphatase:	132 U/L (high)
GGT:	188 U/L (high)
Albumin:	2.9 g/dL (low)
Bilirubin:	3.5 mg/dL (high)
Prothrombin time:	14.9 seconds (high)

Which of his laboratory results suggests that his liver disease is chronic?

a. AST
b. ALT
c. GGT
d. Alkaline phosphatase
e. Albumin

405. You care for a patient who contracted hepatitis C after a blood transfusion many years ago. Her liver disease has progressed, and she now has end-stage disease. Which of the following will be the most likely cause of death in this patient?

a. Liver failure
b. Hepatocellular carcinoma
c. Bleeding varices
d. Encephalopathy
e. Renal failure

406. You are taking care of a 47-year-old woman with hypertension, diabetes, and dyslipidemia. Her examination shows a mild hepatomegaly and her laboratory studies reveal the following:

AST:	120 U/L (normal is 10-40 U/L)
ALT:	154 U/L (normal is 7-56 U/L)
Alkaline phosphatase:	140 IU/L (normal is 44-147 IU/L)
Bilirubin:	1.2 mg/dL (normal 0.3-1.0 mg/dL)
GGT:	61 U/L (normal 9-48 U/L)

She denies alcohol use or abuse. You presume nonalcoholic fatty liver disease (NAFLD). Which of the following is indicated?

a. Recommend a family intervention to help her admit to alcohol abuse
b. More aggressive treatment of her diabetes
c. Consider interferon therapy
d. Consider ribavirin treatment
e. Consider a direct-acting antibody drug (simeprevir or sofosbuvir)

Congestive Heart Failure

407. You have diagnosed a 66-year-old woman with heart failure. She has a history of hypertension, but has never had heart failure before. Which of the following tests is routinely indicated in the initial evaluation of a person with a new diagnosis of heart failure?

a. Echocardiogram
b. Holter monitor
c. Left heart catheterization
d. Treadmill stress test
e. Pharmacologic stress test

For questions 408 to 409, use the following scenario: You are seeing a patient who was discharged from the hospital. She initially presented to the ED with dyspnea and was found to be in heart failure with reduced ejection fraction (HFrEF). Her ejection fraction (EF) was found to be 30%. She was admitted for diuresis and initiation of appropriate first-line therapy.

408. According to the American College of Cardiology/American Heart Association/Heart Failure Society of America (ACC/AHA/HFSA) heart failure guidelines, once this patient's symptoms have been controlled with diuresis, what is the most appropriate first-line therapy for her HFrEF?

a. ACE-inhibitors
b. β-Blockers
c. Calcium channel blockers
d. Nitrates
e. Hydralazine

409. This same patient returns to your office for a follow-up visit 3 months later. She is following her low-sodium diet and taking her medications daily without side effects. She appears euvolemic and vitals today are: heart rate 88 beats/min, blood pressure 130/83 mm Hg, respiratory rate 14 breaths/min, and SpO_2 92%. However, she continues to have considerable dyspnea on exertion and her repeat echocardiogram shows an unchanged EF. What is the next best course of action?

a. Admit her to the hospital for acute diuresis and oxygen
b. Increase the diuretic
c. Add an angiotensin II-receptor blocker (ARB)
d. Add a β-blocker
e. Add metolazone

410. A 62-year-old woman comes to your office complaining of dyspnea. She has a history of COPD, hypertension, and diabetes. She also smokes and drinks heavily. Her evaluation reveals that she has HFrEF. Which of the following interventions will lead to functional improvement in this patient?

a. Optimizing the treatment of her COPD
b. Optimizing the treatment of her hypertension
c. Optimizing her glycemic control
d. Discontinuing cigarette smoking
e. Discontinuing alcohol use

411. You have been treating a 68-year-old man suffering from chronic left HFrEF with furosemide (Lasix), a β-blocker, and an ACE-inhibitor. Despite this therapy, he continues with refractory edema. In his baseline state, he is comfortable at rest, but experiences some symptoms of heart failure with ordinary activity. Which of the following would be the best diuretic to add?

a. Hydrochlorothiazide
b. Triamterene
c. Hydrochlorothiazide and triamterene combined (Dyazide, Maxzide)
d. Metolazone (Zaroxolyn)
e. Spironolactone (Aldactone)

Dementias

For questions 412 to 414, use the following scenario: You are seeing a 74-year-old woman accompanied by her son. He is concerned that his mother has developed problems with her memory since the death of her husband 1 year ago. He reports that she is forgetful, often repeating questions multiple times. She calls him frequently in the middle of the night reporting that there are strangers in her house. If he sleeps at her house, he notes that her sleep is restful but she wakes frequently. Recently, she has begun to get lost while driving and he had to take her keys away. She states that her memory is "impeccable" and feels that her son is being overly critical. Her past medical history is only positive for hypothyroidism and OA. On physical examination, you note that she is not her typically well-kept self; her hair is not combed and she has dirty clothes. She has no focal neurologic deficits. Cranial nerves and muscle strength are normal. Her timed get-up and go testing is normal and she does not have any gait abnormalities. She is alert to person, place, and time. However, her mini-cog is abnormal; she is unable to recall two of the three items you listed and her clock drawing is markedly abnormal.

412. Which of the following is most likely in this patient?

a. Lewy Body dementia
b. Parkinson disease
c. Behavioral variant frontotemporal dementia
d. Alzheimer disease
e. Vascular dementia

413. Which of the following would be most helpful in confirming this diagnosis?

a. History and physical examination
b. MRI of the brain
c. Lumbar puncture
d. Electroencephalogram (EEG)
e. Computed Tomography (CT) of the brain

414. At the end of this visit, the patient's son inquires as to his risk for developing this disorder. Of the following, which is the strongest risk factor for the development of this dementia?

a. Family history
b. Female gender
c. Advancing age
d. Low levels of education
e. Cardiovascular risk factors

415. You are concerned that one of your 65-year-old patients is developing dementia. Which of the following, if present, would lead you to suspect dementia rather than delirium or depression?

a. Acute onset of symptoms
b. Difficulty with concentration
c. Signs of psychomotor slowing
d. Good effort with testing, but wrong answers
e. Patient complaint of memory loss

416. You are caring for a 69-year-old woman with symptoms suggesting Alzheimer disease. Which of the following clinical features of Alzheimer disease is most likely to remain intact until the late stages of the disease?

a. The ability to recall new information
b. Word-finding ability
c. The ability to draw complex figures (intersecting boxes or a clock)
d. The ability to calculate (balance a checkbook)
e. Appropriate social behavior

417. You decide to treat a 72-year-old man for Alzheimer dementia (AD). You choose to use donepezil (Aricept), and begin therapy. With respect to disease progression, which of the following statements best describes donepezil's effect on AD?

a. It dramatically slows the progression of neurodegeneration.
b. It modestly slows the progression of neurodegeneration.
c. It has no effect on the progression of neurodegeneration.
d. It modestly increases the progression of neurodegeneration.
e. It dramatically increases the progression of neurodegeneration.

418. You are seeing an 82-year-old patient with moderately advanced AD. His wife is his primary caregiver and reports that he has had increasing behavioral symptoms over the last 6 months; he paces constantly, is often agitated, and lately, has been resisting the home health worker's care. Despite optimizing nonpharmacologic measures, he has become difficult for her to manage and she would like for you to prescribe something to help with his aggressive behavioral symptoms. He currently takes only blood pressure medication and a statin. Which of the following would be the best initial choice for this patient?

a. Donepezil
b. Sertraline
c. Carbamazepine
d. Memantine
e. Risperidone

Diabetes Mellitus

419. You are interested in providing nutrition classes to your patients at risk for developing type 2 diabetes (T2DM). According to the American Diabetes Association (ADA), which of the following patients is at risk for developing T2DM and should be screened for diabetes?

a. A 46-year-old male patient who has obesity, hypertension, and dyslipidemia who had an A1C of 5.5% last year
b. A 23-year-old female with a BMI of 24 kg/m^2 and whose grandfather was a type 1 diabetic
c. A 22-year-old sedentary male patient with a BMI of 29 kg/m^2 and no past medical history
d. A 33-year-old morbidly obese female who is 3 months postpartum and had gestational diabetes during her pregnancy
e. A 42-year-old Asian American male marathon runner with a BMI of 22 kg/m^2

420. You are evaluating a 36-year-old obese woman who complains of fatigue. She denies polydipsia, polyuria, polyphagia, or weight loss. Which of the following laboratory reports confirms the diagnosis of diabetes?

a. A random glucose reading of 221 mg/dL
b. A random glucose reading of 221 mg/dL, and another, on a later date, of 208 mg/dL
c. A fasting glucose measurement of 128 mg/dL
d. A glucose reading, taken 2 hours after a 75-g glucose load, of 163 mg/dL
e. A hemoglobin A1C of 6.3%

421. An 18-year-old morbidly obese patient in your office is found to have a fasting glucose of 314 mg/dL. Which of the following test results would indicate that he is a type 1 diabetic?

a. Low levels of C-peptide
b. Markedly elevated levels of C-peptide
c. Elevated levels of microalbumin in the urine
d. A markedly elevated hemoglobin A1C
e. The presence of parietal cell antibodies

For questions 422 to 424, use the following clinical scenario: You are managing a 36-year-old woman with a new diagnosis of T2DM. Past medical history includes depression, venous insufficiency, and gestational diabetes with each of her pregnancies. Her fasting plasma glucose is 287 mg/dL, the remainder of her metabolic panel is normal, and her hemoglobin A1C is 9.2%. Urinalysis is normal, but her albumin-to-creatinine ratio is elevated. She has no previous evidence of kidney disease. Her BMI is 33 kg/m² and her blood pressure is 128/76. She denies any symptoms of hyperglycemia, including polydipsia, polyphagia, or blurred vision.

422. What is the most appropriate first course of action for this patient?

a. Admit her to the hospital and start an insulin drip and replace electrolytes as needed
b. Start metformin 1000 mg twice daily
c. Start insulin glargine 0.2 U/kg/d
d. Start metformin and a glucagon-like-peptide 1 (GLP-1) receptor agonist
e. Start metformin and a thiazolidinedione (TZD)

423. At this time, how would you address this patient's positive microalbumin screen?

a. Initiate therapy with an ACE-inhibitor
b. Initiate therapy with an ARB
c. Prescribe a low-protein diet
d. Optimize glycemic control and repeat screening
e. Refer to endocrinology

424. Considering this patient's diagnosis and history, which of the following is true regarding retinopathy prevention and surveillance?

a. A daily aspirin will reduce her retinopathy risk.
b. She should have a dilated eye examination now and quarterly until her A1C is at goal.
c. Lowering her A1C does not reduce retinopathy risk.
d. She should have an annual dilated eye examination beginning at diagnosis.
e. Retinopathy occurs at lower levels of hemoglobin A1C for Caucasian patients.

425. You are seeing an African-American man with newly diagnosed diabetes. His blood pressure at the last visit was 148/76 mm Hg, and at this visit it is 152/82 mm Hg. He has no evidence of CVD or CKD and is not on any antihypertensive agents. Which of the following statements is true regarding the use of an ACE-inhibitor in this patient?

a. An ACE-inhibitor should be added to his regimen because he is diabetic, regardless of his blood pressure.
b. An ACE-inhibitor is the preferred agent to be added to his regimen based on his blood pressure readings.
c. An ACE-inhibitor should not be added to his regimen unless his blood pressure goes above 160 systolic.
d. An ACE-inhibitor should not be added to his regimen unless he has microalbuminuria.
e. An ACE-inhibitor should not be given to this patient if his creatinine is elevated.

426. You are seeing a 75-year-old male patient with a 10-year history of T2DM for his 3-month diabetes follow-up. He takes 20 units of insulin glargine at bedtime and 1000 mg of metformin twice daily. His home glucose readings show fasting sugars in the range of 60 to 130 and postprandial readings in the range of 145 to 210. His A1C today is 8.2%. He has several co-morbidities, including CHF, hypertension, CKD, and a history of a myocardial infarction (MI) 3 years ago. He has had several falls and difficulty with ambulation because of diabetic neuropathy. His daughter is concerned about his episodes of low blood sugar, but he states they don't bother him. What A1C goal would you recommend for this patient?

a. Around 6.5%
b. Around 7.0%
c. Around 7.5%
d. Around 8.0%
e. Around 8.5%

427. A 44-year-old African American with T2DM transfers care to you. Reviewing her records, you find she is on the maximum dose of metformin and her hemoglobin A1C is 7.0%. Review of her baseline laboratory tests reveals normal liver enzymes and a creatinine of 2.3 mg/dL (GFR 35 mL/min/1.73 m^2). Her BMI is 26 kg/m^2. She is hypertensive and is well controlled on a thiazide diuretic and an ACE-inhibitor. Which of the following management options would be the most beneficial?

a. Continue the current regimen
b. Add glyburide
c. Discontinue the metformin and add linagliptin
d. Discontinue the metformin and add dapagliflozin
e. Add sitagliptin

428. You are seeing a 29-year-old woman for a T2DM follow-up visit. She has been taking a GLP-1 receptor agonist for the last 6 months and complains that the side effects are too bothersome and she would like to switch medications. You recommend a dipeptidyl peptidase 4 (DPP-4) inhibitor. Which of the following statements is true about the GLP-1 receptor agonists compared to the DPP-4 inhibitors?

a. Both agents result in a supraphysiologic increase in GLP-1 in the body
b. Both agents have similar effects on bodyweight
c. Both GLP-1 receptor agonists and DPP-4 inhibitors increase glucose-dependent insulin secretion from the pancreas
d. Both GLP-1 receptor agonists and DPP-4 inhibitors increase gluconeogenesis in the liver
e. Both GLP-1 receptor agonists and DPP-4 inhibitors slow gastric emptying

429. You have been treating a 46-year-old woman for T2DM for 2 years with metformin and recently started insulin glargine at night. She is compliant with her diet and medications, and exercises regularly. She is 65 inches tall and weighs 200 lb. Her most recent HbA1C is 9.0% which is elevated from 8.8% 3 months ago. When you added the insulin regimen, she had hypoglycemic episodes, so at her visit 2 weeks ago, you added the sodium-glucose cotransporter 2 (SGLT-2) inhibitor, dapagliflozin to her regimen and stopped her insulin. The patient presents today complaining of a problem that she attributes to the new medication. Which of the following is the most likely complaint?

a. Symptomatic hypoglycemia
b. Edema and weight gain
c. Cough
d. Urinary tract infection
e. GI intolerance

430. You are caring for a patient with T2DM whose measures of control have been worsening despite maximal doses of oral medications. You are considering adding insulin therapy to help with her post-prandial hyperglycemia and want to start a preparation with a rapid onset of action. Which of the following insulin types has the most rapid onset of action?

a. Aspart (NovoLog)
b. Regular
c. Neutral protamine Hagedorn (NPH)
d. Detemir (Levemir)
e. Glargine (Lantus)

431. You are thinking about starting a patient with T2DM on insulin therapy to improve her glucose control. You would like to provide her with steady insulin action without much of a peak time. Which of the following insulin preparations provides the most stable insulin coverage without a peak time of maximum activity?

a. Aspart (Novolog)
b. Lispro (Humalog)
c. Regular
d. NPH
e. Glargine (Lantus)

432. You have maximized oral anti-hyperglycemic therapy for a 56-year-old female patient with T2DM, hypertension, dyslipidemia, and obesity. She works hard at diet and exercise, but her hemoglobin A1C is still elevated at 9.6%. You decide to add insulin to her regimen. She is currently 67 in tall and weighs 100 kg. You decide to start her on 10 units of glargine (Lantus) at night in addition to her current regimen. Which of the following recommendations would you make for this patient regarding self-monitoring of blood glucose (SMBG)?

a. She should test her blood glucose levels any time of day.
b. She should not check her blood glucose levels, as there is no evidence to suggest that it is helpful for patients on only basal insulin.
c. She should check her blood glucose levels, but she doesn't need to bring her glucose log with her to appointments.
d. She should check blood glucose levels once a day, fasting, and receive education about how to make adjustments to her meals and insulin based on these readings.
e. She should check her blood glucose levels fasting, after meals, and at bedtime.

Lipid Disorders

433. You are doing a screening physical examination for a 40-year-old female patient. She does not have diabetes or known coronary artery disease. You calculate her 10-year Atherosclerotic Cardiovascular Disease (ASCVD) risk to be 6.5%. Her low-density lipoprotein (LDL) cholesterol is 165 mg/dL, high-density lipoprotein (HDL) cholesterol is 48 mg/dL, and triglycerides are 193 mg/dL. Given this information, what do you recommend as treatment for her dyslipidemia?

a. Lifestyle modifications such as diet and physical activity
b. Treatment with a low-intensity statin
c. Treatment with a moderate-intensity statin
d. Treatment with a high-intensity statin
e. Treatment with a fenofibrate agent

434. You are caring for a newly established 54-year-old white male patient with T2DM, hypertension, and dyslipidemia. He does not have any clinical ASCVD, but his father died from a MI at the age of 56. He admits he has not been great about following up with a physician and would like to make a greater effort to control his cardiac risks. His blood pressure is well controlled with lisinopril-hydrochlorothiazide. He has never smoked. His 10-year ASCVD risk is calculated at 11.2%. His recent laboratory values are below.

Lab	Result	Lab	Result
Total Cholesterol	168 mg/dL	A1C	8.2%
LDL cholesterol (LDL-C)	120 mg/dL	FPG	128 mg/dL
HDL	41 mg/dL	Cr	1.06 mg/dL
TG	180 mg/dL	eGFR	75 mL/min/1.73m^2

What treatment recommendation do you suggest for his dyslipidemia?

a. Lifestyle modifications such as diet and physical activity
b. Treatment with a low-intensity statin
c. Treatment with a moderate-intensity statin
d. Treatment with a high-intensity statin
e. Treatment with a fenofibrate agent

435. You are caring for a 26-year-old man with dyslipidemia and a family history of early coronary arterial disease. Laboratory analysis reveals a low HDL. Which of the following interventions, if adopted by the patient, would raise his HDL levels to the greatest extent?

a. Eat oat bran
b. Lose weight
c. Start exercising
d. Quit smoking
e. Reduce life stress

436. You have performed a screening lipid profile on an otherwise healthy man. His results indicate elevated triglycerides, a low HDL, a high LDL, an elevated total cholesterol, and an elevated very-low-density lipoprotein (VLDL). You would like to rescreen him in the fasting state. Which of the following laboratory values is likely to decrease in the fasting state?

a. Serum triglycerides
b. HDL
c. LDL
d. Total cholesterol
e. VLDL

437. You have been caring for a 36-year-old man, and identified that he meets criteria for therapeutic lifestyle changes (TLC) to improve his lipid profile. After 4 months of adhering to your recommendations, his LDL is still higher than goal. Which of the following drug classes should be initiated?

a. A statin
b. A bile acid sequestrant
c. Nicotinic acid
d. A fibrate
e. A cholesterol absorption inhibitor

438. You started a 43-year-old female patient of yours on a statin for dyslipidemia. She has no other medical conditions, but does have a family history of coronary heart disease. At a follow-up visit for a different chief complaint, you order a laboratory panel that includes serum transaminases. Her AST is found to be 56 U/L (normal is 10-40 U/L) and her ALT is found to be 115 U/L (normal is 7-56 U/L). Which of the following is most appropriate given these values?

a. Discontinue the statin.
b. Decrease the dose of the statin.
c. Test muscle enzymes (creatine phosphokinase [CPK]) and discontinue the statin if also elevated.
d. Test muscle enzymes (CPK) and decrease the dose of the statin if also elevated.
e. No change is indicated.

439. You have prescribed niacin for a patient with VLDL cholesterol and elevated triglycerides. He reports nonadherence to this regimen because of significant flushing that occurs when he takes the medication. What would you recommend to avoid this side effect?

a. Take the niacin at night
b. Take the niacin with food
c. Take the niacin with milk
d. Take aspirin before taking the niacin
e. Take a proton-pump inhibitor before taking the niacin

440. You are treating a patient who is interested in more "natural" methods to control his cholesterol. He wants to use niacin. Which of the following statements regarding niacin is true?

a. It substantially decreases LDL.
b. It substantially raises HDL.
c. It has no effect on triglycerides.
d. Its side effects generally prevent it from being used.
e. It can't be used in patients who have concurrent diabetes.

441. You are treating a patient with dyslipidemia and clinical ASCVD. She has elevated total cholesterol, LDL-C, and triglycerides. Her HDL is low. Which of the following changes will have the greatest effect on mortality?

a. Increasing HDL
b. Decreasing LDL-C
c. Decreasing triglycerides
d. Decreasing non-HDL cholesterol
e. Decreasing apolipoprotein-A

HIV Care

For questions 442 to 444, consider the following scenario: You are caring for a 26-year-old gay man who recently went to the local health department for anonymous HIV testing. His test was positive, and he is following up with you for initial laboratory testing and recommendations on next steps. As part of his initial testing, you find his CD4 count to be 388 cells/mm^3 and his viral load is below 10,000 copies/mL.

442. During his initial laboratory workup, you identify that he is Hepatitis A and Hepatitis B virus nonimmune. What should you recommend?

a. No vaccinations should be given to this patient.
b. The patient should be vaccinated against Hepatitis A, but not Hepatitis B.
c. The patient should be vaccinated against Hepatitis B, but not Hepatitis A.
d. The patient should be vaccinated against both Hepatitis A and B.
e. The patient should be given immune globulin.

443. As part of his initial evaluation with you, you perform a tuberculin skin test. Which of the following is correct regarding the reading of his skin test?

a. Any induration is indication for treatment.
b. Induration below 5 mm is not indication for treatment.
c. Induration below 10 mm is not indication for treatment.
d. Induration below 15 mm is not indication for treatment.
e. Induration below 20 mm is not indication for treatment.

444. The patient is interested in antiretroviral therapy (ART). Which of the following is most accurate regarding the initiation of ART in this patient?

a. He is a candidate for ART.
b. His CD4 count is too high for him to be considered a candidate for ART.
c. His viral load is too low for him to be considered a candidate for ART.
d. He should not start ART until he has an acquired immunodeficiency syndrome (AIDS)-defining illness.
e. He should only start ART if he is at risk for transmitting HIV to others.

445. You are following a 41-year-old man with HIV who has had a stable CD4 count and undetectable viral load (< 50 copies/mL) for 3 years. His ART regimen consists of efavirenz, tenofovir, and emtricitabine (Atripla, in a single, once-daily pill). His most recent laboratory evaluation revealed a viral load of 187 copies/mL. Which of the following is the appropriate next step?

a. Continue usual monitoring without changing medication regimen
b. Increase the dosage of his Atripla
c. Add an additional medication from a different class of antiretroviral drug
d. Change to Complera (rilpivirine, tenofovir, and emtricitabine in a single, once-daily pill)
e. Refer to an HIV specialist for evaluation

446. You are caring for a 38-year-old woman with HIV for more than 10 years. She has had difficulty continuing her regimen and has only been able to adhere to her ART regimen sporadically. Her viral load is detectable, and her CD4 count is falling. At what CD4 count should you consider prophylaxis against *Pneumocystis jiroveci* pneumonia (PCP)?

a. Less than 500
b. Less than 350
c. Less than 200
d. Less than 100
e. Less than 50

Hypertension

447. You are evaluating a 35-year-old man whose systolic blood pressure (SBP) has been between 140 and 160 mm Hg on three separate occasions in the office, despite lifestyle modifications. He asks you why it is important to follow-up on these findings. According to observational studies, which of the following is true?

a. The risk of CVD increases in a linear fashion between SBP between 140 and 180 mm Hg.
b. An SBP 20 mm Hg higher than normal is associated with a doubling in the risk of death from stroke.
c. An increased risk of CVD is associated with higher SBP at all ages.
d. The relative risk of CVD is lower for this patient than it would be for an elderly person with the same blood pressure.
e. This patient is at greater risk for MI and stroke, but not for heart failure or peripheral artery disease (PAD).

For questions 448 to 452, assume you and your staff have appropriately measured blood pressures of several people in your office. Which of the following categories would these blood pressures fall into? Use the following answer key:

a. Normal blood pressure
b. Elevated blood pressure
c. Stage I hypertension
d. Stage II hypertension
e. Hypertensive crisis

448. A 24-year-old woman with these three consecutive independent readings: 118/78, 126/84, and 112/68.

449. A 36-year-old African-American man with these three consecutive independent readings: 124/86, 130/90, and 122/84.

450. A 52-year-old obese woman with these three consecutive independent readings: 132/92, 129/90, and 134/94.

451. A 43-year-old man with these three consecutive independent readings: 122/82, 124/86, and 118/84.

452. A 33-year-old man with a family history of hypertension with these three consecutive independent readings: 116/72, 122/68, and 128/78.

453. You have diagnosed a 42-year-old patient with hypertension. He is 5 ft 9 in tall, weighs 230 lb, and admits to poor eating habits, drinking four alcoholic beverages daily, and no regular exercise. Which of the following lifestyle modifications, if instituted, will result in the largest SBP reduction?

a. Moderate alcohol consumption to no more than two drinks daily
b. Engage in physical activity for 30 minutes per day, most days of the week
c. Reduce dietary sodium intake to no more than 100 mEq/L per day
d. Adopt a Dietary Approaches to Stop Hypertension (DASH) eating plan (a diet rich in fruits, vegetables, and low-fat dairy products with a reduced saturated and total fat content)
e. Lose 8 to 10 lbs

454. You have seen a 36-year-old African-American man with elevated blood pressure. On one occasion, his blood pressure was 128/84 mm Hg, and on a second occasion, his blood pressure was 138/88 mm Hg. You have encouraged lifestyle modifications including weight loss using exercise and dietary changes. Despite some modest weight loss, at his current visit, his blood pressure is 128/89 mm Hg. Which of the following is the best treatment strategy at this point?

a. Use a thiazide diuretic
b. Use an ACE-inhibitor
c. Use an angiotensin receptor blocker
d. Use a β-blocker
e. Use a two-drug combination of medications

455. You have just diagnosed a 35-year-old man with hypertension. He is otherwise healthy and has no complaints. Which of the following is indicated in the initial evaluation?

a. Uric acid level
b. Resting electrocardiogram
c. Stress test
d. Echocardiogram
e. Renal ultrasound

456. You are treating a 61-year-old man for hypertension. He is not responding well to combination therapy with a thiazide diuretic and a β-blocker. On physical examination, you note an abdominal bruit. Which of the following tests is most likely to help you evaluate him further?

a. CXR
b. MRI or magnetic resonance arteriography (MRA)
c. Urinary metanephrines and vanillylmandelic acid levels
d. Aortic CT scan
e. Echocardiogram

457. Despite lifestyle changes, a 37-year-old patient of yours still has stage I hypertension with SBP more than 10 mm Hg above goal. She has no other medical concerns and no abnormalities on physical examination or initial laboratory evaluation. Which of the following medications is best as an initial first-line monotherapy?

a. A thiazide diuretic
b. An ACE-inhibitor
c. An ARB
d. A calcium channel blocker
e. A β-blocker

458. A 48-year-old male patient suffered from an ischemic stroke. Prior to his stroke, he was untreated for hypertension. After full recovery, he follows up at your office. On examination, his blood pressure is 132/82 mm Hg. Which of the following is true?

a. An ACE-inhibitor should be used to help him achieve a blood pressure less than 130/80.
b. Hydrochlorothiazide should be used to help him achieve a blood pressure less than 130/80.
c. A β-blocker should be used to help him achieve a blood pressure less than 130/80.
d. A β-blocker and hydrochlorothiazide should be used to help him achieve a blood pressure less than 130/80.
e. The usefulness of initiating antihypertensive treatment in this patient is not well-established.

459. A 55-year-old man comes to your office after not being seen by a physician in more than 10 years. He is found to be hypertensive, and his creatinine is found to be 2.3 mg/dL (high). Which medication is most likely to control his blood pressure and decrease the likelihood of progression of his renal disease?

a. A thiazide diuretic
b. An ACE-inhibitor
c. A calcium channel blocker
d. A β-blocker
e. An aldosterone antagonist

460. You diagnosed a 47-year-old woman with hypertension around 6 months ago. Her home blood pressure readings are not at goal, and her blood pressure readings in the office are also not at goal. Of the following, which is the most likely cause of her uncontrolled hypertension?

a. Treatment nonadherence
b. Undiagnosed renal artery stenosis
c. Primary aldosteronism
d. Undiagnosed thyroid disorder
e. Concomitant use of stimulant medications

461. You are monitoring the blood pressure in a 53-year-old patient with stage II hypertension. The patient has no signs or symptoms indicative of secondary hypertension. The patient is not at goal despite maximized dosage of a generic ACE-inhibitor and thiazide diuretic. Which of the following is the appropriate next step?

a. Diagnose the patient with resistant hypertension and refer to specialist
b. Add a third agent from a different class to the regimen
c. Change the ACE-inhibitor to an ARB
d. Change the ACE-inhibitor to a different ACE-inhibitor
e. Change the thiazide diuretic to a loop diuretic

Ischemia and Angina

For questions 462 to 464, use the following answer key:

a. Classic angina
b. Atypical angina
c. Anginal equivalent
d. Nonanginal pain
e. Atypical nonanginal pain

462. A 49-year-old man with a known history of hypercholesterolemia and hypertension complains of chest pain. He describes it as a "heaviness" in the substernal area. It is not associated with activity, but occurs intermittently throughout the day.

463. A 36-year-old man complains of shortness of breath. His symptoms are associated with activity and relieved by rest. He is otherwise healthy.

464. A 44-year-old woman with a known history of asthma complains of chest pain. She reports a stabbing pain that is worse with inspiration. It is not associated with activity and occurs at random times during the day.

465. You are medically treating an 85-year-old woman with stable angina, and choose to use nitrates. Which of the following is the most important consideration when using this medication?

a. Headache as a side effect
b. Fatigue as a side effect
c. Interactions with β-blockers
d. Interactions with calcium channel blockers
e. Development of tolerance

466. You have chosen to treat a 70-year-old man with ischemic heart disease using a β-blocker. Which of the following is the most appropriate endpoint for the use of β-blockers in this case?

a. Use no more than the equivalent of 40 mg twice daily of propranolol
b. Use the amount necessary to achieve a blood pressure of 100/70 mm Hg or less
c. Use the amount necessary to keep the heart rate between 50 and 60 beats/min
d. Increase the dosage until fatigue limits use
e. Increase the amount until angina disappears

Obesity

For questions 467 to 469, use the following answer key:

a. Normal weight
b. Overweight
c. Obesity Class I
d. Obesity Class II
e. Obesity Class III

467. You are discussing weight management with a 28-year-old Caucasian man. He does not exercise in any form, and has a strong family history of obesity. His height and weight make his BMI 27.8 kg/m².

468. You are seeing a Hispanic woman for a work physical examination. She is 31 years old, generally inactive, and has no other medical conditions. Her BMI is 33.4 kg/m².

469. You are caring for a 56-year-old woman with diabetes and hyperlipidemia. Her BMI is 35.8 kg/m².

470. You are caring for a 48-year-old Caucasian woman who has a significant family history of obesity and obesity-related health conditions. She reports that she was at her "ideal" weight in college, where she majored in finance and accounting. Currently, she is single and lives a fairly active life, but she does have a high-stress, executive-level position at work. Given what you know about this patient, which characteristics described in her history put her at risk for overweight or obesity?

a. Her race
b. Her age
c. Her socioeconomic status
d. Her level of education
e. Her marital status

471. The patient described in the question above is interested in a diet that will help her lose weight. Of the following, which type of diet has been consistently shown to be superior to others if long-term weight loss is the desired outcome?

a. Lower-fat diets.
b. The "Adkins" diet (low carbohydrate).
c. The "South Beach" diet (low glycemic index).
d. The "Zone" diet (40% carbohydrates, 30% protein, 30% fat).
e. None have been shown to be superior to others.

472. A 33-year-old woman is seeing you for weight management. At 5 ft 6 in tall and 230 lb, she reports a history of having difficulty with weight since her teenage years. The rest of her medical history is unremarkable. Using conventional dietary techniques, what is her chance of losing 20 lb and maintaining that weight loss for 2 years?

a. 1%
b. 5%
c. 10%
d. 20%
e. 50%

473. You are discussing weight management with an overweight 33-year-old woman. She has tried for years to lose weight, but despite multiple attempts, remains overweight. Which of the following is indicated in the workup of her weight concerns?

a. History and physical alone
b. CBC
c. TSH
d. Serum electrolytes
e. LH to FSH ratio

474. You are caring for an obese 30-year-old woman who would like to consider pharmacotherapy for the treatment of her obesity. Which of the following Food and Drug Administration (FDA)-approved options has been shown to result in the highest weight loss percentage?

a. Orlistat (Xenical)
b. Lorcaserin (Belviq)
c. Phentermine hydrochloride and topiramate (Qsymia)
d. Naltrexone and bupropion hydrochloride (Contrave)
e. Liraglutide (Saxenda)

475. You are evaluating a patient whose BMI is 44 kg/m². You would like the patient to consider weight-loss surgery, specifically a Roux-en-Y gastric bypass. Which of the following is true regarding this procedure?

a. The operative mortality rate for this procedure in the first 30 days is near 5%.
b. Complications from this procedure occur in approximately 40% of the cases.
c. The procedure can be expected to help the patient lose up to 30% of initial body weight.
d. Nutritional deficiencies after surgery are rare.
e. This surgery is reserved for people with BMI greater than 30 kg/m².

Osteoporosis and Other Bone Issues

476. A 49-year-old African-American perimenopausal woman is seeing you after having fractured her wrist. Her past medical history is significant for oral contraceptive use for 20 years, obesity, and Graves' disease leading to current hypothyroidism. She nursed two children for 6 months each. Which component of the patient's history puts her at increased risk for osteoporosis?

a. African-American race
b. Oral contraceptive use
c. Obesity
d. Graves' disease
e. Breast-feeding

477. A 32-year-old woman is seeing you because her mother has been diagnosed with osteoporosis. She asks you what type of exercise will help her prevent the development of the disease. According to recommendations, which of the following exercises should you recommend to help her maintain bone mass?

a. Tennis
b. Swimming
c. Cycling
d. Skating
e. Skiing

478. You are caring for a 48-year-old Caucasian woman with a history of anorexia nervosa in her late twenties. She was an elite track and field athlete in her late teens and early twenties and was considered for the US Olympic team in her prime. Which of the following options is best for primary osteoporosis screening in this woman?

a. History
b. Physical examination
c. Serum calcium
d. Serum human osteocalcin levels
e. Bone density imaging

479. You are evaluating a 76-year-old woman on long-term glucocorticosteroid therapy for polymyalgia rheumatica. Which of the following is the diagnostic imaging test of choice to diagnose osteoporosis?

a. Plain radiographs
b. Single-photon absorptiometry
c. Dual-photon absorptiometry
d. Dual-emission x-ray absorptiometry (DXA) scan
e. Quantitative CT of bone

480. You are treating an elderly postmenopausal woman with osteoporosis. She recently suffered an acute osteoporotic vertebral fracture and is suffering from secondary pain. Which of the following osteoporosis treatments also has analgesic effects with respect to bone pain?

a. Estrogen
b. Combination of calcium and vitamin D
c. Calcitonin
d. Alendronate (Fosamax)
e. Raloxifene (Evista)

481. You have just diagnosed osteoporosis in a postmenopausal woman. She is considering treatment alternatives and wonders about the bisphosphonates. Which of the following is the best description of how this class of medications works?

a. They increase calcium absorption in the GI tract.
b. They block the activity of the cytokines that stimulate bone reabsorption.
c. They bind to bone surfaces to inhibit osteoclast activity.
d. They stimulate osteoblasts and increase bone formation.
e. They mimic estrogen's effect on bone.

482. You are caring for a 56-year-old woman with a several year history of pain and stiffness in her knee joints. She reports that the stiffness is worse after a period of inactivity, and resolves fairly quickly after beginning movement. The pain is described as dull and aching in character, and she says it's aggravated by cold and damp weather. Activity makes the pain worse. On physical examination, you note knee crepitus with passive motion without erythema or significant effusion. You suspect osteoarthritis (OA). Which of the following laboratory tests is most helpful to diagnose OA?

a. ESR.
b. Antinuclear antibody.
c. Rheumatoid factor.
d. Anticitrullinated protein antibody testing.
e. None of the above is helpful to diagnose OA.

483. You are caring for an elderly patient whose OA of the hips is becoming progressively more limiting. Other than using over-the-counter analgesics and anti-inflammatories, he has never been through a formalized treatment program for his OA. Which of the following is true regarding supervised exercise programs for OA of the hips?

a. They have been shown to improve pain control, but not functionality.
b. They have been shown to improve functionality, but not pain control.
c. They have been shown to improve well-being, but not prevention of disability.
d. They have been shown to improve disability, but not overall well-being.
e. They have been shown to improve pain control, functionality, well-being, and prevent disability.

Psychiatric Disorders

484. You are seeing a 32-year-old woman for fatigue. Your differential diagnosis includes major depressive disorder (MDD), but she does not describe a depressed or irritable mood. Which of the following symptoms of depression must be present in order to diagnose an MDD in someone without depressed mood?

a. Sleep changes
b. Loss of interest or pleasure in usually enjoyable activities
c. Guilt or feelings of worthlessness
d. Loss of energy
e. Change in appetite

485. You are caring for a patient who has a problem with alcohol abuse. Upon direct questioning, he says that he drinks because he continually recounts stressful memories from being in the Iraq war. Which of the following medications is the treatment of choice for this disorder?

a. Bupropion
b. Sertraline
c. Alprazolam
d. Valproic acid
e. Venlafaxine

486. You are discussing treatment options for a 43-year-old woman with MDD. Which of the following is a true statement regarding the effectiveness of treatment for depressive disorders?

a. Only about 25% of patients that receive medication alone will find the medication to be effective.
b. Patients who find one medication ineffective are likely to find all medications ineffective.
c. In order to prevent a relapse of depressive symptoms, patients should continue treatment for 3 to 4 months.
d. In general, patients respond best to the combination of medication and counseling.
e. Electroconvulsive therapy (ECT) is ineffective when compared with newer medical therapies.

487. You are treating a 48-year-old man for major depression. His medical history includes a head injury several years ago that has left him with a seizure disorder. Which of the following antidepressants would be contraindicated?

a. Venlafaxine
b. Amitriptyline
c. Mirtazapine
d. Fluoxetine
e. Bupropion

488. You are following a 16-year-old girl with a suspected eating disorder. Which of the following, if present, would help differentiate anorexia nervosa from bulimia nervosa?

a. Binge eating or purging.
b. The use of laxatives, diuretics, or enemas.
c. Self-evaluation is unduly influenced by body weight and shape.
d. Episodic lack of control over eating.
e. Inappropriate behaviors to prevent weight gain.

489. You decide to treat a severely depressed patient with fluoxetine. The response is dramatic and on follow-up he reports that he feels great. He has got a lot of energy—in fact he hasn't slept in 2 days. He just bought a new car despite losing his job. You suspect acute mania. Which of the following is the best choice of medications to control the acute symptoms?

a. Antipsychotics
b. Lithium
c. Valproic acid
d. Carbamazepine
e. Lamotrigine

490. A 26-year-old male college graduate is seeing you for an office visit. He is concerned that he may have attention-deficit hyperactivity disorder (ADHD). Which of the following is true regarding this condition?

a. The symptoms are likely to be more pronounced in adults as compared with children.
b. Children diagnosed with ADHD commonly continue to have symptoms into adulthood.
c. Sleep disturbance is a distinctive feature of adult ADHD.
d. Appetite disturbance is a distinctive feature of adult ADHD.
e. The symptom picture of adult ADHD mimics that in children.

491. You are seeing a 6-year-old boy who is being evaluated for ADHD. Behavioral rating forms completed by his teachers and his parents are consistent with the diagnosis. Which of the following blood tests should you obtain prior to making the diagnosis?

a. No blood tests are necessary.
b. CBC.
c. Sedimentation rate.
d. TSH.
e. Toxicology screen.

492. You are caring for a 33-year-old woman in your office. She is generally healthy but expects to be seen immediately when she asks and demands schedule adjustments to meet her needs. She describes her time as being much more valuable than others, and will become enraged if she has to wait more than a few minutes to see you. You suspect narcissistic personality disorder. Which of the following treatment options is most beneficial?

a. Pharmacologic treatment with an SSRI
b. Pharmacologic treatment with a tricyclic antidepressant
c. Pharmacologic treatment with an antipsychotic
d. Psychotherapeutic intervention
e. Psychotherapeutic intervention plus pharmacologic treatment

493. You are seeing a 24-year-old patient that has been diagnosed with debilitating generalized anxiety disorder (GAD). She has been relatively stable using pharmacotherapy with an SSRI, but has been troubled by associated sexual dysfunction. She got married last month, and now would like to change medications to avoid that side effect. Of the following treatments, which would be the best alternative to treatment with an SSRI in this situation?

a. A benzodiazepine
b. A tricyclic antidepressant
c. Buspirone (BuSpar)
d. A β-blocker
e. An atypical anticonvulsant (like gabapentin or pregabalin)

Thyroid Disorders

494. A 45-year-old woman presents to your office for follow-up. She has a long history of hypothyroidism, and is taking thyroid replacement therapy. She has been on 50 μg of levothyroxine daily for around 1 year, but reports that she's recently felt fatigued and has gained some weight. You obtain a TSH test, and it comes back high at 7.2 mIU/mL. You decide to increase her dosage of levothyroxine in an attempt to get her euthyroid. When should you recheck the TSH to gauge the new dosage?

a. 2 weeks after the dose adjustment.
b. 6 weeks after dose adjustment.
c. 3 months after dose adjustment.
d. 6 months after dose adjustment.
e. TSH should not be used to gauge dose adjustments.

495. You are caring for a 35-year-old man who is complaining of fatigue and an inability to gain weight. Laboratory evaluation reveals a TSH of 6.0 mIU/L (high) but a normal free T$_4$. Which of the following is the best next step?

a. Test for antithyroid peroxidase
b. Test for thyroid autoantibodies
c. Treat with levothyroxine
d. Treat with levothyroxine and T$_3$
e. Monitor at yearly intervals

496. A 26-year-old woman presents with weight gain, lethargy, dry skin, sweatiness, cold intolerance, and thinning hair. You suspect hypothyroidism and order the appropriate laboratory tests. Her TSH is high, and her free T$_3$ and free T$_4$ are both low. Which of the following is the most likely diagnosis?

a. Primary hypothyroidism
b. Secondary hypothyroidism
c. Iodine deficiency
d. Thyroid hormone resistance
e. Subclinical hypothyroidism

497. You are screening a 35-year-old woman who presents with tachycardia, nervousness, tremor, palpitations, heat intolerance, and weight loss. You suspect Graves' disease. What would you expect to find on radionucleotide uptake scanning of the thyroid with Graves' disease?

a. Diffusely decreased uptake
b. Patchy uptake
c. Nodular areas of increased uptake
d. Areas of increased uptake surrounded by hypoactivity
e. Diffusely increased uptake

498. You have confirmed that the patient above has Graves' disease. Which of the following is the treatment of choice?

a. Radioactive iodine
b. Methimazole
c. Propylthiouracil
d. β-blockade
e. Surgery

499. You note a thyroid nodule in a 35-year-old African-American woman who is not demonstrating clinical features of thyroid dysfunction. Which of the following patient characteristics, or features (if present), would increase your suspicion of malignancy?

a. The patient's age
b. The patient's race
c. The patient's sex
d. If the nodule were slowly growing on follow-up
e. If the patient complained of persistent hoarseness

500. When examining a 35-year-old man, you notice a firm 3-cm thyroid nodule. His thyroid studies are normal, and he is clinically euthyroid. An ultrasound is performed, and the nodule appears suspicious for malignancy. What should the next step in the workup be?

a. Follow thyroid studies and continue workup if abnormal
b. Measure thyroid peroxidase antibodies
c. Suppress thyroid with levothyroxine therapy
d. Perform a fine needle aspirate
e. Perform a surgical biopsy

Chronic Conditions

Answers

Adult Sexual Issues

344. The answer is d. The sexual response is divided into four phases. The first is libido (or desire/interest). This phase requires androgens and an intact sensory system. The second phase is arousal (or excitement) and in men, involves erection. Vascular arterial or inflow problems are by far the most common cause, though mood disorders, stressors, and alcohol abuse may all play a role. Lack of attraction to a partner would represent a disorder of desire, not arousal.

345. The answer is b. In patients with decreased sex drive, laboratory workup should be directed by the history and physical examination findings. In a male patient with no other complaints and no physical examination findings, assessment of hormone status is indicated. Testosterone levels should be checked in the morning, when they peak. Free testosterone is a more accurate measure of androgen status, as it is a measure of bioavailable testosterone. The TSH and prolactin levels may be indicated in the presence of other complaints or physical findings. PSA would not be helpful. If this were a female patient, both androgen and estrogen status should be evaluated.

346. The answer is e. Tricyclics and SSRIs frequently cause sexual dysfunction due to a raised threshold for orgasm. Conversely, bupropion actually decreases the orgasm threshold and is least likely to cause sexual dysfunction.

347. The answer is b. Premature ejaculation is the most common sexual dysfunction in men, affecting about 29% of men in the general population. Alprostadil is used for erectile dysfunction, but would not positively affect premature ejaculation. Fluoxetine raises the threshold for orgasm, making it an effective treatment option. Bupropion and sildenafil may decrease the orgasmic threshold and further exacerbate premature ejaculation. Atenolol may cause erectile dysfunction, but would likely not treat premature ejaculation.

348. The answer is d. In men with erectile disorders, obtaining a serum free testosterone level in the morning is appropriate. If the level is low, the level should be confirmed with a second level before testosterone replacement is considered. After a second low measurement is obtained, the next step is to obtain a FSH, LH, and prolactin level. If the FSH and LH are low, but the prolactin is normal, the diagnosis is pituitary or hypothalamic failure. If the FSH and LH are high and the prolactin is normal, the diagnosis is testicular failure. The nocturnal penile tumescence evaluation would be done to eliminate psychologic factors that inhibit arousal in the setting of ED, but would not be helpful to follow up an abnormal testosterone level.

349. The answer is a. Treatment for sexual dysfunction has been studied in many settings by many people. The most effective treatment program found to date for women with primary orgasmic dysfunction is directed self-stimulation. Beginning with basic education in anatomy and physiology, women progress through the stages of tactile and visual self-exploration and manual stimulation. The stop-start technique is a treatment program for premature ejaculation in men. Group therapy can help counteract sexual myths and correct sexual misconceptions, but generally is not used for orgasmic dysfunction. Hypnotherapy may be helpful in situations where relaxation interferes with sexual functioning. Sensate focus involves guided touch of a partner in areas other than the genital area. This is helpful for couples therapy.

Recommended Reading: Adult Sexual Issues

Fitzgerald PA. Endocrine disorders. In: Papadakis MA, McPhee SJ, Rabow MW (eds). *Current Medical Diagnosis & Treatment 2018*. New York, NY: McGraw-Hill.

Mackett CW. Adult sexual dysfunction. In: South-Paul JE, Matheny SC, Lewis EL (eds). *Current Diagnosis & Treatment Family Medicine*. 4th ed. New York, NY: McGraw-Hill.

Naumburg EH, Brown EJ. Sexual dysfunction. In: Smith MA, Shimp LA, Schrager S (eds). *Family Medicine Ambulatory Care and Prevention*. 6th ed. New York, NY: McGraw-Hill.

Addiction

350. The answer is d. Most people who abuse alcohol have completely normal laboratory studies. However, of the tests listed in the question, the GGT is the most sensitive. Elevated GGT is shown to be more sensitive than an elevated MCV, ALT, or AST. The specificity of the GGT is low; it is elevated in nonalcoholic liver disease, diabetes, pancreatitis, hyperthyroidism, heart failure, and anticonvulsant use. The ratio of AST to ALT may help distinguish between alcohol and nonalcohol-related liver diseases, with a ratio of more than 2:1 highly suggestive of alcoholic liver disease. The EtG urine test has recently become popular. It detects recent alcohol consumption, but says nothing about the level of consumption or abuse. Its value is in the monitoring of those patients who are committed to abstinence.

351. The answer is c. Most clinicians agree that psychiatric disorders cannot be reliably assessed in patients who are currently or recently intoxicated. Alcohol is a depressant and may be the main factor in the patient's depressive symptoms. Detoxification and a period of abstinence are necessary before an evaluation for other psychiatric disorders can be effectively completed. It would be premature to treat his depression with a medication until the patient is abstinent.

352. The answer is e. Seizures are a common manifestation of withdrawal from alcohol, occurring in 11% to 33% of patients withdrawing. The Clinical Institute Withdrawal Assessment (CIWA) scale is used to measure withdrawal symptoms. While patients who are actively withdrawing are more at risk for seizures, the scale cannot determine which patients are more likely to experience seizures as a result of their withdrawal. When a patient's score exceeds 10, treatment with benzodiazepines should be initiated and continued until the patient's score is below 8 for 24 hours. Benzodiazepines are the cornerstone of alcohol withdrawal treatment due to their effectiveness in reducing symptoms and their safety profile. Naltrexone is a pure opioid antagonist and is used for opioid detoxification, and potentially to maintain sobriety in alcoholics. Buprenorphine is a partial mu-receptor agonist and helps with opiate withdrawal. Clonidine is an α-adrenergic blocker, and is used for opiate withdrawal to help relieve symptoms. β-Blockers can help with the tachycardia or hypertension associated with withdrawal, but are not considered the cornerstone of therapy. Patients who experience alcohol withdrawal seizures are not at increased risk for recurrent seizures and long-term treatment is not recommended.

353. The answer is b. Drugs used for addiction work in one of four ways. They either cause the body to have a negative reaction to an ingested drug, reduce the reinforcing effects of an ingested drug, block the effects of the drug by binding to the receptor site, or saturate the receptor sites with agonists that do not create the drug's desired effect. Naltrexone, an opiate antagonist, is known to be helpful for both opiate addiction and alcohol addiction. Naltrexone saturates opiate receptor sites and leaves them unavailable for opiate attachment. For alcohol abuse, naltrexone works differently, reducing the reinforcing effect of alcohol (not allowing patients to become "drunk"). At 50 mg daily, this medication has been shown to reduce a patient's desire to drink.

354. The answer is a. Disulfiram causes the body to have a negative reaction to ingested alcohol, regardless of the form. As such, it is a deterrent. The reaction to alcohol that occurs is manifested by flushing, nausea, and vomiting. Importantly, alcohol in cough medicines, mouthwashes, and other forms must be avoided, as the reaction does not discriminate based on from where the alcohol comes. Other medications to prevent relapse include naltrexone (described in question 353), SSRIs, and acamprosate. Although the goal of abstinence cannot be met by medication alone, in selected patients, any of these medications may improve chances for recovery. Acamprosate seems to be the most effective of these medications with twice as many alcoholics remaining abstinent at 12 months compared to those taking placebo. Acamprosate affects both γ-aminobutyric acid (GABA) and glutamine neurotransmission, both of which are important in alcohol's effect on the brain. The effects of this medication appear to be greater and longer lasting than naltrexone. The addition of disulfiram can increase the effectiveness of acamprosate alone.

355. The answer is a. Nicotine-replacement therapy increases the chance that a smoker will quit. Using two forms of nicotine replacement, like a patch and a gum, allows a baseline level of nicotine to be in the patient's system and allows for a bolus during times of craving. This improves quit rates and is recommended if a single form of nicotine replacement is ineffective alone.

356. The answer is d. Behavioral intervention alone is an option for this patient, but you would at least double his success rate if you add medication. First-line therapies include nicotine replacement, bupropion, and varenicline. Although nicotine-containing products are not associated with acute cardiac events, nicotine replacement should be used with caution when working up unstable angina. The patient's seizure disorder contraindicates the use of bupropion. Clonidine is not approved by the FDA for smoking cessation, but several studies have shown that it doubles the rate of abstinence. Varenicline is a selective nicotinic receptor partial agonist. There are no known drug interactions, and it is largely excreted in the urine. Dose modifications would be needed in people with severe renal disease. Common side effects include nausea, insomnia, and abnormal dreams. It is safe in persons with seizure disorders. Varenicline is taken for 1 week before the quit date, and therefore can be taken while a person is still smoking.

357. The answer is e. Twelve-step programs like Alcoholics Anonymous (AA) and NA are among the most effective tools to combat substance use disorders. Although there is a high dropout rate, of those who stay in AA for 1 year, 67% remain sober. Of those that stay 2 years, 85% remain sober, and of those that stay sober for 5 years, 90% remain sober indefinitely. Many people have misconceptions about 12-step programs, and physicians can help patients dispel myths. The programs are spiritual, not religious, and members are not required to be Christian, nor is there any attempt at religious conversion. Referral by a physician is not necessary. They do not solicit members, but do reach out to people that ask for help. They do not engage in research, and there is no formal control or follow-up on members. AA and NA do not provide housing, food, clothing, jobs, or money (although individual members may help each other out), and they are funded completely by member contributions. The organizations do not accept money from outside sources.

358. The answer is a. The pharmacologic options for opiate addiction are increasing. Methadone, an opiate agonist, is an effective cornerstone of treatment for opioid addiction. It saturates opiate receptors and decreases euphoria. However, it cannot be prescribed in a primary care office. Methadone treatment centers are federally regulated. A combination of buprenorphine/naloxone (Suboxone) works by completely blocking opiate receptors (naloxone) and binding to μ-opiate receptors (buprenorphine). There is also a weak kappa antagonist activity with buprenorphine. It is important to know about, as it can be prescribed in the family physician's office, assuming the physician has completed the requisite licensing requirements. Treatment with buprenorphine/naloxone involves three phases: induction, stabilization, and maintenance. Because buprenorphine is a partial opioid agonist, the patient should not have used opioids within the last 12 to 48 hours and should be experiencing some withdrawal symptoms. Suboxone is an oral formulation. The combination serves as a deterrent to abuse because if the combination is crushed and injected it would antagonize the effects of buprenorphine. Induction with Suboxone lasts 3 to 7 days and is complete when an effective dose is found that reduces cravings and limits side effects of Suboxone. Because Suboxone is a partial agonist, it would be ineffective if started while the patient is still using opioids.

359. The answer is b. Opiate withdrawal is well-characterized, and although not life-threatening in otherwise healthy adults, can cause severe discomfort. Symptoms from a short-acting drug like heroin can occur within just a few hours. Withdrawal from longer acting opiates may not cause symptoms for days. Early symptoms include lacrimation, rhinorrhea, yawning, and diaphoresis. Restlessness and irritability occur later, with bone pain, nausea, diarrhea, abdominal cramping, and mood lability occurring even later. Lethargy, slowed movements, and increased sleep are symptoms of opiate use, not withdrawal. Fatigue, depressed mood, and increased appetite are typically experienced by individuals withdrawing from cocaine. Benzodiazepine withdrawal mimics alcohol withdrawal and can begin with symptoms of anxiety, restlessness, and tremor and proceed to psychosis, delirium, and even seizures.

Recommended Reading: Addiction

Greene WM, Gold MS. Drug abuse. In: Kellerman RD, Bope ET (eds). *Conn's Current Therapy, 2018*. Philadelphia, PA: Elsevier.

Mahoney MC, Cummings M. Tobacco cessation. In: South-Paul JE, Matheny SC, Lewis EL (eds). *Current Diagnosis & Treatment Family Medicine*. 4th ed. New York, NY: McGraw-Hill.

Mallin R, Hood Watson K. Alcohol and drug abuse. In: Smith MA, Shimp LA, Schrager S (eds). *Family Medicine Ambulatory Care and Prevention*. 6th ed. New York, NY: McGraw-Hill.

Mallin R, Porter M. Substance use disorders. In: South-Paul JE, Matheny SC, Lewis EL (eds). *Current Diagnosis & Treatment Family Medicine*. 4th ed. New York, NY: McGraw-Hill.

Arthritis and Joint Issues

360. The answer is a. The picture shown demonstrates Heberden nodes (at the distal interphalangeal joints) and Bouchard nodes (at the proximal interphalangeal joints). These abnormalities are commonly classified as osteoarthritis (OA), but are only infrequently associated with pain or disability. Laboratory evaluation will only rarely show an inflammatory process, and an elevated uric acid level would be an incidental finding.

361. The answer is c. Patients with OA of the hands often have normal x-rays until later in the disease process. However, in a patient with Heberden and Bouchard nodes on physical examination, one would expect to see classic changes of OA on plain films. These findings include a loss of joint space, subchondral sclerosis, and osteophyte formation. The presence of calcium deposition in the surrounding cartilage would suggest calcium pyrophosphate disease, or pseudogout. Rheumatoid arthritis (RA) typically produces inflammatory changes including effusions and erosions of the joints. RA is more likely to affect the metacarpal joints than OA.

362. The answer is a. Treatment for OA should be multimodal, including patient education, assistive devices, physical therapy, and pharmacotherapy to achieve improved function and reduced pain. Acetaminophen is recommended as first-line therapy for OA pain. It should be prescribed in dosages of 3 to 4 g/d until pain relief is achieved. NSAIDs such as naproxen are helpful in treating OA pain, but due to their GI and renal side effects, are not recommended as first-line agents. NSAIDs are often used early in the treatment of gout and RA to achieve early pain relief, but they will not alter the course of disease. Methotrexate is the prototypical disease-modifying anti-rheumatic drug (DMARD) but this patient does not have RA. Due to their addictive properties, opiates should be reserved for patients with severe disease who cannot have joint replacement. Corticosteroid injections are often used to reduce inflammation and symptoms, but they are not used first line and would be impractical for this patient with numerous hand joints affected.

363. The answer is c. The patient's history is consistent with an attack of gout. The most common presentation of gout is podagra (an abrupt, intense inflammation of the first metatarsophalangeal (MTP) joint), but any joint can be affected. It is characterized by an abrupt onset of monoarticular symptoms with pain at rest and with movement. The attacks often occur overnight, after an inciting event (excessive alcohol or a heavy meal). The sufferer often cites exquisite pain, with even slight pressure on the joint being quite painful. OA and RA would not occur so abruptly. A stress fracture would likely not be as painful at rest, and cellulitis would generally not be as abrupt or painful. Septic arthritis and gout may be clinically indistinguishable, unless the joint fluid is analyzed.

364. The answer is b. The initial treatment for a first episode of gout is focused on reducing inflammation and this is best achieved with NSAIDs. Indomethacin has traditionally been thought of as the most appropriate therapy for gout, but in reality, most NSAIDs are equally efficacious. IV antibiotics are not appropriate for the treatment of gout, but would be indicated if joint aspiration demonstrated a septic joint. Methotrexate would be indicated if RA is suspected. Colchicine is used in the acute treatment of gout, but its use is limited to one pill every 1 to 2 hours up to a maximum of 1.8 mg and it's not recommended for chronic use. Allopurinol is used as a prophylactic agent to reduce recurrences of gout, but its use is not recommended during an acute flare as it can precipitate crystallization of uric acid in the joint. Additionally, clinicians should withhold prophylactic medication until after the second attack of gout as many patients will not have a second attack or it may take up to a decade for a repeat attack.

365. The answer is d. An evaluation of the joint aspirate is strongly recommended to establish the diagnosis of gout. It is critical to differentiate gout from infectious arthritis which is a medical emergency, and a joint aspirate will do this rapidly and accurately. The sedimentation rates and C-reactive protein are both nonspecific. Serum uric acid levels can be normal or high in the setting of acute gout. A 24-hour urine collection may help determine the most effective treatment for gout, but is not needed for diagnosis. However, the American College of Rheumatology recently revised their guidelines, suggesting therapy begin with xanthine oxidase inhibitors. This obviates the utility of the 24-hour uric acid level.

366. The answer is b. The crystals typical of gout are needle-shaped and have negative birefringence. They are made of monosodium urate monohydrate. The crystals of pseudogout are made from calcium pyrophosphate, are rhomboid-shaped, and demonstrate positive birefringence. Infectious arthritis, OA, and RA would not present with crystals in the joint aspirate. Pseudogout and gout are rarely distinguishable based on symptoms alone and require synovial fluid analysis to accurately make the diagnosis.

367. The answer is c. Infectious arthritis, gout, and pseudogout may all be associated with cloudy joint aspirate fluid. The aspirate fluid obtained from a gout or pseudogout flare may also have a WBC count of 50,000/mm^3 with a high proportion of PMN leukocytes. However, glucose levels fluid aspirated from a knee with gout or pseudogout would be normal.

368. The answer is d. Fluid aspirated from an osteoarthritic knee is characterized by generally clear joint fluid with a WBC count of 2000/mm^3 to

10,000/mm³. The distinguishing factor is the PMN leukocytes. In RA, more than 50% of the WBCs are PMNs, while in OA, less than 50% of the WBCs are PMNs.

369. The answer is a. Extra-articular manifestations of RA can be seen at any stage of the disease. Most common are rheumatoid nodules that can occur anywhere on the body, but usually subcutaneously along pressure points. Vasculitis, dry eyes, dyspnea, or cough can all be seen. Cough and dyspnea may signal respiratory interstitial disease. Cardiac, GI, and renal systems are rarely involved. When a neuropathy is present, it is generally because of a compression syndrome, not as an extra-articular manifestation of the disease.

Recommended Reading: Arthritis and Joint Issues

Johnson BE. Arthritis: osteoarthritis, gout & rheumatoid arthritis. In: South-Paul JE, Matheny SC, Lewis EL (eds). *Current Diagnosis & Treatment Family Medicine.* 4th ed. New York, NY: McGraw-Hill.

Kodner C. Osteoarthritis. In: Smith MA, Shimp LA, Schrager S (eds). *Family Medicine Ambulatory Care and Prevention.* 6th ed. New York, NY: McGraw-Hill.

Asthma

370. The answer is b. Asthma is common, affecting approximately 5% of the population. While there is a genetic component to its development, the strongest identified predisposing factor for its development in children is atopy. In fact, 80% of children with asthma are atopic. The same does not necessarily hold true in adulthood with less than half of asthmatic adults aged 30 years old with evidence of atopy. Obesity is increasingly being recognized as a risk factor as well. Living in poverty and non-white racial group are also important risk factors. Nonspecific predictors include exercise, upper respiratory infections, pneumonia, gastroesophageal reflux disease, changes in weather, stress, and exposure to environmental smoke.

371. The answer is c. It is important to categorize asthma symptoms prior to initiation of treatment based on severity of symptoms. Terms used to describe asthma are intermittent or persistent, and mild, moderate, or severe impairment. Clinicians should assess the degree of daytime symptoms, nighttime symptoms, impairment of activities, and, if on therapy, how often they are using their short-acting β_2-agonist therapy. The recommended reading at the end of this section includes a publication from the National Heart, Lung and Blood Institute that describes classification and treatment guidelines for an initial visit, follow up visits and a step-wise approach for long term management of asthma. This can be accessed at: https://www.nhlbi.nih.gov/files/docs/guidelines/asthma_qrg.pdf. Based on this information, the patient in this question has moderate symptoms in all categories, but is not yet on medication. Therefore, her asthma would be considered moderate persistent.

372. The answer is c. PFT is essential to the diagnosis and management of asthma. The FEV_1 is reduced in patients with obstructive defects. The FVC, or the amount of air a patient can exhale during the entire test, is also low in patients with obstructive defects. An FEV_1 of 60% to 80% of predicted or an FEV_1/FVC of 75% to 80% are consistent with moderate persistent asthma. Peak flow meters use the peak expiratory flow rate (PEFR) to parallel the FEV1 and they are quite useful in the home management of asthma, but they are not a component of the in-office PFT. A reading of 60% to 80% would be consistent with moderate persistent asthma. The volume-time curve is used to measure the validity of the patient's efforts on the PFT and should be at least 6 seconds to ensure a valid test attempt.

373. The answer is d. For patients more than 12 years of age with moderate persistent asthma, therapy should be initiated at step 3. These patients need to have daily control of inflammation. The preferred regimen is maintenance therapy with either a low-dose inhaled corticosteroid plus a long-acting β_2-agonist or a medium-dose inhaled corticosteroid alone. All patients should be given a short-acting β_2-agonist rescue inhaler for acute/quick relief. The alternative regimen for this step would be to use a low-dose inhaled corticosteroid plus a leukotriene receptor antagonist.

374. The answer is c. Asthma is classified by its severity, and by assessing daytime and nighttime symptoms. Patients with symptoms less than twice a week, with brief exacerbations, and with nighttime symptoms less than twice a month are classified as having "mild intermittent" asthma. There is no "moderate intermittent" classification. The "mild persistent" classification refers to symptoms more than twice a week but less than once a day, with symptoms that sometimes affect usual activity. Nighttime symptoms occur more than twice a month. The "moderate persistent" classification is characterized by daily symptoms and use of short-acting inhaler, with exacerbations that affect activity and may last for days. Nighttime symptoms occur at least weekly. "Severe persistent" asthma is characterized by continual symptoms that limit physical activities, with frequent exacerbations and nighttime symptoms.

375. The answer is a. For a patient with mild persistent asthma, intensification to step 2 therapy is indicated. The preferred therapy for step 2 is the addition of a low-dose inhaled corticosteroid, the alternative regimen is the use of a leukotriene receptor antagonist, cromolyn, or theophylline. A medium-dose inhaled corticosteroid or a low-dose inhaled corticosteroid plus a long-acting bronchodilator would be indicated for step 3 therapy. A medium-dose inhaled corticosteroid plus a leukotriene receptor antagonist would be indicated for step 4 therapy.

376. The answer is b. The goal of asthma control therapy is to maintain long-term control of symptoms with the least amount of medication to prevent remodeling of the lungs and increased risks of morbidity/mortality. When patients have a step-up or step-down to their therapy, it is recommended they receive follow-up within 2 to 6 weeks or if their condition worsens. The peak flow readings are used to direct the patient's care using a home device that measures PEFR. Peak flow measurements parallel the FEV_1 and are an easy and inexpensive way to monitor asthma control. Readings fall in either the green (PEFR 80% to 100%), yellow (PEFR 50% to 80%), or red zone (PEFR $\leq$ 50%). PEFR in the green zone indicates a patient should continue their current course of therapy and does not trigger follow-up care. Yellow zone readings are a warning and should precipitate additional medicine or a call to their physician. Red zone readings are more worrisome and the patient should use their inhaler and either call their physician or go to the ED.

377. The answer is b. In this case, the patient has had mild intermittent asthma, but is becoming persistent and requires a step-up in therapy. Since he is intolerant of inhaled steroids, a leukotriene modifier is the best choice. They have been shown to improve lung function and reduce the need for rescue therapy. Long-acting β-agonists should not be used as monotherapy since they have been shown in studies to have a small but statistically significant increased risk of severe or fatal asthma attacks. Cromolyn therapy has been replaced by newer agents, mainly because of compliance issues. Theophylline and oral steroids would not be indicated in this case.

378. The answer is e. Multiple studies have shown that infections with viruses and bacteria predispose to acute asthma exacerbations. However, the use of empiric antibiotics is not recommended. There is no consistent evidence to support improved clinical outcomes. Antibiotics should be considered in cases where there is a high likelihood of acute bacterial respiratory infection, as in the case of high fever, purulent sputum production, or radiographic evidence of lower respiratory or sinus infection.

Recommended Reading: Asthma

Dabelic A. Respiratory problems. In: South-Paul JE, Matheny SC, Lewis EL (eds). *Current Diagnosis & Treatment Family Medicine.* 4th ed. New York, NY: McGraw-Hill.

Data from National Heart, Lung, and Blood Institute, National Asthma Education and Prevention Program. Expert panel report 3: Asthma Care Quick Reference. Bethesda, MD: National Heart, Lung, and Blood Institute; Revised September 2012. NIH publication no. 12-5075. https://www.nhlbi.nih.gov/files/docs/guidelines/asthma_qrg.pdf. Accessed September 7, 2018.

MacClements J. Asthma. In: Smith MA, Shimp LA, Schrager S (eds). *Family Medicine Ambulatory Care and Prevention.* 6th ed. New York, NY: McGraw-Hill.

Back Pain

379. The answer is c. Spondylolisthesis is an anterior displacement of vertebrae in relation to the one below. It is the most common cause of low back pain in patients younger than age 26, especially athletes. Imaging should be used selectively in low back pain and it should be avoided in patients with acute low back pain without a history or examination findings concerning for serious pathology. Patients with radicular pain or mild neurologic deficits do not require imaging unless the deficit is severe, progressive, or suggestive of cauda equine syndrome (saddle anesthesia, bladder or bowel incontinence). Patients more than 50 years of age, those with a history of cancer, patients with worsening of pain at night, or those with unexplained weight loss have a greater risk of underlying malignancy and should be considered for imaging. Similarly, a fever, immunosuppression, or injection drug use suggest and increased risk of infection. While weight gain and obesity can worsen low back pain, it is not a reason to order imaging. Pain that worsens with activity and improves with rest is suggestive of mechanical low back pain and does not necessitate imaging. An inciting event such as trauma should also cause a clinician to consider early imaging.

380. The answer is a. It is recommended that patients with low back pain maintain usual activities, as dictated by pain. Prolonged bed rest has not been shown to be effective in returning people to their usual activities sooner. NSAIDs are effective for short-term symptomatic pain relief. Opioids may be indicated in pain relief for those who have failed NSAIDs, but are significantly sedating. Short-acting opioids should only be used acutely to avoid the risk of addiction. If patients with chronic low back pain require opioids to maintain function, long-acting opioids should be considered. Steroids can be considered in those with acute disk herniation. Epidural corticosteroid injections may be useful to treat sensory and radicular pain associated with low back pain but facet joint injections have not been shown to be more effective than placebo.

381. The answer is b. MRI is indicated for people whose pain persists for more than 6 weeks despite normal radiographs and with no response to conservative therapy. Flexion/extension films would not be helpful in identifying more concerning causes of pain. EMG is not indicated without neurologic involvement. A bone scan and/or ESR should be considered in those with symptoms consistent with cancer or infection.

382. The answer is c. Treatment for chronic low back pain is challenging. NSAIDs are effective but can cause side effects if used chronically. Muscle relaxants do not exhibit any direct effect on skeletal muscle and owe their efficacy to sedation. They have not been shown to add benefit when added to NSAIDs. Opioid agents may be necessary for acute flares of pain, but should not be used for chronic pain because of the risk of dependency. Low-dose tricyclic antidepressants can be useful in the treatment of chronic pain and do serve as adjuvants to other analgesics. There is no evidence that SSRIs improve pain or function in chronic back pain. There is no evidence that injections into facet joints or trigger points improve pain relief or function.

Recommended Reading: Back Pain

Criswell DF. Low back pain. In: Smith MA, Shimp LA, Schrager S (eds). *Family Medicine Ambulatory Care and Prevention.* 6th ed. New York, NY: McGraw-Hill.

Webb CW. O'Connor FG. Low back pain in primary care: an evidence-based approach. In: South-Paul JE, Matheny SC, Lewis EL (eds). *Current Diagnosis & Treatment Family Medicine.* 4th ed. New York, NY: McGraw-Hill.

Chronic Obstructive Pulmonary Disease

383. The answer is c. Chronic and progressive dyspnea is the cardinal symptom for patients with COPD, but cough is often the presenting symptom. Upon clinical diagnosis, office spirometry is necessary to make the diagnosis, assess the disease severity, and monitor response to treatment. CBC may be indicated to screen for polycythemia or to assess acute illness in the febrile patient with COPD, but is not necessary. Arterial blood gas measurements should only be obtained if the FEV_1 is found to be less than 50% predicted. A high-resolution CT scan is not a routine part of care unless the diagnosis is in doubt, or a procedure is being considered. ECGs may show changes due to COPD, but are not routinely indicated in the evaluation.

384. The answer is c. An accurate assessment of a patient's airflow limitation using office spirometry plus a measure of their symptoms is essential to categorizing a patient's COPD and risk for future exacerbations. The GOLD divides patients into GOLD stages 1, 2, 3, and 4. Patients with GOLD 1 or 2 categorization are at low risk for future exacerbations while patients in GOLD 3 or 4 are at high risk for future exacerbations and treatment modalities are selected to reduce this future risk and improve symptoms. Nocturnal oximetry, smoking pack-years, and CXR changes are not part of the GOLD classification system.

385. The answer is e. Office spirometry is helpful to diagnose COPD and assess its severity. While all the answer choices are common measurements of airflow, the more sensitive measure to diagnose COPD is the FEV_1 to FVC ratio. It is considered normal if it is 70% or more of the predicted value based on the patient's gender, age, and height. When a patient's FEV1/FVC is less than 70%, the FEV_1 is useful to assist in the classification of the patient's COPD; FEV_1 is more than or equal to 80% predicted in GOLD 1, FEV_1 is between 50% and 80% predicted in GOLD 2, FEV_1 is between 30% and 50% in GOLD 3, and FEV_1 is less than 30% in GOLD 4 disease. The TLC is not often used in the routine management of COPD, but is an important marker for restrictive disease.

386. The answer is e. The single most important intervention in smokers with COPD is to encourage smoking cessation. However, the only drug therapy that has been shown to improve the natural history of COPD progression is supplemental oxygen in those patients that are hypoxemic. Benefits of oxygen therapy include longer survival, reduced hospitalizations, and better quality of life. Bronchodilators do not alter the course of the disease or decline in function, and COPD is generally not a steroid-responsive disease. Antibiotics can be useful to treat infection and exacerbation, but no convincing evidence exists to support their use chronically.

387. The answer is e. In COPD patients with increases in dyspnea, sputum volume, and sputum purulence, the use of antibiotics is recommended. Antibiotics are also recommended in any patient with COPD requiring mechanical ventilation but not necessarily for a drop in SpO_2. The use of antibiotics in the setting of these cardinal symptoms has been shown to reduce the risk of death.

388. The answer is d. The Reduction in the Use of Corticosteroids in Exacerbated COPD trial (REDUCE) randomized patients with an acute COPD exacerbation and a history of smoking to a 5-day or 14-day course of glucocorticoids. All patients received antibiotics, inhaled β-agonists, and inhaled antimuscarinics. The 5-day group received less than half the dose of glucocorticoids, had a shorter hospitalization, and no difference in the rate of readmission.

Recommended Reading:
Chronic Obstructive Pulmonary Disease

Dabelic A. Respiratory problems. In: South-Paul JE, Matheny SC, Lewis EL (eds). *Current Diagnosis & Treatment Family Medicine.* 4th ed. New York, NY: McGraw-Hill.

Leuppi JD, Schuetz PK, Bingisser R, et.al. Short-term vs conventional glucocorticoid therapy in acute exacerbations of chronic obstructive pulmonary disease: the REDUCE randomized clinical trial. *JAMA.* 2013;309(21):2223-2231.

Vogt HB. Chronic obstructive pulmonary disease. In: Smith MA, Shimp LA, Schrager S, (eds). *Family Medicine Ambulatory Care and Prevention.* 6th ed. New York, NY: McGraw-Hill.

Renal Disease

389. The answer is d. Weight, diabetes, and hypertension, by themselves, do not indicate the presence or absence of renal insufficiency. However, most cases of chronic renal failure are caused by diabetes and hypertension (60%), so those should be recognized as significant risk factors. The serum creatinine level can be normal in elderly people with chronic renal insufficiency, because they generally have less muscle mass. Therefore, the best indicator of the presence of renal failure is the calculated or estimated glomerular filtration rate or GFR. The other tests mentioned are not sufficient tests, and normal values in these tests do not indicate that the patient does not have renal insufficiency.

390. The answer is e. The National Kidney Foundation's staging system categorizes CKD into five progressive stages based on the GFR. The stages are below:

Stages of Chronic Kidney Disease based on GFR

Stage	GFR (mL/min/1.73 m^2)
1	≥ 90
2	60-89
3a	45-59
3b	30-44
4	15-29
5	< 15 (or dialysis)

This patient has a normal BUN and creatinine. However, her GFR is significantly decreased and falls in the stage 3a category. Her microalbumin/Cr ratio is also elevated, indicating microalbuminuria; however, this does not affect her staging due to an already abnormal GFR.

Primary prevention for CKD includes optimizing control of cardiac risk factors, including diabetes, hypertension, and lipids. However, this patient already has stage 3a CKD and, unfortunately, the disease is likely to progress even with optimal control of these conditions. Patients with CKD should avoid nephrotoxic drugs, such as NSAIDs. However, avoidance of these drugs prevents further injury, but does not slow the progression of CKD. The addition of a thiazide diuretic can be helpful to control hypertension in patients with CKD, but does not prevent the progression of CKD. Likewise, a statin will affect the patient's cardiovascular risk but is unlikely to affect the progression of the CKD. ACE-inhibitors or ARBs have been shown to slow the progression of proteinuric CKD through the reduction of hyperfiltration injury to the nephrons.

391. The answer is d. The patient's laboratory values and clinical picture is consistent with moderate renal failure (National Kidney Foundation stage 3a). At this point, nephrology referral is indicated. Renal replacement therapy (transplant or dialysis) is indicated for severe renal insufficiency (GFR < 15 mL/min). Increasing the ACE and diuretic therapy are both options, but should not replace the need for a nephrology referral.

392. The answer is d. The long-term complications of CKD are many. There is a higher risk for CVD in this population as compared with the general population. In fact, most patients with stage 3 CKD die, primarily due to CVD, before reaching the need for dialysis. The reason for this is unclear, but may be related to the uremic milieu, underlying comorbidities, and the hesitancy to perform diagnostic procedures in the setting of CKD.

393. The answer is d. This patient has end-stage renal disease (ESRD) and will likely require dialysis in the near future due to his worsening GFR. However, GFR and Cr are not the most critical deciding factors in when to start dialysis. Emergent dialysis is usually initiated when renal impairment leads to fluid overload, electrolyte and/or acid-base abnormalities, or severe symptoms such as seizures, nausea/vomiting, or pericarditis. Ideally, the primary care physician and nephrologist should work together to plan for nonemergent dialysis when ESRD is imminent. This patient is not experiencing severe symptoms. He does have hyperkalemia, which can lead to cardiac conduction abnormalities and arrhythmias. An EKG should be performed to rule out conduction abnormalities such as peaked T waves. If the EKG is normal, stopping his ACE-inhibitor (which can cause hyperkalemia) and adding a loop diuretic is appropriate. If the EKG is abnormal, cardiac monitoring is the next best step. This patient has an A1C above normal, but with his advancing age and multiple comorbidities, it is recommended to relax glycemic goals to avoid the dire consequences of hypoglycemia. Patients with ESRD often have anemia due to decreased erythropoietin levels. However, there is no benefit in starting erythropoietin-stimulating agents until hemoglobin levels are less than 9 g/dL. A parathyroid scan is not indicated unless the patient is refractory to treatments.

394. The answer is a. Metabolic bone disease is common as CKD progresses. The declining GFR leads to increased phosphorus retention. Calcium tends to bond with phosphorus, depositing in soft tissue and leading to hypocalcemia and hyperparathyroidism. Decreased intake and/or absorption of vitamin D also contributes to secondary hyperparathyroidism. Phosphorus level reduction through dietary phosphorus restriction is the initial treatment in ESRD. Foods rich in phosphorus include soda, eggs, dairy, nuts, beans, meat, and processed foods. In patients with GFR less than 20 mL/min/1.73 m², dietary restriction alone is rarely sufficient. Phosphorus binders, such as calcium carbonate or acetate, should be utilized to achieve a phosphorus level less than or equal to 5.5 mg/dL. Vitamin D and calcium supplementation can assist in the management of metabolic bone disease but are not the initial steps. The patient does have secondary hyperparathyroidism, but ESRD is the likely cause and does not require additional investigation by an endocrinologist at this time. Cinacalcet suppresses parathyroid hormone production, but is not the first step in treatment of hyperparathyroidism and can result in severe hypocalcemia.

Recommended Reading: Renal Disease

Dirkx TC, Woodell T, Watnick S. Kidney disease. In: Papadakis MA, McPhee SJ, Rabow MW (eds). *Current Medical Diagnosis & Treatment 2018.* New York, NY: McGraw-Hill.

Chronic Pain

395. The answer is b. Adjunctive medications often supplement the benefits from analgesics and can be very effective treating neuropathic pain. Both antidepressants and anticonvulsants have been used to treat chronic pain as described in this question, but the anticonvulsants, particularly gabapentin, have become the mainstay of treatment for neuropathic pain. If the patient did not respond to gabapentin or pregabalin, an antidepressant can be considered.

396. The answer is a. Tramadol is a novel analgesic that has serotonergic, noradrenergic, and opioid agonist effects. In the absence of a history of opioid abuse, it does not pose the same level of concern for abuse and dependence as opioids, and is therefore a reasonable option for people who need breakthrough pain relief but do not want to use true opioid medications. While muscle relaxants may be considered in this scenario, this patient's history does not mention muscle spasms. Therefore, a muscle relaxant is less likely to offer benefit.

397. The answer is e. Interventional pain management techniques are considered for patients who fail conservative therapy when there is specific pathology identified. Lumbar epidural steroid injections are effective for treating spinal stenosis and herniated disks when people want to delay more aggressive surgical intervention. If this person wanted to avoid surgery completely, treating the pain with anticonvulsants or an antidepressant may be considered.

398. The answer is b. Postherpetic neuralgia is especially difficult to treat, especially if it persists for a period of time after the resolution of the acute outbreak. The anticonvulsants pregabalin and gabapentin both have indications for treating pain associated with postherpetic neuralgia.

399. The answer is c. Antidepressants can be an excellent adjunctive analgesic. Efficacy has been demonstrated for fibromyalgia, chronic headaches, and neuropathic pain. Because depressive symptoms (loss of energy, anhedonia, sleep disturbances, and depressed mood among others) are common in patients with chronic pain, they should be considered when there are concomitant symptoms and conditions for which antidepressants have shown to be beneficial for pain relief. Tricyclics and medications with dual serotonin and norepinephrine activation (venlafaxine and duloxetine) are generally seen as being most beneficial.

400. The answer is a. NSAIDs are an excellent first-line medication for mild to moderate pain, especially when there is an inflammatory component suspected. One NSAID is not superior to another, and periodic substitution of one with another in the class may afford an improved response. Celecoxib (a cyclooxygenase-2 [COX-2] inhibitor) may have a better side effect profile, but should not be a first-line agent except in elderly patients or in patients who have failed first-line NSAIDs. Tramadol is a centrally acting synthetic opioid agonist. It binds to μ-opioid receptors and inhibits serotonin and norepinephrine reuptake. It should not be a first-line option. While tricyclic antidepressants like amitriptyline and anticonvulsants like gabapentin may work well in neuropathic pain, they are less well-studied in nociceptive pain and therefore are not good first-line agents.

401. The answer is c. There are many agents to choose from to treat chronic neuropathic pain. If the pain is unresponsive to NSAIDs, one can choose a trial of a COX-2 inhibitor, but studies have shown that tricyclic antidepressants like amitriptyline are more efficacious. Anticonvulsants like gabapentin would be another option. Tramadol and opioids may work to control the pain, but may increase risk of addiction and would not be best as a next step in this case.

402. The answer is c. In chronic nonmalignant pain, there is evidence that continued escalating opioid doses results in worsened analgesic response. This is because *N*-methyl-D-aspartate. (NMDA) receptors in nerve cells are upregulated and lead to tolerance, while pain receptors become increasingly more sensitive to stimuli. In situations of tolerance to medication, it is appropriate to switch from one opioid agent to another, usually starting at half the equivalent dose of the alternative medication. Stopping the opioid would result in withdrawal, and increasing the dose would be inappropriate because of the physiologic effects described above. There is no evidence to support the addition of a second anticonvulsant, and although antidepressants have been shown to help in chronic pain, it is more likely that changing opioid would provide better pain control.

Recommended Reading: Chronic Pain

Glick RM, Marcus DA. Chronic pain management. In: South-Paul JE, Matheny SC, Lewis EL (eds). *Current Diagnosis & Treatment Family Medicine*. 4th ed. New York, NY: McGraw-Hill.

Rabow MW, Pantilat SZ, Steiger S, Naidu RK. Palliative care & pain Management. In: Papadakis MA, McPhee SJ, Rabow MW (eds). *Current Medical Diagnosis & Treatment 2018*. New York, NY: McGraw-Hill.

Temporal MP. Chronic (persistent) pain. In: Smith MA, Shimp LA, Schrager S (eds). *Family Medicine Ambulatory Care and Prevention*. 6th ed. New York, NY: McGraw-Hill.

Chronic Liver Disease

403. The answer is e. Determining the cause of liver disease has important implications for treatment. The most important aspect of diagnosing alcoholic liver disease is the documentation of chronic alcohol abuse. However, alcohol use is sometimes denied by the patient. Alcoholic hepatitis is associated with the classic laboratory findings of a disproportionate elevation of AST compared to ALT with both values usually being less than 300 IU/L. This ratio is generally greater than 2.0, a value rarely seen in other forms of liver disease, including those listed in this question (viral or autoimmune hepatitis or hematochromatosis). In alcoholic liver disease, the GGT is elevated, often to more than eight times the upper limit of normal.

404. The answer is e. Laboratory studies that represent acute hepatocellular injury include AST, ALT, LDH, and alkaline phosphatase. Laboratory values that represent hepatic function include albumin, bilirubin, and pro-thrombin time. Tests of hepatic function are more suggestive of chronic disease as opposed to acute injury.

405. The answer is c. Patients with untreated, chronic hepatitis C are at risk for progression to cirrhosis. In cirrhotic patients, varices occur second-ary to chronic high pressure in the portal veins. Bleeding from varices is the most common cause of death in cirrhotic patients. The other potential causes of death listed are less common. Hepatocellular carcinoma occurs at a rate of about 3% to 5% per year in patients with cirrhosis from hepatitis C.

406. The answer is b. NAFLD is a relatively recently described condition, but is the most common liver disease in the United States. It encompasses a wide spectrum of disease, with liver histology being similar to patients with hepatitis related to alcohol, but without the requisite history. For some reason, this condition impacts women more than men. It may be part of "syndrome X" that includes obesity, diabetes mellitus, dyslipidemia, and hypertension. Seventy-five percent of people will have hepatomegaly on clinical examination, with a smaller percentage (25%) demonstrating splenomegaly. Although there are no pathognomonic laboratory markers, elevations of AST and ALT are common with an AST:ALT ratio of less than 1. Evidence of steatosis may be seen on a hepatic ultrasound. Treatment for this condition includes weight reduction, treatment of diabetes, and treatment of lipid disorders. There is no current evidence that supports any specific pharmacologic therapy.

Recommended Reading:
Chronic Liver Disease

Matheny SC, Long K, Roth JS. Hepatobiliary disorders. In: South-Paul JE, Matheny SC, Lewis EL (eds). *Current Diagnosis & Treatment Family Medicine*. 4th ed. New York, NY: McGraw-Hill.

Potter MC, Egan M. Cirrhosis. In: Smith MA, Shimp LA, Schrager S (eds). *Family Medicine Ambulatory Care and Prevention*. 6th ed. New York, NY: McGraw-Hill.

Congestive Heart Failure

407. The answer is a. Routine laboratory testing in a person with the new diagnosis of heart failure includes an electrocardiogram, a CBC, a urinalysis, serum creatinine, potassium and albumin levels, and thyroid function studies. An echocardiogram is imperative to help identify structural abnormalities of the heart and to measure the ejection fraction (EF), thereby differentiating between heart failure with reduced ejection fraction (HFrEF) and heart failure with preserved ejection fraction (HFpEF) as well as between right and left ventricular heart failure. Holter monitoring is not routinely warranted, as it would not identify a cause for heart failure, but would be used to identify an arrhythmia. Catheterization or stress testing may be important if ischemia or ischemic cardiomyopathy is identified as a cause, but is not a routine initial test.

408. The answer is a. The ACC/AHA/HFSA guidelines recommend therapy based on their four categories of heart failure. Stage A includes patients at risk for heart failure but without structural heart disease or symptoms. Stage B includes patients with structural heart disease (atherosclerosis, valvular disease) without signs or symptoms of heart failure. Patients in stage C heart failure have current or prior symptoms of heart failure and structural heart disease, while stage D patients have refractory heart failure. In contrast, the New York Heart Association (NYHA) functional classification categorizes patients based on the degree of symptoms they *currently* have. All NYHA classes fall into the ACC/AHA/HFSA stages C or D. Class I patients have no limitation of activity. Class II patients have slight limitations, are comfortable at rest, but have fatigue, palpitations, dyspnea, or angina with ordinary activity. Class III patients are also comfortable at rest, but less-than-ordinary activity causes symptoms. Class IV patients have symptoms at rest and increased symptoms with even minor activity. For this question, many clinical trials have shown that ACE-inhibitors decrease symptoms, improve quality of life, decrease hospitalizations, and reduce mortality in patients with Stage C (NYHA class II to IV) HFrEF. In addition, they slow the progression to heart failure among asymptomatic patients with HFrEF. All patients with heart failure should be prescribed an ACE-inhibitor unless they have a contraindication. β-Blockers are helpful, but not necessarily as a first-line agent, and should be reserved for patients who are euvolemic. Nitrates and hydralazine can be used in patients who do not tolerate ACE-inhibitors, although they lack evidence to show that they improve prognosis. ARBs are generally utilized in patients who cannot tolerate ACE-inhibitors. Some calcium channel blockers (nifedipine, diltiazem, and nicardipine) may worsen systolic dysfunction.

409. The answer is d. This patient is euvolemic and has normal oxygen saturation and does not have any indication for acute, inpatient treatment. In patients who continue to be symptomatic with an EF less than 35% and are already euvolemic and on an ACE or ARB, the next step is the addition of a β-blocker. Studies have shown that three β-blockers (bisoprolol, metoprolol, and carvedilol) can reduce symptoms, improve quality of life, and reduce mortality. The concomitant use of ACEs and ARBs is not recommended due to the increased risk of hyperkalemia. Metolazone is useful in patients with refractory edema, but this is not the case with this patient.

410. The answer is e. Many noncardiac comorbid conditions may affect the proper diagnosis and clinical course of heart failure. All of the interventions in this question should be done, but only discontinuing alcohol use has actually been shown to improve function significantly. Optimally treating COPD is important, as exacerbations from heart failure are often difficult to distinguish from COPD exacerbations. Optimally treating diabetes and hypertension will minimize the negative effects of these conditions on the heart, but will not improve damage already done. Cigarette smoking should be discontinued, but generally does not lead to functional improvement. Those with alcoholic cardiomyopathy actually see improvement of the left ventricular function with abstinence.

411. The answer is d. Some patients have difficulty maintaining optimal fluid balance, and a second diuretic is needed. In this case, adding metolazone can significantly increase diuresis in the outpatient treatment of heart failure with volume overload. Prolonged therapy should be avoided; it is often only needed 1 or 2 times a week. Hydrochlorothiazide would not enhance diuresis, nor would triamterene. Spironolactone can be used, but is usually only considered for NYHA class III or IV patients or those with a serum potassium level less than 5.0 mmol/L.

Recommended Reading: Congestive Heart Failure

Bashore TM, Granger CB, Jackson KP, Patel MR. Heart disease. In: Papadakis MA, McPhee SJ, Rabow MW (eds). *Current Medical Diagnosis & Treatment 2018*. New York, NY: McGraw-Hill.

Diller PM, Bernheisel CR. Congestive heart failure. In: Smith MA, Shimp LA, Schrager S (eds). *Family Medicine Ambulatory Care and Prevention*. 6th ed. New York, NY: McGraw-Hill.

Yancy CW, Jessup M, Bozkurt B, et al. 2017 ACC/AHA/HFSA Focused Update of the 2013 ACC/AHA Guidelines for the Management of Heart Failure: A Report of the American College of Cardiology/ American Heart Association Task Force on Clinical Practice Guidelines and the Heart Failure Society of America. *J Am Coll Cardiol.* 2017 [epub ahead of print]. Accessed at http://www.acc.org/latest-in-cardiology/ten-points-to-remember/2017/04/27/15/50/2017-acc-aha-hfsa-focused-update-of-hf-guideline.

Dementias

412. The answer is d. Dementias often have overlapping features, sometimes making it difficult to delineate early in the course of the disease. Lewy body dementia is characterized by visual hallucinations, fluctuating attention, and gait/motor/sleep disturbances. Similarly, Parkinson disease is associated with fluctuating attention, gait/motor/sleep disturbances, cogwheel rigidity, and a pill-rolling tremor. Cognitive impairment occurs early in Lewy Body disease while it has a much later onset in Parkinson. Frontotemporal dementia typically presents with behavioral, personality, and language changes. Vascular dementia has a stepwise progression in a patient with a history of stroke or significant vascular risk factors, such as hypertension or diabetes. This patient has no vascular history, has had a steady decline that is focused on memory and cognition. Nocturnal confusion is present, but without evidence of disordered sleep.

413. The answer is a. Currently, there are no laboratory or imaging studies of sufficient accuracy to confirm the diagnosis of Alzheimer dementia (AD). Diagnosis of AD includes five steps: history, cognitive assessment, physical examination, laboratory testing (to rule out other causes of cognitive impairment), and establishing a working diagnosis. Neither EEG nor lumbar puncture would add to the diagnosis of AD, but may be useful if the presentation suggests other disorders such as delirium or infection.

414. The answer is c. Epidemiologic studies have identified several genetic and environmental risk factors for Alzheimer disease. Increasing age is the strongest risk factor. The prevalence doubles every 5 years after the age of 65, with up to 50% of individuals aged 85 to 90 years old meeting criteria for the disease. Family history is another major risk factor, and individuals with a first-degree relative with the disease are 4 times more likely to develop the disease themselves. Other risk factors include female gender, low levels of education, cardiovascular risk factors, and a history of head trauma.

415. The answer is d. Dementia is often difficult to distinguish from delirium or depression in the elderly. However, delirium is generally acute in onset and associated with a loss of concentration. Dementia's onset is insidious, and concentration is less likely to be a problem. Depression is associated with psychomotor slowing, while dementia is generally not. While people with dementia may complain of memory loss, it is far more likely that the patient's family will complain of the patient having memory loss in dementia. Depressed patients usually present themselves complaining of memory loss. Depressed and delirious patients will generally show poor effort in testing, while demented patients will generally display good effort, but get wrong answers.

416. The answer is e. Often, memory disturbances are the presenting symptom in Alzheimer disease. Remote memories are well-preserved initially, with the ability to recall new information being lost early in the illness. Difficulty with word-finding is also noted early. Decreased ability to recognize and draw complex figures is an early sign of problems, as is the loss of the ability to calculate. Social propriety and interpersonal skills often remain strikingly preserved until late in the illness.

417. The answer is c. Three cholinesterase inhibitors are approved for the treatment of Alzheimer disease. They include donepezil (Aricept), galantamine (Reminyl), and rivastigmine (Exelon). They reduce the metabolism of acetylcholinesterase, thereby prolonging its action at cholinergic synapses. They are associated with modest improvements in cognition, behavior, activities of daily living, and global measurements of functioning. However, they do not change the progression of neurodegeneration.

418. The answer is a. Behavioral symptoms are common in Alzheimer disease as it progresses. Managing behavioral symptoms can often be accomplished with good communication skills and support. However, when medication is needed, the first step should be a cholinesterase inhibitor such as donepezil; studies have demonstrated benefit in controlling aberrant behaviors. SSRIs can have a mild to moderate effect on mood, but are unlikely to affect aggressive behavior. Anticonvulsants and antipsychotic medications such as carbamazepine and risperidone are helpful in reducing agitation and aggressiveness in AD, but come with significant side effects and should be used after trialing a cholinesterase inhibitor.

Recommended Reading: Dementias

Sloane PD, Kaufer DI. Alzheimer's disease. In: Kellerman RD, Bope ET (eds). *Conn's Current Therapy 2018*. Philadelphia, PA: Elsevier.

Diabetes Mellitus

419. The answer is d. The ADA recommends screening all persons older than 45 years for diabetes every 3 years. Screens should start earlier in people with risk factors including a sedentary lifestyle, family history of diabetes in a first-degree relative, hypertension, overweight or obesity (BMI $\geq$ 25 kg/m^2 or $\geq$ 23 kg/m^2 in Asian Americans), high-risk ethnic groups (African American, Hispanic, Native American), a previous history of impaired glucose tolerance, abnormal lipids (especially elevated triglycerides and low HDL), a history of CVD, and women with polycystic ovary syndrome, a history of gestational diabetes, or a birth of a child greater than 9 lb.

420. The answer is c. The diagnosis of diabetes may be made by random glucose measurements more than 200 mg/dL with classic signs of diabetes (polydipsia, polyuria, polyphagia, weight loss), a fasting glucose greater than 126 mg/dL, a hemoglobin A1C level of more than or equal to 6.5%, or a glucose reading greater than 200 mg/dL 2 hours after a 75-g glucose load. All results should be confirmed with repeat testing.

421. The answer is a. In the past, young adults diagnosed with diabetes were primarily type 1 (T1DM). However, the epidemic of obesity in the United States has increased the rate of T2DM in people less than 20 years old from 5% to 30% over the last decade. C-terminal peptide is cleaved from natively produced insulin. Fasting C-peptide levels are markedly elevated in patients with T2DM, but in people with T1DM, C-peptide levels should be low due to the absence of native insulin. Microalbuminuria, markedly elevated hemoglobin A1C and peripheral neuropathy can all occur in type 1 or 2 diabetes. T1DM is caused by autoimmune destruction of the pancreatic islet cells and the antibody glutamic acid decarboxylase (GAD 65) is most commonly used to diagnose T1DM. Parietal cell antibodies are not associated with T1DM, but with pernicious anemia.

422. The answer is d. The ADA recommends dietary modifications and pharmacologic therapy at diagnosis of T2DM based on A1C and glucose levels. For patients with an A1C less than 9%, consider monotherapy; for patients with an A1C more than or equal to 9%, consider dual therapy, and for patients with an A1C more than or equal to 10%, blood glucose more than or equal to 300 mg/dL, or marked symptoms, consider combination injectable therapy. Patients with diabetic ketoacidosis or hyperosmolar hyperglycemia should be treated inpatient with an initial insulin drip and close monitoring. This patient has a normal urinalysis/electrolytes and is asymptomatic, so it is unlikely she has either condition. Dual therapy should be considered for this patient. In the absence of CVD, the ADA recommends metformin plus a second agent selected based on consideration of drug-specific effects and patient factors. A GLP-1 receptor agonist would be an appropriate choice for this patient due to their neutral or negative effects on bodyweight. TZDs tend to cause fluid retention and should not be used in patients with congestive heart failure. In her case, it would likely negatively affect her venous insufficiency. Insulin alone is not an appropriate initial therapy, but may be appropriate in combination with metformin.

423. The answer is d. All patients with T2DM should be screened annually for albuminuria with a urinary albumin-to-creatinine ratio through a random urine collection. However, two of three specimens in a 3- to 6-month period of time should be abnormal before considering a patient to have albuminuria. When albuminuria is confirmed, patients with T2DM should be treated with an ACE-inhibitor (or an ARB if they are intolerant of ACEs) to slow the progression toward ESRD. Referral to nephrology is indicated when the GFR falls below 60, or when the albumin-to-creatinine ratio exceeds 300 mg/g, or if the cause of the kidney disease is unclear. Patients with albuminuria should limit dietary protein intake to 0.8g/kg bodyweight/day. However, this patient has only had one positive albumin-to-creatinine ratio and the most appropriate therapy at this time would be to optimize her glycemic control and repeat the screening in 3 months.

424. The answer is d. Diabetic retinopathy is the leading cause of blindness in the United States. The risk increases with the length of time that the patient has had diabetes, and the condition worsens with increasing hemoglobin A1C levels. However, African-American patients develop retinopathy at lower levels of A1C. In type 2 diabetics it can be seen at diagnosis, and yearly dilated eye examinations are recommended beginning at the time of diagnosis. In patients with T1DM, dilated eye examinations should begin 5 years after diagnosis. More frequent examinations may be indicated in patients when eye pathology is present. Aspirin has no effect on eye complications.

425. The answer is d. ACE-inhibitors are clearly the first choice for blood pressure control in diabetic patients with CKD. They control blood pressure effectively, help prevent progression of renal disease, and are indicated in the presence of coronary disease and CHF. Although compelling, there is insufficient evidence to recommend ACE-inhibitors in all diabetic patients. According to the Eighth Joint National Committee (JNC-8) guidelines, African-American patients with T2DM **without** albuminuria and blood pressure readings between 140/90 and 160/100 mm Hg should receive either a thiazide-type diuretic or a calcium channel blocker alone or in combination as initial treatment. If albuminuria is present, an ACE or an ARB should be considered first. Among these four classes of medication, the ADA guidelines don't specify a preferred initial agent unless albuminuria is present, then they recommend an ACE or ARB preferentially. ACE/ARBs can be used irrespective of creatinine levels, though potassium should be monitored as creatinine rises.

426. The answer is e. The ADA recommends an A1C glycemic target of less than 7% for nonpregnant adults; however, providers may suggest less stringent goals for individual patients if this cannot be achieved without significant hypoglycemia. Less stringent goals may also be appropriate for patients with a history of severe hypoglycemia, limited life expectancy, advanced microvascular or macrovascular complications, extensive comorbid conditions, or long-standing diabetes that is difficult to control. This patient is elderly, with multiple comorbidities and evidence of hypoglycemia. The presence of hypoglycemia, especially severe or asymptomatic hypoglycemia, should prompt the clinician to raise this patient's glycemic targets to avoid hypoglycemia, because it is associated with increased morbidity and mortality. His current A1C is 8.2% and the only answer choice that is less stringent is 8.5%.

427. The answer is c. The decline of renal function can make maintaining glycemic control a challenging endeavor. Metformin, due to the risk of lactic acidosis, should be avoided in patients with a GFR less than 45 mL/min/1.73 m². This patient has good glycemic control, but her declining renal function demands a change in her regimen. Sulfonylureas (glyburide, glipizide, and glimepiride) should also be avoided in patients with significant renal impairment, due to their renal clearance and the increasing risk of hypoglycemia. Sodium glucose cotransporter 2 (SGLT-2) inhibitors (dapagliflozin, canagliflozin, and empagliflozin) should be avoided or discontinued in patients with a GFR of 30 to 60 mL/min/1.73 m². DPP-4 inhibitors have varying degrees of utility and dosing adjustment in patients with renal impairment, but linagliptin is not cleared by the kidneys and, therefore, requires no dosing adjustment in CKD.

428. The answer is c. GLP-1 is a gut hormone that, when stimulated by an oral glucose load, stimulates insulin secretion. This "incretin" effect is diminished in patients with T2DM. Native GLP-1 has a half-life of only a few minutes due to breakdown by the enzyme DPP-4, while GLP-1 receptor agonists are resistant to the effects of DPP-4 and result in supraphysiologic levels of GLP-1 in the body. DPP-4 inhibitors, in contrast, prolong the action of physiologic GLP-1, restoring levels comparable to healthy controls. This results in drug classes with varying efficacy and side-effect profiles. Both DPP-4 inhibitors and GLP-1 receptor agonists increase glucose-dependent insulin secretion from the pancreas and decrease glucagon production in the liver. However, the GLP-1 receptor agonists slow gastric emptying, increase satiety, and have a weight loss effect. This slowed gastric emptying is also responsible for the most frequent adverse reactions of nausea and vomiting. The DPP-4 inhibitors have a weight-neutral profile with an absence of GI side effects.

429. The answer is d. SGLT-2 inhibitors block renal reabsorption of glucose, causing urinary excretion of excess glucose. The most common side effects of SGLT-2 inhibitors are orthostatic hypotension, urinary tract infections, and vaginal yeast infections. Hypoglycemia can occur with any antihyperglycemic agent, but is not a prominent side effect of SGLT-2s.

Edema and weight gain are common side effects of TZDs, while cough occurs in some patients who take ACE-inhibitors. GI intolerance, including nausea and vomiting or diarrhea, is common with metformin and GLP-1 receptor agonists.

430. The answer is a. It is important to thoroughly understand the action of the different types of insulin preparations in order to make therapeutic decisions about diabetic patients and their control. Aspart, lispro (Humalog), and glulisine (Apidra) have the most rapid onset of action, between 15 and 30 minutes. Regular insulin has an onset between 30 and 60 minutes. NPH has an onset between 1 and 2 hours, as does glargine (Lantus) and detemir (Levemir).

431. The answer is e. It is important to thoroughly understand the action of the different types of insulin preparations in order to make therapeutic decisions about diabetic patients and their control. Lispro's activity peaks early, between 30 and 90 minutes after injection. Aspart's activity peaks around 1 and 3 hours after injection. Regular insulin peaks between 2 and 4 hours after injection. NPH peaks 5 to 7 hours after injection. Glargine (Lantus) and Detemir (Levemir) do not have a predictable peak, and last for around 20 and 24 hours. Insulin degludec (Tresiba) has an effective duration of 42 hours.

Drug	Onset of Action	Peak (hours)	Duration (hours)	Cost
Rapid-acting				
Lispro (Humalog)	15 minutes	0.5–1.5	2–4	
Aspart (NovoLog)	15 minutes	1–3	3–5	$$
Glulisine (Apidra)	15 minutes	1–1.5	5	$$$
Inhaled insulin (Afrezza)	12–15 minutes	< 1	2–5	
Short-acting				
Regular (Humulin)	30 minutes	2–4	5.8	$
Intermediate				
NPH (Novolin)	1–3 hours	5–7	16–18	$
Long-acting				
Glargine (Lantus)	1 hour	None	24	$$$
Detemir (Levemir)	1 hour	None	20	$$$

(Reproduced with permission from South-Paul JE, Matheny SC, Lewis EL. CURRENT Diagnosis & Treatment: Family Medicine, 4th Ed. New York, NY: McGraw-Hill Education; 2015: Table 36-4, p. 388.)

432. The answer is d. Patients with T2DM may require insulin therapy if diet, exercise, and oral hypoglycemic agent do not provide appropriate control.

A low initiating dose of insulin glargine is commonly used, estimating 0.1 U/kg of body weight, as an addition to the current regimen. The dose can be titrated over time to meet fasting blood glucose targets. The utility and frequency of SMBG is dependent on the type of regimen the patient is prescribed and what they do with the information. For T2DM patients on intensive basal-bolus insulin regimens, clinical trials show testing up to 6 to 10 times/day is associated with lower A1C levels. For T2DM patients on basal insulin and/or oral agents, the evidence is not as clear. Generally, patients on basal insulin should check at least fasting blood glucose levels and use those levels to make adjustments to their basal insulin dose; this is associated with lower A1Cs. Several studies have not shown much benefit to SMBG in noninsulin treated patients. The most important factors of whether SMBG lowers blood glucose are educating about and acting on the information. Therefore, patients should receive education about how to manage their blood glucose levels and clinicians should review and make recommendations on their patients' levels.

Recommended Reading: Diabetes Mellitus

American Diabetes Association. Standards of Medical Care in Diabetes—2018. Diabetes Care. 2018; 41(suppl 1): S1-118. Accessed at https://professional.diabetes.org/content-page/standards-medical-care-diabetes.

Rockafellow SD, Richardson CR, Mengel MB. Diabetes mellitus. In: Smith MA, Shimp LA, Schrager S (eds). *Family Medicine Ambulatory Care and Prevention.* 6th ed. New York, NY: McGraw-Hill.

Vail B. Diabetes mellitus. In: South-Paul JE, Matheny SC, Lewis EL (eds). *Current Diagnosis & Treatment Family Medicine.* 4th ed. New York, NY: McGraw-Hill.

Lipid Disorders

433. The answer is a. Recent guidelines describe four groups of patients who benefit from statin therapy for ASCVD prevention: (1) patients with clinical ASCVD, such as coronary artery disease, stroke, transient ischemic attack (TIA), or peripheral artery disease (PAD); (2) patients with primary elevations of LDL-C more than or equal to 190 md/dL; (3) patients aged 40 to 75 with diabetes and LDL-C between 70 and 189 mg/dL and without clinical ASCVD; or (4) patients without clinical ASCVD or diabetes with an LDL-C between 70 and 189 mg/dL AND an estimated 10-year ASCVD risk more than or equal to 7.5%. Recommendations regarding intensity of statin level are based on these groups, but this patient does not benefit from statin therapy at this time. Lifestyle modifications are recommended as the mainstay of all prevention efforts for patients with dyslipidemias or risk factors for ASCVD.

434. The answer is d. According to the ACC/AHA blood cholesterol guidelines, for the prevention of ASCVD events this patient should receive a high-intensity statin based on his risk factors. Patients with clinical ASCVD, patients with diabetes and 10-year ASCVD risk more than or equal to 7.5%, and patients with an LDL-C more than or equal to 190 mg/dL benefit from a high-intensity statin. Patients 40 to 75 years old with diabetes and an LDL-C between 70 and 189 mg/dL or patients 40 to 75 years old with a 10-year ASCVD risk more than or equal to 7.5%, and those with clinical ASCVD who are more than 75 years old or cannot tolerate a high-intensity statin receive benefit from a moderate-intensity statin. While his triglycerides are elevated, treating them with a fenofibrate agent would not be expected to improve his health outcome. Use of a high-intensity statin will be likely to lower this patient's LDL-C by approximately 50%.

435. The answer is c. Several lifestyle modification efforts are known to increase HDL cholesterol. By losing weight, a person can expect to raise HDL by 5 to 10 points. Smoking cessation has the same approximate effect. Adopting an exercise program is even more effective, raising HDL by up to 15 points. Eating oat bran and decreasing life stress can lower LDL, but is not likely to raise HDL. Additionally, alcohol, in moderation, raises HDL cholesterol.

436. The answer is a. Blood lipids change acutely in response to food intake. The triglyceride level is lowest in the fasting state and rises by an average of 50 mg/dL postprandially. As the triglyceride level rises, the total and LDL cholesterol each fall. Thus total and LDL cholesterol tend to be higher when fasting. HDL varies little whether fasting or not.

437. The answer is a. The National Cholesterol Education Program ATP III guidelines recommend that medications should be added to TLC after 3 months if LDL goals are not achieved, even in lower risk patients. Given their track record, statin agents are the drugs of first choice.

438. The answer is e. The primary side effects seen with statin agents include myopathy and increased liver enzymes. Rhabdomyolysis occurs in less than 0.1% of cases, but elevated transaminases occur more commonly. Discontinuation of the agent is required only if liver enzymes increase to more than 3 times normal (and that occurs in only 1% of patients on statins). Routine monitoring of serum aminotransferase levels is no longer recommended by the FDA since hepatic side effects will most often trigger an evaluation, and the effects are reversible. Routine monitoring of muscle enzymes is not supported by evidence, but unexplained pain in large muscle groups should prompt an investigation for myopathy.

439. The answer is d. Niacin is associated with a prostaglandin-mediated flushing effect. Aspirin (81-325 mg) blocks much of the flushing that is associated with sustained-release niacin preparations. Taking niacin at night, with food, on an empty stomach or with milk, or with a proton-pump inhibitor will not impact the side effects. Initiating niacin at a low dose (100 mg daily) and slowly titrating up can also decrease flushing. Only 50% to 60% of patients can tolerate the full-dose of Niacin; extended-release dosing is better tolerated.

440. The answer is b. Niacin was the first lipid-lowering agent associated with decreased total mortality. It moderately decreases LDL, can increase HDL by 20% to 25%, and moderately decreases triglycerides. It causes a prostaglandin-mediated flushing that patients often describe as "hot flashes." This side effect can be easily moderated by having the patient take an NSAID or aspirin at least an hour before taking the niacin. Although niacin can increase blood sugar, it is safe for diabetics to use.

441. The answer is b. Numerous studies have demonstrated the benefits of lowering LDL-C on all-cause and cardiovascular mortality. Non-HDL cholesterol is the sum of HDL and VLDL cholesterol; while reductions in VLDL are considered beneficial, there are no studies evaluating its effect on mortality. Niacin increases HDL and lowers VLDL and has been shown to reduce cardiovascular events and mortality, but not to the extent that lowering LDL does. Additionally, raising HDL doesn't seem to have an added benefit to lowering LDL cholesterol. Apolipoprotein A is protective against CVD and lowering it would negatively affect outcomes. The effect of lowering triglycerides is not well understood; studies have shown higher risks of

CVD in patients with elevated triglycerides. However, the current data do not support lowering triglycerides for CVD prevention.

Recommended Reading: Lipid Disorders

Baron RB. Lipid disorders. In: Papadakis MA, McPhee SJ, Rabow MW (eds). *Current Medical Diagnosis & Treatment 2018.* New York, NY: McGraw-Hill.

Reamy BV. Dyslipidemias. In: South-Paul JE, Matheny SC, Lewis EL (eds). *Current Diagnosis & Treatment Family Medicine.* 4th ed. New York, NY: McGraw-Hill.

Stone NJ, Robinson JG, Lichtenstein AH, et al. A Report of the American College of Cardiology/American Heart Association Task Force on Practice Guidelines. *Circulation.* 2013;01. Available at http://circ.ahajournals.org/content/circulationaha/early/2013/11/11/01.cir.0000437738.63853.7a.full.pdf.

Wells TD, Cox AM, Smith MA, Crouch MA. Dyslipidemias. In: Smith MA, Shimp LA, Schrager S (eds). *Family Medicine Ambulatory Care and Prevention.* 6th ed. New York, NY: McGraw-Hill.

HIV Care

442. The answer is d. In the United States, an estimated 1.2 million people are living with HIV disease, and approximately 20% of these individuals do not know their HIV status. Worldwide, AIDS is now the leading cause of death for persons aged 15 to 59 years. In some African countries, HIV is such a problem that average life expectancy has been reduced by more than 20 years. When a person is newly diagnosed with HIV, a complete physical examination and laboratory assessment should be conducted. A CD4 count should be done at the initial visit, then every 3 to 6 months after. A plasma HIV RNA (viral load) should be done at the initial visit, before starting antiretroviral therapy (ART), and every 3 months while on ART. A full hepatitis panel should be conducted on all newly diagnosed patients, and if the patient is found to be Hepatitis A and/or Hepatitis B nonimmune, vaccination is indicated.

443. The answer is b. In patients with HIV who have a tuberculin skin test, 5 mm induration is the cutoff for treatment of latent tuberculosis infection. This is also true of people with recent contact with an individual with active TB, a person with a CXR consistent with prior healed TB, or anyone receiving immunosuppressive therapy. For people with no risk factors for TB and a normal immune system, induration of greater than or equal to 15 mm is positive. Induration greater than or equal to 10 mm is considered positive in injection drug users, people with certain clinical conditions (diabetes, renal failure, some hematologic disorders), recent immigrants, persons from medically underserved populations and residents of high-risk settings (prisons, nursing homes, or other long-term care facilities), and laboratory personnel working with mycobacteriology.

444. The answer is a. Guidelines for recommending antiretroviral treatment have changed over the years as treatment regimens have changed and more evidence has been gathered. The most current guidelines state that in settings where ART exists and is available, all patients who are motivated and ready to start therapy should start regardless of CD4 count or viral load. This is because HIV infection causes a generalized heightened level of immune activation and inflammation which may increase the incidence of illness and disease independent of CD4 count or HIV progression. There is evidence to suggest that HIV accelerates the aging process with premature loss of bone density and neurocognitive decline. Adding to those benefits, recent studies have shown that HIV transmission significantly decreases for those taking ART, validating a "treatment as prevention" public health strategy.

445. The answer is a. After initiation of ART in a patient with HIV, the CD4 count and viral load should be assessed every 3 to 6 months. If a patient has been on a long-term stable regimen, the 6-month interval is appropriate. An increase in viral load to detectable levels after achieving suppression may be a sign of treatment failure, but low viral loads (< 200 copies/mL) are common and considered harmless "blips" in treatment. The patient can continue to be followed. However, if there is persistent viremia, clinicians should consider consultation with an HIV specialist. The management of true treatment failure is extremely complex and will require resistance testing.

446. The answer is c. Prophylaxis against opportunistic infections should occur in HIV-infected patients when the CD4 cell count decreases to specific threshold values. Below 200, the provider should recommend prophylaxis against *P jiroveci* pneumonia (PCP). Below 100, the provider should recommend prophylaxis against toxoplasmosis. Below 50, the provider should recommend prophylaxis against *Mycobacterium avium-intracellulare* complex (MAC).

Absolute CD4 Count	Opportunistic Infection/ Malignancy	Specific OI Prophylaxis Recommended
Above 300	Vaginal candidiasis Tuberculosis Skin disease Fatigue Bacterial pneumonia Herpes zoster	No specific opportunistic infection prophylaxis
Below 300	Oral hairy leukoplakia Thrush Fever, diarrhea, weight loss	
Below 200	Kaposi's sarcoma Non-Hodgkin's lymphoma PCP CNS lymphoma	Pneumocystis prophylaxis with Bactrim (1 tablet daily)
Below 100	Toxoplasmosis Esophageal candidiasis Cryptococcosis	Toxoplasma prophylaxis with Bactrim DS (1 tablet daily)
Below 50	Cytomegalovirus (CMV) Mycobacterium avium complex (MAC) CNS lymphoma	MAC prophylaxis with Azithromycin (1200 mg weekly)

(*Reproduced with permission from South-Paul JE, Matheny SC, Lewis EL.* CURRENT Diagnosis & Treatment: Family Medicine, *4th Ed. New York, NY: McGraw-Hill Education; 2015: Table 55-3, p. 587.*)

Recommended Reading: HIV Care

Mathad IS, Westergaard R, Gupta A. HIV disease. In: Bope ET, Kellerman RD (eds). *Conn's Current Therapy, 2017.* Philadelphia, PA: Elsevier.

Prasad R. HIV primary care In: South-Paul JE, Matheny SC, Lewis EL (eds). *Current Diagnosis & Treatment Family Medicine.* 4th ed. New York, NY: McGraw-Hill.

Saberi P, Mahoney M, Goldschmidt RH. Human immunodeficiency virus and acquired immunodeficiency syndrome. In: Smith MA, Shimp LA, Schrager S (eds). *Family Medicine Ambulatory Care and Prevention.* 6th ed. New York, NY: McGraw-Hill.

Hypertension

447. The answer is b. Many observational studies have demonstrated graded associations between higher SBP and increased CVD risk. Risks for

CVD increase in a log-linear fashion with SBP levels less than 115 mm Hg to more than 180 mm Hg and from diastolic blood pressure (DBP) levels less than 75 mm Hg to more than 105 mm Hg. In addition, blood pressure 20 mm Hg higher than normal is associated with a doubling in the risk of death from stroke, heart disease, or other vascular disease. Studies have also shown that higher SBP is associated with increased risk of angina, MI, HF, stroke, PAD, and abdominal aortic aneurysm. The increased risk of CVD associated with higher SBP has been reported across a broad age spectrum, from 30 years to more than 80 years of age. Interestingly, the relative risk of incident CVD associated with higher SBP is smaller at older ages.

448. The answer is a.

449. The answer is c.

450. The answer is d.

451. The answer is c.

452. The answer is b.

Categorizing blood pressure is important to help determine treatment options. The stage is determined after appropriately taking two or more blood pressure readings on two or more occasions and averaging those readings. A table outlining the classifications is below. If the SBP and DBP are in two separate categories, the blood pressure should be designated in the higher category. The newer categorization eliminates the category of "prehypertension."

Reading	Classification
Less than 120/80 mm Hg	Normal
Systolic between 120 and 129 AND diastolic less than 80	Elevated
Systolic between 130 and 139 mm Hg OR diastolic between 80 and 89 mm Hg	Stage 1
Systolic at least 140 mm Hg OR diastolic at least 90 mm Hg	Stage 2
Systolic over 180 mm Hg and/or diastolic over 120 mm Hg	Hypertensive crisis

453. The answer is d. Lifestyle modifications can help to manage hypertension. Weight reduction is beneficial, and SBP can fall up to 4 to 5 mm Hg for each 4 kg of weight lost. A DASH diet can lower blood pressure between 8 and 14 mm Hg. Dietary sodium reduction, increased exercise, and moderation of alcohol can be expected to lower SBP between 3 and 6 mm Hg.

454. The answer is a. The patient in this question has stage I hypertension (SBP between 130 and 139 mm Hg, or diastolic blood pressure between 80 and 89 mm Hg). Since lifestyle modifications have not helped, the next step is to institute drug therapy. The most effective first-line treatment for preventing the occurrence of CVD is either an ACE-inhibitor, an ARB, a calcium channel blocker, or a thiazide diuretic. In the African-American hypertensive population, a calcium channel blocker or a thiazide diuretic is recommended.

455. The answer is b. Baseline laboratory screening is important to assess for end-organ damage and identify patients at high risk for cardiovascular complications. The routine tests for a newly diagnosed hypertensive patient include hemoglobin and hematocrit, sodium, potassium, creatinine, fasting glucose, calcium, a fasting lipid profile, urinalysis, a TSH, and a resting electrocardiogram. An echocardiogram and a uric acid level are optional. Other tests are not indicated unless physical examination or history makes them likely to be positive.

456. The answer is b. The prevalence of renovascular disease as the cause in a person with hypertension alone is around 5%. The patient described in the question has physical examination findings consistent with renal artery stenosis. Imaging options include MRI/MRA, CT scan, and ultrasound. The preferred method depends on capabilities of the institution. Urinary metanephrines and vanillylmandelic acid levels would help rule out pheochromocytoma. A CXR would be helpful if coarctation of the aorta were suspected. An aortic CT would help to or quantify an aortic aneurysm, and an echocardiogram would help to identify left ventricular hypertrophy or systolic dysfunction.

457. The answer is a. 2017 ACC/AHA guidelines recommend that low-dose diuretics are the most effective first-line treatment for preventing the occurrence of cardiovascular morbidity and mortality. The use of ACE-inhibitors, ARB, calcium channel blockers, or thiazide diuretics can also be used as first-line therapy. β-Blockers are not recommended as first-line therapy unless the patient has ischemic heart disease or heart failure.

458. The answer is e. 2017 ACC/AHA guidelines indicate that for secondary stroke prevention, the usefulness of initiating antihypertensive treatment is not well established for blood pressures less than 140/90. For previously treated adults, a goal of 130/80 is reasonable.

459. The answer is b. Several clinical trials have documented the benefit of ACE-inhibitors in patients with hypertension and CKD. ARBs are also beneficial. His blood pressure goal should be less than 130/80.

460. The answer is a. The three most common causes of uncontrolled hypertension in patients who are diagnosed with the disease are patient nonadherence, inadequate therapy, and inappropriate therapy. Other secondary causes of hypertension are possible, but less likely than nonadherence, and while use of some medications may make blood pressure control difficult, nonadherence is more common.

461. The answer is b. Most patients with hypertension do not reach their blood pressure goal with a single medication, and most need a second from a different class. If a patient is not at goal with two medications at maximized dosage, the addition of a third agent from another class is the best next step. Changing to a different brand within the same class may help in some cases, but using a third class is likely to be more effective. Changing to a different class (rather than adding a medication from a third class) is not likely to help the patient reach his/her blood pressure goal.

Recommended Reading: Hypertension

Eversen AE, Eaton CB. Hypertension. In: Smith MA, Shimp LA, Schrager S (eds). *Family Medicine Ambulatory Care and Prevention.* 6th ed. New York, NY: McGraw-Hill.

Whelton PK, Carey RM, Aronow WS, et al. 2017 ACC/AHA/AAPA/ABC/ ACPM/AGS/APhA/ASH/ASPC/NMA/PCNA guideline for the prevention, detection, evaluation, and management of high blood pressure in adults: executive summary: a report of the American College of Cardiology/American Heart Association Task Force on Clinical Practice Guidelines. *Hypertension.* 2017.

Ischemia and Angina

462. The answer is b.

463. The answer is c.

464. The answer is d.
Angina is not one type of pain. Rather it is a constellation of symptoms. Understanding the best way to describe the pain ensures that you and your colleagues understand one another. Chest pain may fit one of the following categories:

- Typical (classic) angina: This will present as ill-defined chest pressure, heaviness, or a squeezing sensation. The location is generally substernal or left sided. It may radiate to the jaw, back, or down the arm. It generally begins gradually and lasts only a few minutes, and stress or exertion may be aggravating factors. Classic angina is usually relieved by rest or by nitroglycerine.
- Atypical angina: This has some, but not all the features of classic angina. For example, there may be a sense of heaviness, but it won't be precipitated by exercise or relieved by rest. Or, the pain may have an atypical character (like stabbing pain or sharp pain), but the precipitating or relieving features may be anginal.
- Anginal equivalent: This is when an atypical symptom (usually shortness of breath) fits all the features of angina, but there is no chest pain.
- Nonanginal pain: This has neither the character nor the precipitating/relieving factors of classic angina.
- Atypical nonanginal pain: This is not used as a descriptor for chest pain.

465. The answer is e. Nitrates improve myocardial blood flow and oxygen demand via endothelial vasodilation. Tolerance is the most significant issue to consider when using nitrates for stable angina. Tolerance can develop within 1 day when long-acting nitrates are given. When using a patch, it is important to have intervals of 10 to 12 hours without the patch to retain the antianginal effect. Headache and fatigue may be important side effects, but are more of a nuisance than an important consideration. Nitrates can be used with β-blockers and calcium channel blockers. Nitrates should be avoided in persons taking erectile dysfunction medications like sildenafil. Since both medications are vasodilatory, the combination can cause a sudden and potentially serious blood pressure drop.

466. The answer is c. β-blockade decreases heart rate, contractility, and blood pressure, reducing oxygen demand and therefore angina symptoms. All β-blockers, regardless of their selectivity, are equally effective in treating angina. About 20% of patients do not respond. Many family physicians are reluctant to increase the dose to the most effective levels. In general, the dose should be adjusted to achieve a heart rate of 50 to 60 beats/min.

Recommended Reading: Ischemia and Angina

Lee DF, Aggarwal L, Hixon AL. Ischemic heart disease and acute coronary syndrome. In: Smith MA, Shimp LA, Schrager S (eds). *Family Medicine Ambulatory Care and Prevention*. 6th ed. New York, NY: McGraw-Hill.

Tobin K, Eagle K. Angina pectoris. In: Bope ET, Kellerman RD (eds). *Conn's Current Therapy, 2017*. Philadelphia, PA: Elsevier.

Obesity

467. The answer is b.

468. The answer is c.

469. The answer is d.
More than 97 million adults in the United States are overweight or obese. The percentage of overweight adults in the United States is around 66.3%. Obesity is a disorder of excess body fat resulting in an increased risk for adverse health conditions. In 1997, the World Health Organization recommended adoption of BMI as a standard for the assessment of body fat. It is calculated by dividing a person's weight in kilograms by their height in meters squared. The classifications for obesity are:

- Normal weight: BMI between 18.5 and 24.9 kg/m^2
- Overweight: BMI between 25 and 29.9 kg/m^2
- Obesity Class I: A BMI between 30 and 34.9 kg/m^2
- Obesity Class II: A BMI between 35 and 39.9 kg/m^2
- Obesity Class III: A BMI greater than or equal to 40 kg/m^2.

BMI by itself cannot estimate obesity in some subgroups of individuals. These include competitive athletes and bodybuilders (who may have a misleadingly high BMI but a low total body fat), pregnant women, children, and adolescents (excessive calorie intake will usually manifest in additional height and weight, so appropriate weight-to-height ratios must be assessed using age and gender specific tables).

470. The answer is b. Risk factors for obesity include race, age, inactivity, socioeconomic status, and marital status. Regarding race, higher percentages of black and Hispanic Americans meet the criteria of overweight or obesity than in their non-Hispanic white counterparts. In fact, 76% of blacks over 20 meet the criteria for being overweight, 76% of Mexican Americans meet the criteria for being overweight, and 64% of non-Hispanic whites meet the criteria for being overweight. Regarding socioeconomic status and education level, in industrialized countries, a higher prevalence of obesity is seen in those with lower educational levels and low income. Regarding marital status, a tendency to gain weight is seen after marriage and parity. Regarding age, the prevalence of obesity increases with age, and is particularly apparent between the ages of 40 and 60.

471. The answer is e. Diet control is the cornerstone of obesity management. There are many dietary approaches to controlling one's diet, but no specific diet has consistently been shown to be superior to others related to long-term weight loss outcomes. The key is to create a calorie deficit below what is needed to maintain weight—and as long as that occurs, the composition of the diet is secondary.

472. The answer is d. Unfortunately, only 20% of patients will lose 20 lbs and maintain the weight loss for 2 years using conventional dietary techniques. Only 5% can maintain a 40-lb weight loss. Those who are successful report continued close contact with their health care provider. Most successful programs are multidisciplinary and include a low-calorie diet, behavior modification, exercise, and social support.

473. The answer is a. The history and physical examination are of utmost importance when evaluating the obese patient. Less than 1% of obese patients have a secondary nonpsychiatric cause for their obesity. Hypothyroidism and Cushing syndrome are important examples that can generally be detected by history and physical (but would need additional testing if historical features or physical findings point in that direction). However, laboratory evaluation is necessary to assess the medical consequences of obesity. Testing should include fasting glucose, LDL, HDL, and triglyceride levels. Should the patient present with global symptoms such as skin changes, hair loss, abnormal menstrual cycles, or atypical fat distribution, laboratory evaluation should include a workup of endocrine disorders.

474. The answer is c. There are five FDA-approved medications for weight loss. Orlistat blocks fat absorption in the gut, and can result if a 2 to 4 kg greater weight loss than placebo. In other studies, Lorcaserin, a selective serotonin receptor agonist, leads to weight loss of about 3% of initial weight. The combination of naltrexone and bupropion demonstrates a 2%

to 4% weight reduction compared with placebo at 1 year. Liraglutide is an injectable incretin, and has been shown a 3.7% to 4.5% weight loss compared to placebo at 1 year. In clinical trials, the combination of phentermine hydrochloride and topiramate resulted in up to 9.8% more weight loss compared to placebo. All of these options have side effects, and the choice of medication used should depend on specific patient factors.

475. The answer is b. Bariatric surgery is an increasingly more common treatment option for severe obesity. In the United States, the most common procedure performed is the Roux-en-Y gastric bypass. The procedure can result in substantial weight loss, up to 50% of the initial weight in some studies. Complications are common and occur with about 40% of the cases. Operative mortality is actually quite low, (0% to 1% in the first 30 days). Nutritional deficiencies are common postoperatively, and patients require life-long supplementation. Because of the risks of the surgery, bariatric surgery is limited to those with a BMI more than 40 kg/m^2, or more than 35 kg/m^2 if there are obesity-related comorbidities present.

Recommended Reading: Obesity

Baron RB. Nutritional disorders. In: Papadakis MA, McPhee SJ, Rabow MW (eds). *Current Medical Diagnosis & Treatment 2018*. New York, NY: McGraw-Hill.

Hariharan RR, Reed BC, Edmonson SR. Obesity. In: Smith MA, Shimp LA, Schrager S (eds). *Family Medicine Ambulatory Care and Prevention*. 6th ed. New York, NY: McGraw-Hill.

Osteoporosis and Other Bone Issues

476. The answer is d. Osteoporosis is a public health problem affecting more than 40 million people. It results in approximately 1,500,000 fractures annually in women in the United States alone, not to mention the fractures that occur in men. The direct expenditures for osteoporotic fractures have increased in the last 10 years from around $5 billion to around $15 billion. The disease occurs because of poor acquisition of bone mass or accelerated bone loss. African Americans are less at risk than Caucasians or Asians. There is no evidence that oral contraceptive use increases risk. Obesity is considered to be protective because of increased estrogen production, as long as the person is not sedentary. Hyperthyroidism is a common cause of accelerated bone loss. Breast-feeding is a significant drain on calcium stores, but studies have shown that the associated bone mineral loss is completely reversed within 12 months of weaning.

477. The answer is a. Weight-bearing activity is known to retard bone loss. While there have been no randomized clinical trials comparing the effect of various activities on bone mass, recommended activities include walking, jogging, weight lifting, aerobics, stair climbing, field sports, racquet sports, court sports, and dancing. For women who have been very sedentary, any increase in activity may have a positive effect on bone mass. That said, swimming is questionable, as it is not weight-bearing. There is no data on cycling, skating, or skiing. To be beneficial, the duration of exercise should be between 30 and 60 minutes at a time, and the frequency should be 3 to 4 times weekly.

478. The answer is e. Primary osteoporosis refers to deterioration of bone mass not associated with other chronic illnesses or problems. History and physical are neither sensitive enough nor sufficient for the diagnosis of primary osteoporosis. While decreased serum calcium may indicate malabsorption or a vitamin D deficiency, it is not useful as a diagnostic tool for osteoporosis. Measures of bone turnover, like serum human osteocalcin levels, are of research interest, but are not useful for screening. Imaging studies are best. The United States Preventive Services Task Force (USPSTF) recommends screening for osteoporosis in women aged 65 years and older and in younger women whose fracture risk is equal to or greater than that of a 65-year-old white woman who has no additional risk factors.

479. The answer is d. Plain radiographs are not sensitive enough to diagnose osteoporosis until total density has decreased by 50%. Single- and dual-photon absorptiometry provide poor resolution and are less accurate than other methods. DXA and quantitative CT are the most widely used screening techniques. Quantitative CT is most sensitive, but results in substantially greater radiation exposure than DXA. For this reason, DXA is the diagnostic test of choice. Bone densitometry provides a T-score (the number of standard deviations above or below the mean matched to young controls) and a Z-score (the number of standard deviations above or below the mean-matched to age-matched controls). Z-scores are of little value to clinicians. A T-score more than 2.5 standard deviations below the mean (a score of −2.5 or lower) indicates osteoporosis.

480. The answer is c. Calcitonin directly inhibits osteoclastic bone resorption and is considered a reasonable treatment alternative for patients with established osteoporosis in whom estrogen-replacement therapy is not recommended. It has the unique characteristic of producing an analgesic effect with respect to bone pain and is often prescribed for patients who have suffered an acute osteoporotic fracture. For some reason, the increase in BMD associated with the use of calcitonin may be transient. Therefore, calcitonin should be thought of as a more acute treatment, with other medications being the mainstay of chronic therapy.

481. The answer is c. Bisphosphonates work by binding to the bone surface and inhibiting osteoclastic activity. Therefore, less bone is lost during the remodeling cycle. Vitamin D increases absorption of calcium in the GI tract. Estrogen and selective estrogen receptor modulators (raloxifene or Evista) work by blocking the activity of cytokines. Fluoride stimulates osteoblasts, but does not result in the formation of normal bone.

482. The answer is e. The diagnosis of osteoarthritis rests on clinical grounds. Laboratory testing should be used selectively to rule out other diagnoses or help guide treatment decisions. There are no specific blood tests to order as part of the routine diagnosis of osteoarthritis. Even radiographs aren't extremely helpful. While a number of radiographic features are common in osteoarthritis, there may be relatively poor correlation between observed radiographic changes and symptoms. The absence of radiographic findings does not rule out osteoarthritis, and the presence of typical radiographic findings does not guarantee that osteoarthritis is the source of a patient's complaints.

483. The answer is a. At-home or supervised exercise programs have been shown to provide benefits in terms of pain control, functionality, overall well-being and prevention of disability for osteoarthritis of the knees. Interestingly, for osteoarthritis of the hips, exercise programs have been shown to reduce pain, but have not shown the improvements in other areas.

Recommended Reading: Osteoporosis and Other Bone Issues

DeCastro A, Carek PJ. Osteoporosis. In: Bope ET, Kellerman RD (eds). *Conn's Current Therapy, 2017.* Philadelphia, PA: Elsevier.

Kodner C. Osteoarthritis. In: Smith MA, Shimp LA, Schrager S (eds). *Family Medicine Ambulatory Care and Prevention.* 6th ed. New York, NY: McGraw-Hill.

Manard WT, Schamp RO. Osteoporosis. In: Smith MA, Shimp LA, Schrager S (eds). *Family Medicine Ambulatory Care and Prevention*. 6th ed. New York, NY: McGraw-Hill.

Newstadt DH. Osteoarthritis. In: Bope ET, Kellerman RD (eds). *Conn's Current Therapy, 2017*. Philadelphia, PA: Elsevier.

South Paul JE. Osteoporosis. In: South-Paul JE, Matheny SC, Lewis EL (eds). *Current Diagnosis & Treatment Family Medicine*. 4th ed. New York, NY: McGraw-Hill.

Psychiatric Disorders

484. The answer is b. Depression is common. It is the seventh most common outpatient diagnosis in family medicine, and despite the frequency with which we see it in our population, it is likely often undiagnosed and undertreated. MDD is the most severe form of depression. It is characterized by at least 2 weeks of five or more of the following symptoms:

- Depressed mood
- Loss of interest or pleasure in daily activities (anhedonia)
- Weight gain or loss
- Insomnia or hypersomnia
- Psychomotor agitation or slowing
- Fatigue or loss of energy
- Feelings of guilt or worthlessness
- Inability to concentrate
- Thoughts of death or suicidal ideation.

Either depressed mood or anhedonia must be present as one of the symptoms.

485. The answer is b. Posttraumatic stress disorder (PTSD) used to be classified as an anxiety disorder, but in DSM-5 has been reclassified as a trauma- and stressor-related disorder. People who suffer from it re-experience a traumatic event. Drugs and alcohol are commonly used by the patient to self-treat. The only class of medications that are FDA approved to treat PTSD is the SSRIs. They are therefore considered the pharmacological treatment of choice for the condition.

486. The answer is d. Physicians have various treatment options for depression. Studies have shown that the combination of medication and therapy offers the best treatment outcomes. However, antidepressants alone are effective in about 50% to 60% of patients with major depression. If a patient fails to respond to one medication, he or she may respond to another. At least 80% of patients with major depression will respond to at least one antidepressant medication. In order to prevent relapse, treatment should continue for 6 to 12 months. ECT has a high rate of therapeutic success, but is reserved for those who do not respond to other modes of treatment.

487. The answer is e. While many of the newer antidepressants are well-tolerated, physicians should be familiar with the adverse effects and contra-indications for their use. Hypertension is a relative contraindication to ven-lafaxine. Patients experiencing hypersomnia and motor retardation should avoid mirtazapine. Patients who report agitation and insomnia should avoid bupropion and venlafaxine. Mirtazapine and tricyclic antidepressants like amitriptyline are less preferred for patients with obesity. Bupropion is contraindicated for patients with seizure disorder.

488. The answer is d. Eating disorders are psychologic disorders in which the person afflicted has an altered perception of body weight or shape and disturbances of eating behavior. Distinguishing between anorexia and buli-mia may be important from a treatment standpoint. Some characteristics are common to both eating disorders, while other characteristics may help to differentiate them. Both disorders involve self-evaluation that is unduly influenced by body weight and/or shape. While binge eating or purging are considered characteristics of bulimia, there is a binge eating/purging subtype of anorexia that involves that behavior as well. Both bulimics and binge eating/purging subtypes of anorexics may use diuretics, enemas, and laxatives. Both engage in inappropriate behaviors to prevent weight gain. However, bulimics sense a lack of control over eating during episodes of binging, while anorexics often feel a strong sense of control. This is a char-acteristic that may help distinguish the two.

489. The answer is a. In some bipolar patients, the diagnosis is made after the initiation of an antidepressant allows the patient to cycle into a manic phase. All the medications listed in this answer can be used to help bipolar disorder, but only the antipsychotics will be of benefit in the acute phase. Choices include olanzapine, risperidone, or aripiprazole. Lithium, valproic acid, carbamazepine, and lamotrigine are all excellent options for mainte-nance once the acute mania is under control, and can be started during the acute episode, but are not as effective controlling acute symptoms.

490. The answer is b. Of children diagnosed with ADHD, 60% to 75% will continue to exhibit symptoms into adulthood. In adults, symptoms of ADHD may be more subtle, and symptoms may actually change. Deficits in executive function tend to be more salient (poor organization or time management) and the "hyperactivity" of childhood may be replaced by restlessness or difficulty relaxing. Patients with impulsivity as a child may replace that with difficulty monitoring behavior or modulating emotional intensity.

491. The answer is d. When screening for ADHD, a thorough history and physical should be completed, and behavioral rating forms should be reviewed. Laboratory testing should be obtained to rule out other causes of symptoms, and include blood chemistries, a TSH, and a lead level. Most children with ADHD will have normal laboratory values, but these tests can exclude other causes of symptoms.

492. The answer is d. Personality disorders are grouped into three categories or "clusters" based on DSM-5. Cluster A is odd, eccentric personality disorders and includes paranoid, schizotypal, and schizoid personality disorders. Cluster B is dramatic, emotional, erratic personality disorders, and includes antisocial, borderline, histrionic, and narcissistic personality disorders. Cluster C is anxious, fearful personality disorders, and includes avoidant, dependent. and obsessive-compulsive personality disorders. Although they are common (with a prevalence of around 8% in the general US population), many do not rise to the level of creating problem or concern for the person and are either undiagnosed or untreated. When diagnosed, treatment can be a challenge. Some medications can be effective for specific disorders (for example, avoidant personality disorder can be treated with SSRIs, and obsessive-compulsive personality disorders may become less compulsive with SSRIs), but medications are not helpful for patients with narcissistic, antisocial, or histrionic personality disorders. Cognitive behavioral psychotherapy, which challenges irrational beliefs, can be helpful with narcissistic personality disorder, but should be conducted by an extremely experienced therapist, and usually requires a multiyear commitment.

493. The answer is c. SSRIs are the first-line therapy for most anxiety disorders, with the exception of situational anxiety. Sexual dysfunction is a common side effect, and if that becomes problematic for patients, family physicians should be prepared with other treatment options. While benzodiazepines are excellent choices for panic attacks or intermittent anxiety, the potential for abuse and dependence make them a poor choice for GAD.

Tricyclics may be considered after a failed trial of SSRIs, but because of their side-effect profile, their adherence is low. They are more commonly used when there is comorbid chronic pain or insomnia. Buspirone has an unknown mechanism of action, but has been shown to be as effective as benzodiazepines for GAD. It has a delayed onset of action (around 2 weeks), but in the patient described in this question, the levels of the SSRI will be decreasing while serum levels of buspirone are increasing. β-Blockers are primarily used to relieve autonomic symptoms of situational anxiety, but not for GAD. Atypical anticonvulsants may be used to augment therapy in cases of refractory anxiety, but are not the primary treatment options.

Recommended Reading: Psychiatric Disorders

Faulkner RA, Garcia LT. Depression. In: Smith MA, Shimp LA, Schrager S (eds). *Family Medicine Ambulatory Care and Prevention*. 6th ed. New York, NY: McGraw-Hill.

Michels PJ, Steadman MS. Anxiety disorders. In: South-Paul JE, Matheny SC, Lewis EL (eds). *Current Diagnosis & Treatment Family Medicine*. 4th ed. New York, NY: McGraw-Hill.

Novac A. Mood disorders, depression, bipolar disease and mood dysregulation. In: Bope ET, Kellerman RD (eds). *Conn's Current Therapy, 2017*. Philadelphia, PA: Elsevier.

Raj KS, Williams N, DeBattista C, Psychiatric disorders. In: Papadakis MA, McPhee SJ, Rabow MW (eds). *Current Medical Diagnosis & Treatment 2018*. New York, NY: McGraw-Hill.

Reed BC. Eating disorders. In: Smith MA, Shimp LA, Schrager S (eds). *Family Medicine Ambulatory Care and Prevention*. 6th ed. New York, NY: McGraw-Hill.

Searight HR, Gafford J, Evans SL. Attention deficit hyperactivity disorder. In: Smith MA, Shimp LA, Schrager S (eds). *Family Medicine Ambulatory Care and Prevention*. 6th ed. New York, NY: McGraw-Hill.

Thyroid Disorders

494. The answer is b. Thyroid disorders are common, with hypothyroidism being much more common than hyperthyroidism, nodular disease, or thyroid cancer. The incidence of hypothyroidism is 7% of women and 3% of men aged 60 to 89 years. Once diagnosed, the TSH level is the most important measure to gauge the dose of thyroid replacement therapy. Dose of thyroid replacement therapy will vary depending on age, weight, cardiac status, and severity of the condition. Once therapy is adjusted, a TSH level should be checked in 6 weeks and therapy should be titrated to keep the TSH in the normal range.

495. The answer is e. Subclinical hypothyroidism is distinguished by an elevated TSH and a normal free T_4. This condition occurs in 4% to 8% of the general population. It will progress to clinical hypothyroidism at a rate of 2% to 5% per year. Risk for progression includes the presence of thyroid autoantibodies, old age, a female gender, and a TSH level greater than 10 mIU/L. Patients who do not progress are considered euthyroid with a reset thyrostat, and they should be monitored clinically and biochemically on an annual basis. Antithyroid peroxidase levels would help to diagnose autoimmune thyroiditis, but would not be helpful in this case. Starting thyroxine would be appropriate if the TSH was greater than 10 mIU/L, but not if the levels were only slightly elevated.

496. The answer is a. Primary hypothyroidism is common, usually a result of Hashimoto thyroiditis or after Graves' disease. In this case, the TSH would be elevated, and the free T_3 and T_4 would be low. Secondary hypothyroidism is related to hypothalamic or pituitary dysfunction. Iodine deficiency is a cause of primary hypothyroidism. Subclinical hypothyroidism is when the TSH is elevated, but the T_3 and T_4 are normal. Thyroid hormone resistance would present with the TSH, T_3, and T_4 all being elevated.

497. The answer is e. Once hyperthyroidism is identified, radionucleotide uptake and scanning of the thyroid is useful to determine whether the problem is due to Graves' disease or another cause. In scans of patients with Graves' disease, there is increased uptake on radionucleotide imaging with diffuse hyperactivity. Nodules demonstrate limited areas of uptake on a radionucleotide scan with surrounding hypoactivity. In subacute thyroiditis, uptake is patchy and decreased overall.

498. The answer is a. Radioactive iodine is the treatment of choice for Graves' disease in adults who are not pregnant. Methimazole is the drug of choice in patients who choose antithyroid drug therapy, except during the first trimester of pregnancy when propylthiouracil is preferred. β-Blockade is not a treatment, but can be given to patients with symptomatic thyrotoxicosis or patients with resting heart rates of more than 90 beats/min. Surgery is reserved for patients in whom medication and radioactive iodine ablation are not acceptable, or in patients where a large goiter is compressing nearby structures or is disfiguring.

499. The answer is e. Several features of the history are associated with an increased risk of malignancy in a thyroid nodule. These include prior history of head and neck irradiation, or a family history of endocrine cancers. Also included are age less than 20 years or more than 70 years, male gender, and rapid growth of the nodule. Physical findings that raise clinical suspicion include a nodule with a firm consistency, cervical adenopathy, and symptoms like persistent hoarseness, dysphonia, or dysphagia.

500. The answer is d. Once a thyroid nodule is found, the next step in the workup is obtaining a TSH assay and ultrasonography of the thyroid. If the nodule appears suspicious on the basis of shape, size, margins, position, or echogenic pattern, a fine needle aspiration (FNA) should be performed irrespective of the patient's TSH level. If the patient had an elevated TSH and the nodule did not appear suspicious, thyroid peroxidase antibodies can be measured, and treatment of hypothyroidism can be initiated. If the FNA reveals malignant cells, surgical intervention is indicated.

Recommended Reading: Thyroid Disorders

Allweiss P, Hueston WJ, Carek PJ. Chapter 37: Endocrine disorders. In: South-Paul JE, Matheny SC, Lewis EL (eds). *Current Diagnosis & Treatment Family Medicine.* 4th ed. New York, NY: McGraw-Hill.

Index